Introduction to the Optics of the Eye

Introduction to the Optics of the Eye

David A. Goss, O.D., Ph.D., F.A.A.O.
Professor of Optometry, Indiana University, School of Optometry, Bloomington

Roger W. West, O.D., Ph.D.
Professor of Optometry, Northeastern State University, School of Optometry, Tahlequah, Oklahoma; Associate Medical Staff Member, W.W. Hastings Hospital, Tahlequah

BUTTERWORTH
HEINEMANN

Boston   Oxford   Auckland   Johannesburg   Melbourne   New Delhi

Library of Congress Cataloging-in-Publication Data

Goss, David A., 1948–
    Introduction to the optics of the eye / David A. Goss, Roger W. West.
        p. ; cm.
    Includes bibliographical references and index.
    ISBN 0-7506-7346-X (alk. paper)
    1. Physiological optics. I. West, Roger W. II. Title.
    [DNLM: 1. Eye—anatomy & histology. 2. Optics. 3. Refractive Errors. WW 101 G677i 2001]
    QP475 .G57 2001
    612.8'4—dc21   2001025677

British Library Cataloguing-in-Publication Data
A catalogue record for this book is available from the British Library.

The publisher offers special discounts on bulk orders of this book.
For information, please contact:

Manager of Special Sales
Butterworth–Heinemann
225 Wildwood Avenue
Woburn, MA 01801-2041
Tel: 781-904-2500
Fax: 781-904-2620

For information on all Butterworth–Heinemann publications available, contact our World Wide Web home page at: http://www.bh.com

10 9 8 7 6 5 4 3 2 1

Printed in the United States of America

To

Virginia A. Goss,
caring and proud mother

Ann E. West,
loving and understanding wife

Contents

Preface

It is unfortunately the case that many clinical ophthalmologists look upon optics with a feeling approaching horror. . . . This feeling of antipathy is indeed a pity for, apart from the inherent interest of the subject, most ophthalmologists (if we exclude those who live in their particular super-specialties above the clouds) spend much of their time on the prescription of spectacles or contact lenses. Indeed, of all aspects of medicine this practice gives to more people more comfort and increased efficiency than any other medical technique.

—Sir Stewart Duke-Elder, 1970

The eye is an organic structure, and as such it shares the vagaries of all biological tissue. It varies among individuals, it is imprecise, it is susceptible to environmental influences during its development, and it is changed by age and disease. Yet it is still an optical instrument and, as such, can be treated and understood in terms of the physical sciences that deal with optics and light. This dichotomy makes the eye of interest to readers whose backgrounds vary over an unusual range of fields such as biology, engineering, physics, and health care, as well as, of course, to the merely curious reader.

This book provides a readable introduction to the optics of the human eye that is accessible to this wide audience, regardless of each reader's particular knowledge or interests. However, we feel that this book will be particularly useful to clinicians, whether they be students or well-established practitioners. Duke-Elder wrote the words quoted above in the preface to the fifth volume of his famous *System of Ophthalmology* series of books. It speaks eloquently to the importance of understanding the optics of the eye. Although Duke-Elder was writing about ophthalmologists, the same could be said of many optometrists.

It is our hope that this book will give readers a greater appreciation of the part optics plays in the visual process and in vision care. We intend that its depth be sufficient to give the reader a useful background in each of its areas, and to prepare the reader who desires further information to get better use out of the more comprehensive and difficult books on this subject. Chapters 1 and 2 cover basic geometrical and physical optics to assist those who feel the need to review. Chapters 3 through 5 include the basic optics of the eye, the retinal image, and measurement of the optical components. These chapters have been kept broad and should be of interest to both clinicians and nonclinicians. A major emphasis of this book is the application of visual optics to clinical vision care. This information is contained mostly in Chapters 6 through 9, which cover the development, measurement, and management of refractive errors, along with various aspects of ocular accommodation. In Chapter 10 we offer a section on the often unappreciated heritage of visual optics.

In order to maintain readability, our emphasis is on concepts rather than details about specific experiments. We avoid extensive references to the primary literature. Instead, we cite mainly review papers and reference books, although we have included some papers of special interest from the primary literature. Readers seeking additional information can refer to the cited literature and to the recommended reading list at the end of each chapter.

Because computers are now available to virtually everyone, concepts are probably more important than computational skills. Nevertheless, we feel that people who are new to the field of optics can gain a better feel for raytracing by working through several computational problems. Therefore, there are numerous worked examples in this book. Where computations are long, we have placed them in an appendix to the corresponding chapter. Our method of calculating vergences is not the method adopted in many computer programs, but we believe that it gives the best intuitive feel for what is being done with these calculations. For those who wish to do extensive calculations, optical design software is widely available.

Epigrams at the start of the chapters show that natural philosophers and scientists hundreds of years ago considered the issues covered in these pages. Most of these epigrams were taken from *A Natural History of Vision,* by Nicholas J. Wade (MIT Press, Cambridge, MA, 1998), an enlightening book that uses quotations from important scientific publications extending from ancient Greece to the mid-nineteenth century to show advancements in the knowledge of vision.

Most of the work on this book was completed while David Goss was on sabbatical. I (D. G.) thank Indiana University for granting the sabbatical and I thank the administration, faculty, and staff of the Northeastern State University College of Optometry for their wonderful hospitality. We thank Arthur Bradley, Richard Castillo, Ron Everson, Doug Penisten, Tom Salmon, Larry Thibos, and Hank Van Veen for reviewing portions of the manuscript. Line drawings were produced by John McKenna, Indiana University School of Optometry class of 2001. We thank Jay Galst for providing photographs from his collection of medals commemorating notable persons in optical science and vision care. We also thank Karen Oberheim of Butterworth–Heinemann for her enthusiasm for this project. As usual, we bear the responsibility for any errors.

David A. Goss
Roger W. West

Introduction to the Optics of the Eye

Chapter 1

Geometrical Optics

A visual ray proceeds along a straight line and may be naturally bent only at a surface which forms a boundary between two media of different densities . . . the bending takes place not only in the passage from rarer and finer media to denser . . . but also in the passage from a denser to a rarer . . . this type of bending does not take place at equal angles but . . . the angles, as measured from the perpendicular, have a definite relationship. —Ptolemy, A.D. 150 (From Wade NJ. *A Natural History of Vision.* Cambridge, MA: MIT Press, 1998;19.)

In this chapter we provide a review of geometrical optics. Although one chapter cannot do justice to a field as extensive as geometrical optics, the material in this chapter should provide sufficient background for understanding the optics of the eye. To expand on some areas, the reader can consult the cited references and the Further Reading list at the end of the chapter.

REFRACTION

The speed of light in a vacuum is constant (symbolized by c). When traveling through matter, light slows down. How much the light slows down in a given medium is represented by that medium's index of refraction (n) where:

$$n = \frac{c}{c_m} = \frac{\text{Velocity of Light in a Vacuum}}{\text{Velocity of Light in a Medium } (m)}$$

$n_{vac} = 1.000$

$n_{air} = 1.00029$ (approximately the vacuum value)

$n_{water} = 1.334$

$n_{glass} = 1.523$ (ophthalmic crown glass)

Light has a wave nature and its travel can be described most accurately as the progression of its *wavefronts*. However, rather than draw the wavefronts, it is easier to draw lines (*rays*) that are perpendicular to the wavefronts and show the direction in which the light energy is traveling.

Single Flat Refractive Surfaces

If a *ray* is traced toward a flat surface at an angle of incidence (i), on entering the surface the ray will be redirected at an angle of refraction (r). The angular amount of refraction is described by Snell's law (Figure 1.1):

$$n_1 \sin i = n_2 \sin r$$

Example

$n_1 = 1.334$ (water), $n_2 = 1.523$ (glass), $i = 30°$

$$n_1 \sin i = n_2 \sin r$$

So,

$$\sin r = \left(\frac{n_1}{n_2}\right) \sin i$$

$$= \left(\frac{1.334}{1.523}\right) \sin 30°$$

$$= 0.438$$

$$r = \sin^{-1} 0.438 = 25.97°(i > r)$$

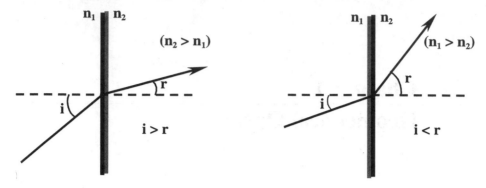

Figure 1.1. Rays that strike a flat interface at an angle of incidence (*i*) will be refracted at an angle of refraction (*r*). The interface separates refractive indices n_1 and n_2.

Plates with Parallel Sides

When a ray goes through a plate with plane (flat) parallel sides, it emerges parallel to the entering ray. If the angle of incidence $i \neq 0$, however, the ray is displaced from where the ray would have been in the absence of the plate (Figure 1.2).

Prisms

A prism is a transparent substance with two plane surfaces inclined at an apical angle (*A*). A plate is a special case of a prism whose $A = 0$. When $A > 0$, a traversing ray no longer exits parallel to the enter-ing ray. Prisms are used to disperse light into a spectrum, but also to change the direction of rays and the locations of images.

The deviation of a *ray* is toward the prism's base (the side opposite the apical angle), but the devia-tion of an *image* is toward the apex. When looking at an object first without and then through a prism, the eye must turn in the direction of the prism's apex to maintain fixation (Figure 1.3).

The number of degrees that a prism deviates a ray from its original direction (the total deviation [d_T]) is the sum of the deviations induced by each surface (Figure 1.4). If the prism is thin (i.e., *A* is small) the prism power $d_T \approx A(n_2 - 1)$, which for n_2 near 1.50 is about $0.5A$. In ophthalmic optics prism power (d_T)

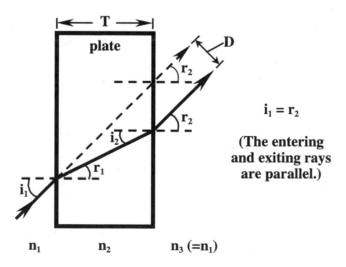

Figure 1.2. Rays that strike the first surface of a flat parallel plate at an angle of incidence i_1 will after two refractions leave the second surface at an angle of refraction r_2, which equals i_1. The entering and exiting rays are parallel but the exiting ray is displaced laterally by a distance *D*.

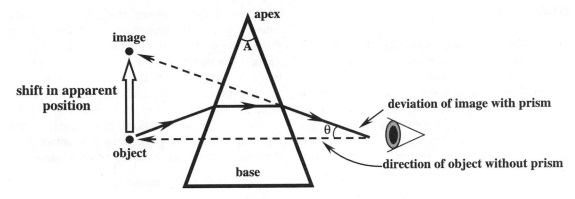

Figure 1.3. Inserting a prism in the line of sight causes an apparent movement of an object in the direction of the apex of the prism.

is measured in *prism diopters* (Δ). Specifically, 1^Δ equals the lateral displacement of 1/100 of the distance from the prism to the plane (e.g., a screen) on which the displacement is measured. Thus, at 1 meter the displacement given by a 1^Δ prism is 1 cm. There are 0.57 degrees per prism diopter or 1.74 prism diopters per degree for small angles.

Lenses (Two Curved Surfaces)

Lenses can be roughly modeled as two prisms. A biconvex converging lens is similar to two prisms placed together base to base. A biconcave diverging lens is similar to two prisms placed together apex to apex. However, with a lens, the prismatic angle *A* changes in a continuous manner from cen-

ter to edge so that rays traversing more peripheral parts of the lens will be refracted more strongly, so that all rays are directed either toward or from one image point.

OBJECTS AND IMAGES

Light going through an optical system (e.g., a lens) is categorized as object light or image light. In ray-tracing diagrams the rays are shown as being directed toward or away from *point* objects and images. However, *extended* objects and images can also be raytraced if they are treated as collections of object and image points. Extended objects are often represented as arrows to show their lateral size.

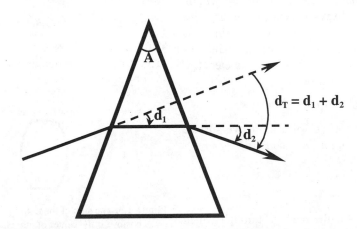

Figure 1.4. The total angle of deviation d_T of a ray as it traverses a prism is equal to the sum of the deviations caused by each refractive surface.

Object Light

Object light is associated with light entering an optical system. An object point represents the center of curvature of the wavefronts entering the lens and is further classified as real or virtual. An object point is *real* (O_R) if light entering the system is diverging. An object is *virtual* (O_V) if light entering the optical system is converging. No object is physically present at O_V but O_V still represents the center of curvature of wavefronts before they enter the lens.

Image Light

Image light is associated with light leaving an optical system. An image point represents the center of curvature of wavefronts leaving the lens and is also classified as real or virtual. An image point is *real* (I_R) if the light leaving the system is converging. An image is *virtual* (I_V) if the light leaving the system is diverging. No image is physically present at I_V but I_V still represents the center of curvature of wavefronts after they leave the lens.

THE GAUSS EQUATION

The distance between an object and its lens surface is symbolized by ℓ, and the distance between an image and its lens surface is symbolized by ℓ'. *Vergence* (L or L'), a measure of wavefront curvature, is the reciprocal of the distance (ℓ) from an object or distance (ℓ') to an image, each multiplied by the refractive index that the ray is physically within. Diverging rays are always associated with negative distances and negative vergences. Converging rays are always associated with plus distances and plus vergences. If distances are measured in meters (m) the vergence unit is the *diopter*:

$L = n_1/\ell$ and $L' = n_2/\ell'$

The dioptric power (F) of a refractive surface can be calculated from n_1, n_2, and r:

$$F = \frac{(n_2 - n_1)}{r_m}$$

where n_1 is the n for the medium through which light travels to enter the refractive surface (object light), n_2 is the n for the medium through which

light travels after crossing the refractive surface (image light), and r equals the radius of curvature of the refractive surface (border between n_1 and n_2) in meters. The sign of r is plus if the center of curvature (C) is to the side of the refractive surface with the image rays, and minus if C is to the side of the refractive surface with the object rays (Figure 1.5).

The *Gauss equation* allows image locations and sizes to be determined given the dioptric power of the refractive surface and object locations and sizes:

$L + F = L'$ in full becomes

$$(n_1/\ell) + \frac{(n_2 - n_1)}{r} = (n_2/\ell')$$

The magnification $m = I/O$ is found by

$$m = L/L' = \frac{n_1/\ell}{n_2/\ell'}$$

Example: Plus Power Surface

$n_1 = 1.50$, $n_2 = 2.00$, $r = +5$ cm, $\ell = -50$ cm (object distance)

Find the position of the image and its magnification (Figure 1.6A).

$$F = \frac{n_2 - n_1}{r} = \frac{(2.00 - 1.50)}{+5}(100) = +10 \text{ D}$$

$\ell = -50$ mm, $L = n_1/\ell = 1.50(100)/(-50)$
$= -3.00 \text{ D} = L$

$L + F = L', -3.00 + (+10.00) = +7.00 \text{ D}$
$= L'$

$L' = n_2/\ell', \ell' = n_2/L' = 2.00(100)/(+7.00)$
$= +28.6 \text{ cm} = \ell'$

$m = L/L' = (-3.00)/(+7.00) = -0.43 \ x = m$

Thus, the image is 28.6 cm to the right of the interface; it is real, inverted, and 0.43 times the size of the object.

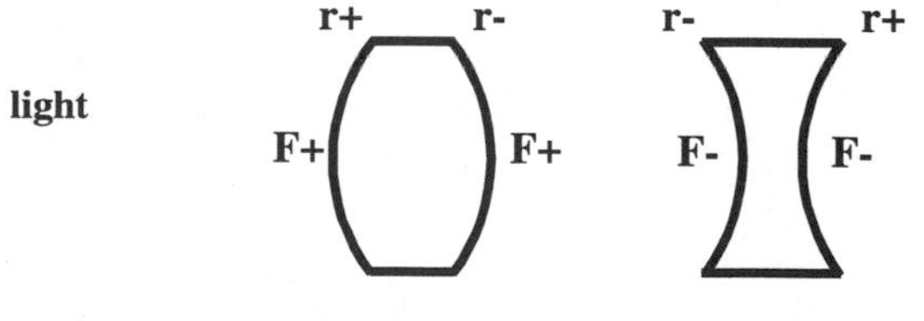

Figure 1.5. The sign of the radius of curvature for a surface (r) is positive if the center of curvature is downstream from the direction in which light is traveling and negative if it is upstream from the direction in which light is traveling.

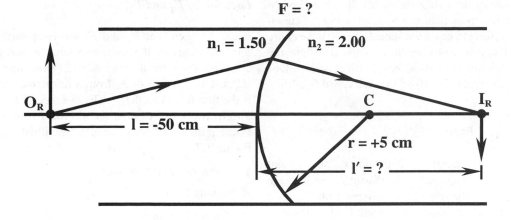

(A)

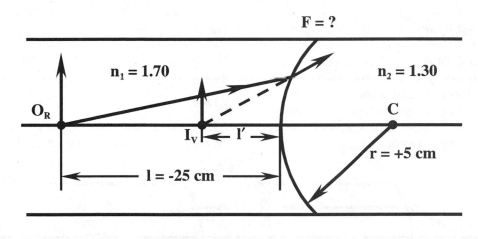

(B)

Figure 1.6. (**A**) A real object is located to the left of a single refractive surface and produces a real image to the right of the surface. (**B**) A real object is located to the left of a single refractive surface and produces a virtual image to the left of the surface.

Example: Minus Power Surface

$n_1 = 1.70$, $n_2 = 1.30$, $r = +5$ cm, $\ell = -25$ cm

Find the image distance (ℓ') and m (Figure 1.6B).

$$F = \frac{n_2 - n_1}{r} = \frac{(1.30 - 1.70)}{-5}(100) = -8.00 \text{ D}$$

Even though the surface has a plus radius, $n_2 - n_1$ is minus so the surface has a minus power.

$\ell = -25$ cm, $L = n_1/\ell = 1.70(100)/(-25)$
$= -6.80$ D $= L$

$L + F = L'$, $-6.80 + (-8.00) = -14.80$ D $= L'$

$L' = n_2/\ell'$ so $\ell' = n_2/L' = 1.30(100)/(-14.80)$
$= -8.78$ cm $= \ell'$

Minus implies I_V is to the left of the interface but the image rays are to the right in n_2, so n_2 is used in $\ell' = n_2/L'$.

$m = L/L' = (-6.8)/(-14.80) = +0.46 \ x = m$

The image is virtual, 8.78 cm to the *left* of the interface, erect, and 0.46 times as large as the object.

REFRACTIVE SURFACES AND RAY DIAGRAMS

Optical Axis

Most lenses have spherical surfaces and the optical axis is the imaginary line connecting the centers of curvature of the two surfaces. Usually, if an optical system has more than one lens, all centers of curvature are made to lie on the same line so that the entire optical system has one optical axis. If a light ray coincides with the optical axis, it strikes each surface perpendicularly ($i = 0$) and is undeviated ($r = 0$).

First Focal Point

The first focal point (F_1) is the on-axis object point that results in an infinitely distant on-axis image point. Thus, the object rays diverge from F_1 for a plus power or converge toward F_1 for a minus power and the image rays leave the system virtually parallel.

Second Focal Point

The second focal point (F_2) is the on-axis image point that results when rays enter a refractive surface from a distant axial point object. Thus, the object rays enter the system virtually parallel and converge toward F_2 for a plus power or diverge from F_2 for a minus power.

Location of F_1 and F_2

It can be seen that F_1 and F_2 are necessarily on opposite sides of the refractive surface and their corresponding focal lengths will have opposite signs. The distance of F_1 from a refractive surface is the first focal length (f_1). The distance of F_2 from a refractive surface is the second focal length (f_2). Focal points and focal lengths are illustrated in Figure 1.7.

1. $f_2 = n_2/F$ and $f_1 = -n_1/F$

   Solving for F:

   $$F = n_2/f_2 = -n_1/f_1$$

   So if

   $$n_1 \neq n_2, f_2 \neq -f_1 \quad f_2 = -(n_2/n_1)f_1$$

   Therefore, if

   $$n_2 > n_1$$

   then

   $$|f_2| > |f_1|$$

2. Another useful relationship is $f_1 + f_2 = r$. Then, the distance between F_1 and the refractive surface

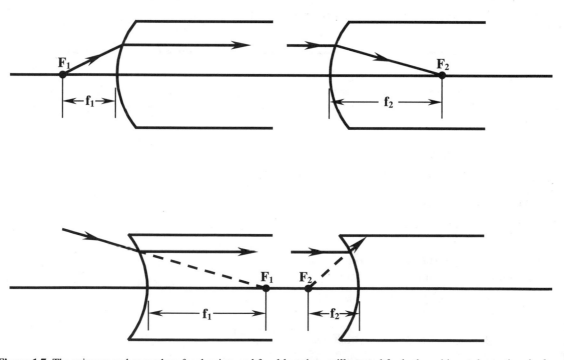

Figure 1.7. The primary and secondary focal points and focal lengths are illustrated for both positive and negative single refractive surfaces.

(RS) equals the distance between F_2 and the center of curvature (C). Knowing this simplifies drawing raytrace diagrams (Figure 1.8). That is, if

$$f_1 = -5 \text{ and } f_2 = +10$$

then

$$r = f_1 + f_2 = -5 + (+10) = +5$$

Predictable Rays for Single Refractive Surfaces

If the locations of F_1 and F_2 are drawn on graph paper relative to the refractive surface, three predictable rays can be traced from an object point to the corresponding image point. Any two of these rays will suffice to locate the image point. The image point is located where these rays cross in image space. The three predictable rays allow us to find *off-axis* image points from *off-axis* object points. If the point on an extended object most distant from the optical axis is used, we can compare the size of the image and object (magnification) and determine whether the image point is on the same or opposite side of the optical axis as the object point (whether the image is erect or inverted).

The predictable rays are the following:

1. A ray that goes through an object point while traveling parallel to the optical axis also goes through the corresponding image point in a direction that lines up with F_2.
2. A ray that goes through an object point in a direction that lines up with F_1 exits parallel to the optical axis and goes through the corresponding image point.
3. A ray that goes through an object point in a direction that lines up with the center of curvature (C) will pass through the lens undeviated

and go through the corresponding image point. This ray is called a *nodal ray*.

These rays are labeled 1, 2, and 3 in Figure 1.9.

When the objects or images are virtual, forward or backward extensions of the rays go through the virtual objects and images. The extensions are drawn (in Figure 1.9) as dashed lines to indicate that these rays do not correspond to light that is physically present.

The next example is a graphical raytrace for the problem worked out algebraically in an earlier example. For accurate results, the refracting surface must be drawn flat but its curvature (concave or convex) is noted by the location of the center of curvature (C) of its radius and it can be illustrated by adding "wings" to the edge of the refracting surface where rays will not be traced.

Example

$n_1 = 1.70$, $n_2 = 1.30$, $r = +5$ cm, $\ell = -25$ cm, $F = -8$ D (previously calculated) (see Figure 1.9).
Then

$$f_2 = \frac{n_2}{F} = \frac{1.30}{-8}(100) = -16.25 \text{ cm}$$

$$f_1 = -\frac{n_1}{F} = -\frac{1.70}{-8}(100) = +21.25 \text{ cm}$$

Check:

$$f_1 + f_2 = r, +21.25 + (-16.25) = +5$$

Note that the analysis leaves the image rays within the material of refractive index n_2 even though the virtual image (I_v) is to the left of the surface.

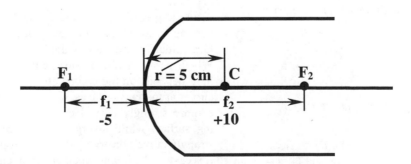

Figure 1.8. F_1, F_2, and C are shown for a positive power single refractive surface.

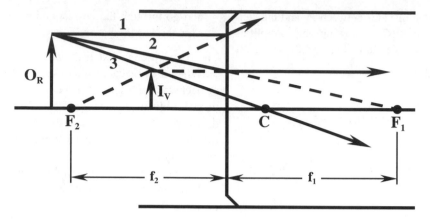

Figure 1.9. Predictable rays for a real object to the left of a negative single refractive surface. The image is virtual and to the left of the surface.

Two Refracting Surfaces

The preceding analyses of refracting surfaces leave the image rays within the material of refractive index n_2. However, the most common use of the refracting surface equations is to trace rays into a lens through the first refracting surface and out through a second refracting surface (or a series of refracting surfaces) to obtain the image for the complete lens. This simply involves a repetition of the Gauss equation in which each successive surface uses the image (I) from the previous surface as its object (O).

The total magnification (m_T) resulting from the rays going through both lenses is the product of the magnifications for lens 1 and lens 2.

$$m_T = (m_1)(m_2) = (h_1'/h_1)(h_2'/h_2) = h_2'/h_1$$

since

$$h_2 = h_1'$$

Or,

$$m_T = (m_1)(m_2) = (I_1/O_1)(I_2/O_2) = I_2/O_1$$

since

$$O_2 = I_1$$

Then,

$$m_T = (L_1/L_1')(L_2/L_2') = (\ell_1'/\ell_1)(\ell_2'/\ell_2)$$

Example: Given $F_1 = +14$ D, $F_2 = -13$ D, $n_1 = n_3 = 1.00$, $n_2 = 1.50$, $d = 5$ cm, and $\ell_1 = -25$ cm, find ℓ_2' and m_T (Figure 1.10).

First Refracting Surface

$$\ell_1 = -25 \text{ cm}, L_1 = n_1/\ell_1 = (1.00/-25)(100)$$
$$= -4.00 \text{ D}$$

$$L_1 + F_1 = L_1', -4.00 + (+14.00) = +10.00$$
$$= L_1'$$

$$\ell_1' = n_2/L_1' = (1.50/+10)(100) = +15 \text{ cm}$$
(I_1 is 15 cm to the right of surface 1.)

Second Refracting Surface: Distance of O_2 from second surface $\ell_2 = \ell_1' - d$

$$\ell_2 = +15 - 5 = +10 \text{ cm}, L_2 = n_2/\ell_2$$
$$= (1.50/+10)(100) = +15 \text{ D}$$

$$L_2 + F_2 = L_2', +15 + (-13) = +2 \text{ D}$$

$$\ell_2' = n_3/L_2' = (1.00/+2)(100) = +50 \text{ cm}$$

$$m_T = (L_1/L_1')(L_2/L_2') = (-4/+10)(+15/+2)$$
$$= -3 x$$

I_2 is real, 50 cm to the right of the second surface, inverted, and three times as large as the original object O_1.

In the preceding example the lens has one converging (convex) and one diverging (concave) surface. Such lenses are called *meniscus lenses*. Whether thin meniscus lenses converge or diverge light depends on the comparative steepness of the curves at the two surfaces. Converging lenses have a more strongly curved converging than diverging surface while diverging lenses have a more strongly curved diverging than converging surface. It is easy to determine whether a thin lens with both converging and diverging surfaces has a net

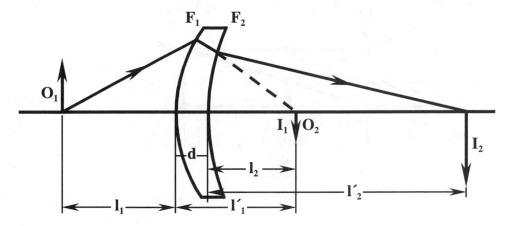

Figure 1.10. A raytrace through a thick lens. Rays from a real object in front of two refractive surfaces produce a real image to the right of the second surface.

convergence or divergence. If the center is thicker than the edge, it is converging. If the edge is thicker than the center, it is diverging.

THIN LENSES

If a thick lens is made sufficiently thin, it can be treated as a single refractive surface with a dioptric power F, but with air to each side (n_1 and n_2 = 1.000). (Such a case is a low power spectacle lens.) Then, the Gauss equation gives:

$L + F = L'$ or $(1/\ell) + F = (1/\ell')$, where ℓ and ℓ' are again in meters.

Example

$\ell = +20$ cm, $F = -3$ D

Locate the image (Figure 1.11).

$L = 1/\ell = 100/(+20) = +5$ D

$L + F = L'$, $+5 + (-3) = +2$ D $= L'$

$\ell' = 1/L' = 100/(+2) = +50$ cm

$m = L/L' = +5/+2 = +2.5x$

A plus ℓ' indicates converging light so the image is 50 cm to the *right* of the lens.

A plus m indicates the image is erect relative to the object.

Systems Containing Two Thin Lenses

If the object rays are imaged after going through two lenses instead of just one, graphically or algebraically solve for the image for lens 1 (I_1). Then use I_1 as the object for lens 2 (O_2) and solve for the image produced by lens 2 (I_2). The position of I_2, which is the image for the entire system, can be described by its distance from lens 2 (ℓ_2'). Raytracing through two thin lenses is illustrated in the next example. Note that the powers of the two thin lenses are the same as the surface powers of the thick lens in Figure 1.10. Also, the object distance from the first surface is the same for both examples.

Example: Given two thin lenses $F_1 = +14$ D and $F_2 = -13$ D separated by $d = 3.33$ cm, and an object is $\ell_1 = -25$ cm in front of the first lens, find ℓ_2' and M_T (Figure 1.12).

First Refracting Surface

$\ell_1 = -25$ cm, $L_1 = n_1/\ell_1 = (1.00/-25)(100)$
$= -4.00$ D

$L_1 + F_1 = L_1'$, $-4.00 + (+14.00) = +10.00$
$= L_1'$

$\ell_1' = n_2/L_1' = (1.00/+10)(100) = +10$ cm
(I_1 is 10 cm to the right of surface 1.)

Second Refracting Surface: Distance of O_2 from second surface $\ell_2 = \ell_1' - d$

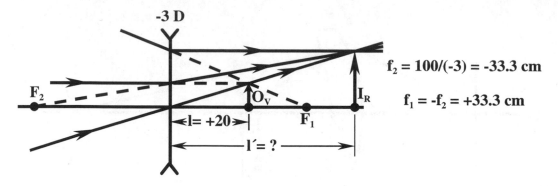

$$f_2 = 100/(-3) = -33.3 \text{ cm}$$

$$f_1 = -f_2 = +33.3 \text{ cm}$$

Figure 1.11. Although all lenses have two refractive surfaces, if the lens is thin enough the total refraction may be drawn or calculated as though caused by a single surface.

$\ell_2 = +10 - 3.33 = +6.67$ cm, $L_2 = n_2/\ell_2$
$= (1.00/+6.67)(100) = +15$ D

$L_2 + F_2 = L_2{}', +15 + (-13) = +2$ D

$\ell_2{}' = n_3/L_2{}' = (1.00/+2)(100) = +50$ cm

$M_T = (L_1/L_1{}')(L_2/L_2{}') = (-4/+10)(+15/+2)$
$= -3 \ x$

I_2 is real, 50 cm to the right of the second surface, inverted, and three times as large as the original object O_1. This is the same result as that found for the thick lens in Figure 1.10.

Note from a comparison of Figure 1.10 and 1.12 that a thick lens can be modeled as two thin lenses. The powers of the two thin lenses are the same as the respective surface powers of the thick lens. However, the separation of the two thin lenses must be the thickness of the thick lens divided by its refractive index. In the above example, d for the

thick lens was 5 cm so the separation for the two thin lenses must be $d = 5$ cm/1.50 = 3.33 cm.

Two Thin Lenses in Contact

When two thin lenses (1 and 2) are separated by a distance d, it is important to note that the vergence of O_2 at lens 2 will change from the vergence of I_1 at lens 1 over the distance (d) between the lenses even though I_1 and O_2 are at the same location. Object vergence (L_2) at lens 2 *will not* equal the image vergence ($L_1{}'$) at lens 1 because there is a loss or gain of curvature as the wavefront travels the distance (d) between the lenses. However, if the distance (d) between the thin lenses is 0, then:

$F_1 + F_2 = F_T$ and

$L_1 + F_T = L_2{}'$ (only if $d = 0$)

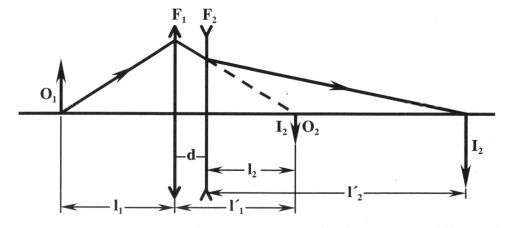

Figure 1.12. A raytrace through the two thin lenses. This system models the single thick lens illustrated in Figure 1.10.

Predictable Rays for Thin Lenses

The focal points F_1 and F_2 are always equally distant from but on opposite sides of a thin lens.

$$f_1 = -1/F_1 \text{ and } f_2 = 1/F_2$$

If we follow the convention in which light travels from left to right,

1. F_1 is a real object (O_R) to the left of a converging lens but a virtual object (O_V) to the right for a diverging lens.
2. F_2 is a real image (I_R) to the right of a converging lens but a virtual image (I_V) to the left for a diverging lens.

Three rays going through a lens from an object point to an image point can be drawn graphically and are *predictable rays*. Any two of these can be used to find the image point that corresponds to an off-axis object point. These rays are numbered 1, 2, and 3 in Figure 1.13.

1. A ray that goes through an object point while traveling parallel to the optical axis also goes through the corresponding image point in a direction that lines up with F_2.
2. A ray that goes through an object point in a direction that lines up with F_1 exits parallel to the optical axis and goes through the corresponding image point.
3. A ray that goes through an object point and also goes through the optical center of a *thin* lens (where the lens intersects the optical axis) will pass through the lens undeviated and go through the corresponding image point. This ray is the *nodal ray* for a thin lens.

FOCAL LENGTHS AND POWERS OF MULTIPLE THIN OR THICK LENS SYSTEMS

A series of refractive surfaces can be combined to make complex systems. Since each lens surface has its own power and focal points F_1 and F_2, how do we define powers and focal lengths for a system of two or more refracting surfaces?

Back Vertex Power

If parallel light is incident on the first surface of a system, then the focal length (f_2) of the system can be defined conveniently as the distance between the last surface and the point of focus (F_2). This distance is called the *back focal length (f_b)*. $F_v = 1/f_b$ is called the *back vertex power.* This is the power that a single thin lens would require to have the same focal point F_2 if it is placed at the same location as the back surface of the system (Figure 1.14).

f_b = back focal length

$F_v = 1/f_b$ = back vertex power (where f_b is in meters)

Front Vertex Power

If light is incident on the first surface of a system such that parallel light leaves the last surface, then the axial position of an object that would do this is defined as F_1 and its distance from the first lens or surface is f_f *(front focal length)*. $F_n = -1/f_f$ is called the *front vertex power* or *neutralizing power*. This is the power that a single thin lens would require to have the same focal point F_1 if it is placed at the same location as the front surface of the system (Figure 1.15).

f_f = front focal length

$F_n = -1/f_f$ = front vertex power or the neutralizing power (where f_f is in meters).

F_v and F_n are not true dioptric powers in the sense that they can be used in the Gauss equation $L + F = L'$. Only use F_v and F_n when parallel light is entering or exiting the system.

REFLECTION

Plane (Flat) Mirrors

When rays are traced toward a mirror surface at an angle of incidence (i) to the normal, the light is reflected from the surface at an angle of reflection (s) on the opposite side of the normal that equals the angle of incidence.

Although no light is physically present behind the mirror, a point object in front of a plane mirror will form an image that appears to be as far behind the mirror as the object is in front of the mirror. The location of images can be determined by locating the point images of representative point objects,

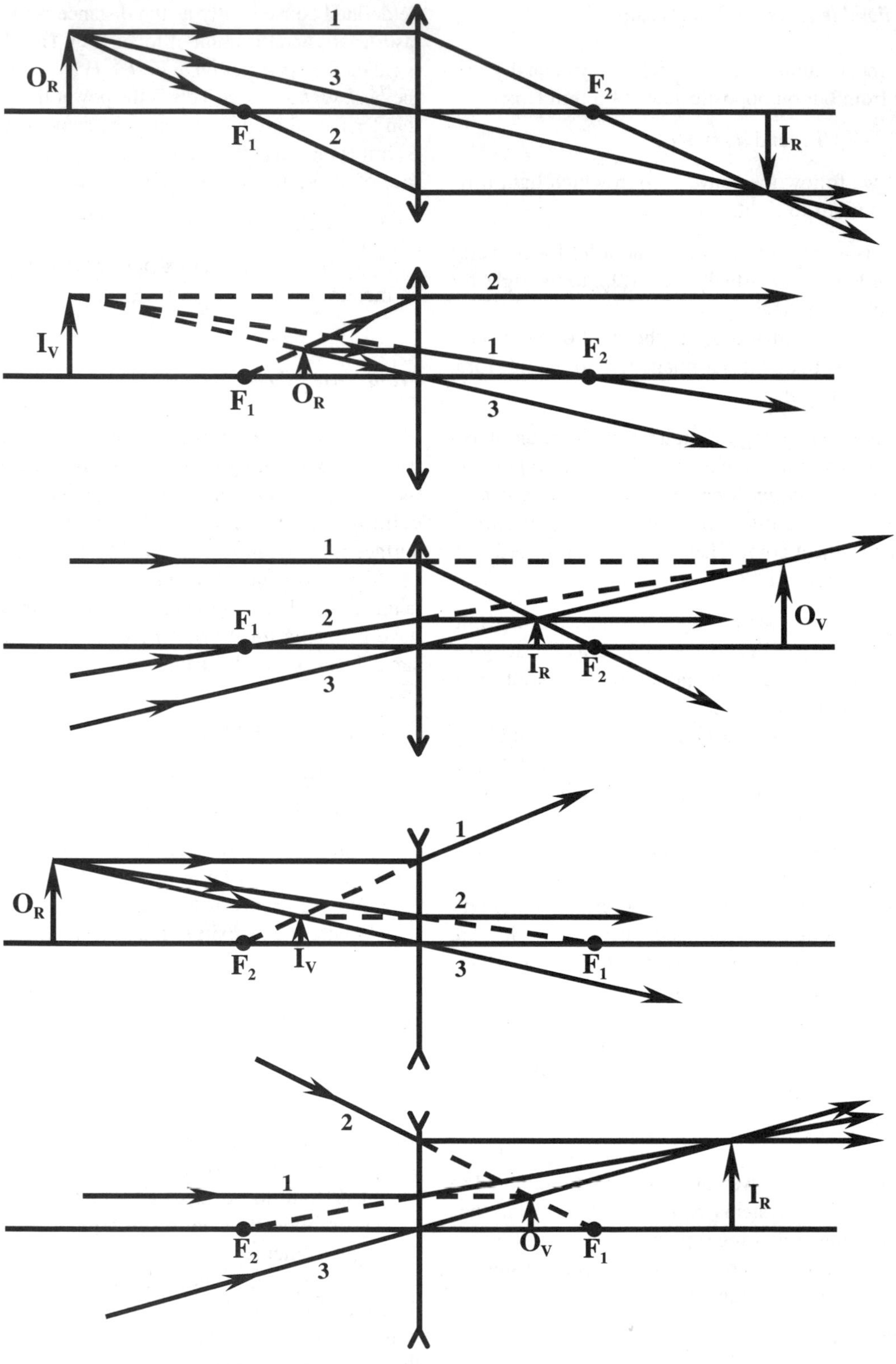

Figure 1.13. Examples of predictable rays traced through plus and minus thin lenses. The numbers correspond to the rays itemized in the text.

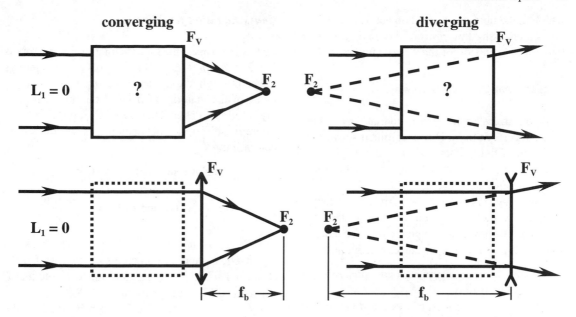

Figure 1.14. Back vertex power and focal length for converging and diverging systems. The distance between the last surface of the system and its focal point is the back focal length f_b. The vergence of the rays as they leave the last surface is the back vertex power F_V. F_V can be simulated by a single thin lens of power F_V, which replaces the system and is located at the last surface.

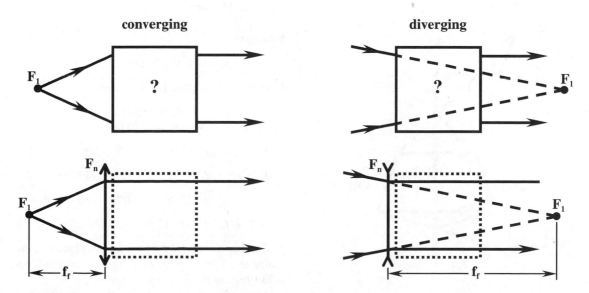

Figure 1.15. Front vertex power and focal length for converging and diverging systems. The distance between the first surface of the system and its focal point is the front focal length f_f. The vergence of the rays as they enter the first surface is the front vertex power or neutralizing power F_n. F_n can be simulated by a single thin lens of power F_n, which replaces the system and is located at the first surface.

which make up the extended object. If the object is off-center from the mirror, the rays are traced toward an extension of the mirror (Figure 1.16).

Images from Curved Mirrors

Curved mirrors act like lenses in that they can converge or diverge light. However, mirrors reverse the direction of light, whereas lenses don't. This gives a reversal as to which side of the element real or virtual images are located.

Following reflection, light's direction of travel is reversed, so the signs given to image distances are reversed. However, the vergence rule for assigning signs to object or image distances still applies:

- If the object or image rays are *converging,* the vergence is *plus.*
- If the object or image rays are *diverging,* the vergence is *minus.*

It is helpful to remember the following rules:

- *Concave mirrors* converge light. They have plus power, plus focal lengths, and plus radii of surface curvature.
- *Convex mirrors* diverge light. They have minus power, minus focal lengths, and minus radii of surface curvature.

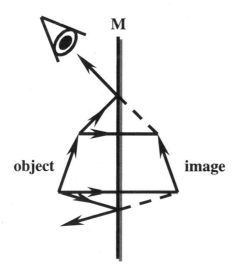

Figure 1.16. For a flat mirror, each point in an extended image is as far behind the mirror as its corresponding object point is in front of the mirror.

Gauss Equation for Mirrors

Just as for lenses, the Gauss equation for mirrors is $L + F = L', m = L/L'$. Since object and image rays travel through the same space, $n_1 = n_2$ and the index of the material in front of the mirror is simply referred to as n. Thus, $L = n/\ell$, and $L' = n/\ell'$. There *is* a difference between lenses and mirrors in determining F.

- F_{lens} (for one surface) $= -n_1/f_1 = n_2/f_2$.

$$\left(\text{Also, } F_{\text{lens}} \text{ (for one surface) } = \frac{n_2 - n_1}{r_1}.\right)$$

- $F_{\text{mirror}} = n/f$. Since light is folded back on itself, F_1 and F_2 coincide so $f_1 = f_2 = f$ without a subscript or sign difference. (Note that F can still be plus or minus.)
- $f_{\text{mirror}} = r/2$. The focal length is one half the radius of curvature of the mirror's surface.

Thus, if r is minus (convex mirror), f is minus. If r is plus (concave mirror), f is plus. Then, $F = n/f = n/(r/2)$, but $f = r/2$ regardless of what n is. (The power F depends on n, but f does not.)

F for a mirror is referred to as *catoptric power* (reflective power) and is measured in diopters just as for lenses.

Concave Mirrors

Example

$$r = +10 \text{ cm, } \ell = -20 \text{ cm}$$

Find I and m (Figure 1.17):

$$f_m = r/2 = +10/2 = +5 \text{ cm, } F_m = n/f_m = (1.00/+5)(100) = +20 \text{ D}$$

$$\ell = -20 \text{ cm, } L = n/\ell = (1.00/-20)(100) = -5 \text{ D}$$

$$L + F_m = L', (-5) + (+20) = -15 \text{ D}$$

$$\ell' = n/L' = (1.00/-15)(100) = +6.67 \text{ cm}$$

$$m = L/L' = -5/+15 = -0.33x$$

The image is 6.67 cm in front of the mirror, real (since the light is plus, converging), inverted, and 0.33 times as large as the object.

It is left as an exercise for the reader to show that if an object is −4 cm in front of this mirror (*O* between *F* and mirror), the image is 20 cm *behind*

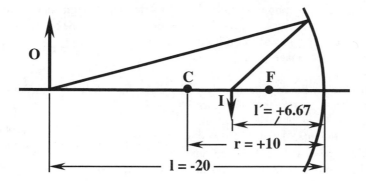

Figure 1.17. In this concave mirror, a real object is located farther from the mirror than its center of curvature.

the mirror as a virtual image that is erect and 5 times as large as the object. This is how a shaving mirror works.

Convex Mirrors

Example

$r = -20$ cm, $\ell = -20$ cm

Find I and m (Figure 1.18).

$f_m = r/2 = -20/2 = -10$ cm, $F_m = n/f_m$
$= (1.00/-10)(100) = -10$ D

$\ell = -20$ cm, $L = n/\ell = (1.00/-20)(100) = -5$ D

$L + F_m = L'$, $(-5) + (-10) = -15$ D

$\ell' = n/L' = (1.00/-15)(100) = -6.67$ cm

$m = L/L' = -5/-15 = +0.33x$

The image is 6.67 cm behind the mirror, virtual, erect, and 0.33 times as large as the object.

It is left as an exercise for the reader to show that if an object is +5 cm behind this mirror (a virtual object), the image is 10 cm *in front* of the mirror as a real image that is erect and 2 times as large as the object.

Graphical Raytracing for Mirrors

There are *four* predictable rays for mirrors. Only two of these four possible rays need to be drawn to find the location, size, and orientation of the image. The four predictable rays for mirrors are the following:

1. A ray drawn through an object point and parallel to the optical axis also goes through the corresponding image point in a direction that lines up with F.
2. A ray drawn through an object point in a direction that lines up with F exits parallel to the optical axis and goes through the corresponding image point.

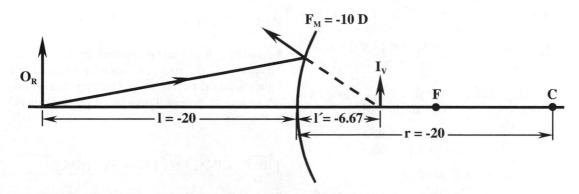

Figure 1.18. A convex mirror that has a real object in front of it.

3. A ray drawn through an object point in a direction that lines up with the center of curvature (C) of the mirror's surface will reflect on itself and also pass through the image point. This is the nodal ray for mirrors.
4. The fourth predictable ray has no corresponding type in lens diagrams. A ray that is drawn through an object point and that also strikes the vertex of the mirror (the intersection of the mirror with the optical axis) will be reflected an equal angle to the opposite side of the optical axis and will go through the corresponding image point.

These rays are shown in Figure 1.19.

Just as lenses do, mirrors have object locations where $m = +1$ or -1:

1. $m = -1x$ when the object is $2f$ from the mirror at the center of curvature (C). Then the image is at the same location as the object and is the same size but inverted.
2. $m = +1x$ when the object is *at* the mirror. Then the image is superimposed on the object, is the same size, and is erect.

Mirror-Refractive Surface Combinations

A system that uses both lenses and mirrors is referred to as *catadioptric*. *Thick* lenses with reflection off the back surface are referred to as *mangin mirrors*. The back surface may be silvered deliberately to make it reflective or the reflection may be the unwanted partial reflection obtained from all optical surfaces (ghost reflections).

Example: For a spectacle lens in air, $r_1 = +15$ cm, $r_2 = +10$ cm, n of lens $= 1.50$, and the lens is 0.5 cm thick. If a window is 50 cm from the lens, where is the ghost image of the window from the back surface of the lens as viewed from the front of the lens? (See Figure 1.20.)

$F_1 = (n_2 - n_1)/r_1 = [(1.50 - 1.00)/(+15)](100)$
$= +3.33$ D (*lens power for surface 1*)

$F_2 = (n_3 - n_2)/r_2 = [(1.00 - 1.50)/(+10)](100)$
$= -5.00$ D (*lens power for surface 2*)

(Not needed in this problem.)

$F_m = n_2/f_m = n_2/(r_2/2) = [1.50/(-10/2)](100)$
$= -30$ D (*mirror power for surface 2*)

(Note that the sign changes to minus because this surface is now a *convex mirror*.)

$\ell_1 = -50$ cm, $L_1 = n_1/\ell_1 = (1.00/-50)(100)$
$= -2.00$ D

$L_1 + F_1 = L_1', -2 + (+3.33) = +1.33$ D
$= L_1'$

$\ell_1' = n_2/L_1' = (1.50/+1.33)(100) = +112.50$ cm $= \ell_1'$ (distance of I_1 from first surface)

$\ell_2 = \ell_1' - d = +112.50 - 0.5 = +112.00$ cm $= \ell_2$

$L_2 = n_2/\ell_2 = (1.50/+112.00)(100) =$ $+1.339$ D $= L_2$

$L_2 + F_m = L_2', +1.339 + (-30) = -28.66$ $= L_2'$

$\ell_2' = n_2/L_2' = (1.50/-28.66)(100) = -5.23$ cm $= \ell_2'$ (distance of I_2 to the right of surface 2)

$\ell_3 = \ell_2' - d = -5.23 - 0.5 = -5.73$ (distance of I_2, which becomes O_3 to the right of surface 1)

$n_2/\ell_3 = (1.50/-5.73)(100) = -26.16$ D $= L_3$

$L_3 + F_3 = L_3'$ (where $F_3 = F_1$) $-26.16 +$ $(+3.33) = -22.83$ D $= L_3'$

$\ell_3' = n_1/L_3' = (1.00/-22.83)(100) = -4.38$ cm $= \ell_3'$ (distance of I_3 behind front surface of lens)

$m = (L_1/L_1')(L_2/L_2')(L_3/L_3')$
$= (-2/+1.33)(+1.34/-28.66)(-26.16/-22.83)$
$= +0.08x = m$

The image of the window is 4.38 cm behind the front surface of the spectacle lens, is erect, and is 0.08 times as large as the window.

Purkinje Images

Other examples of images formed by mangin mirrors are Purkinje images, which are reflections of a light source off the surfaces of the cornea and crystalline lens of the eye. Purkinje images are covered in Chapter 3.

THE EQUIVALENT LENS SYSTEM

The equivalent lens system is a mathematical model that uses a single thin lens to describe image

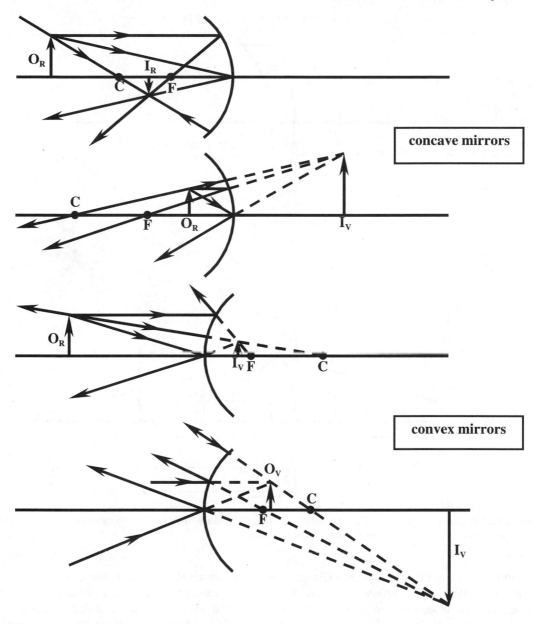

concave mirrors

convex mirrors

Figure 1.19. Examples of predictable rays for concave and convex mirrors. The numbers on the rays correspond to those rays itemized in the text.

formation by a thick lens or a combination of lenses. The equivalent lens system is defined by three pairs of *cardinal points*:

1. First and second focal points (F_1 and F_2).
2. First and second principal points (P_1 and P_2).
3. First and second nodal points (N_1 and N_2).

We have already covered the first of these pairs (F_1 and F_2) and we will now cover the last two.

Primary (P_1) and Secondary (P_2) Principal Points and Planes

It is possible, for computational purposes, to replace a complex system (having more than one surface) with just *one* thin lens of a power F_e (the equivalent power). However, the equivalent thin lens must have *two locations*. The location of the thin lens for entering object rays is P_1 (the *first principal plane*)

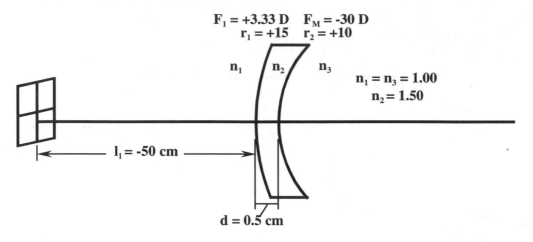

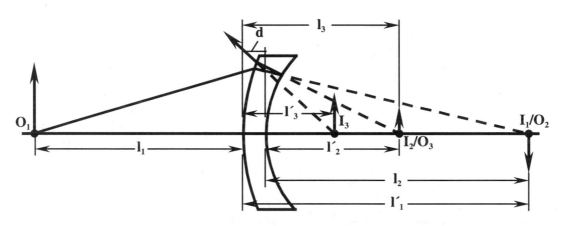

Figure 1.20. Example of a mangin mirror problem. Light from an object in front of a meniscus spectacle lens is reflected off the back surface to produce a virtual image behind the lens.

and the location of the thin lens for exiting image rays is P_2 (the *second principal plane*). These planes cross the optical axis at the *first* and *second principal points* (also called P_1 and P_2).

F_1 and F_2 can be defined for a complex optical system as shown in the Figure 1.21. (The following figures show a single thick lens but the system may actually consist of many lenses, thin or thick.)

If a ray goes through F_1 and through the optical system, it will exit the last surface parallel to the optical axis. The actual route taken by the ray is shown by a solid line. However, if the entering and exiting rays are extended within the system along their entering and exiting directions (dashed lines), they will meet on the first principal plane (P_1). The point where the plane crosses the optical axis is the

first principal point (P_1). The distance from P_1 to F_1 is the *first equivalent focal length* (f_{e1}). P_1 is located where the equivalent thin lens of power F_e would be placed to intercept incoming object rays in the equivalent thin lens system. The necessary power of the equivalent thin lens would then be $F_e = -n_o/f_{e1}$.

If a ray parallel to the optical axis is sent into an optical system, it will focus at F_2. The actual route taken by the ray is shown by a solid line. However, if the entering and exiting rays are extended within the system along their entering and exiting directions (dashed lines), they will meet on the second principal plane (P_2). The point where the plane crosses the optical axis is the second principal point (P_2).

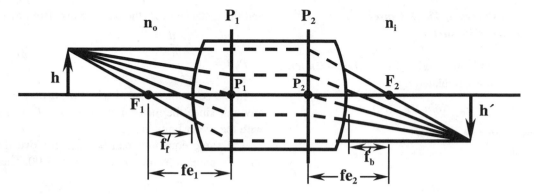

Figure 1.21. Once the equivalent system is determined for a thick lens, the path for any object ray can be traced through the original system.

The distance from P_2 to F_2 is called the *second equivalent focal length* (f_{e2}). P_2 is where the equivalent thin lens of power F_e would be placed for exiting image rays. Its necessary power would then be $F_e = n_i/f_{e2}$.

For a thick lens in air $F_e = -1/f_{e1} = 1/f_{e2}$, and $f_{e1} = -f_{e2}$. (But f_f usually does not equal f_b.)

Gauss Raytracing Using Cardinal Points

In the accompanying figures, the complex systems have been drawn as single thick lenses. However, a combination of many lenses can also be replaced by two principal planes (P_1 and P_2), and the first and second focal points (F_1 and F_2).

Up to this point the objects and images have been in an index of 1.00 but we can extend this to any index. If we allow the object rays to be in a medium of index n_o and the image rays to be in a medium of index n_i, then the equivalent power $F_e = -n_o/f_{e1} = n_i/f_{e2}$, where f_{e1} is the distance between P_1 and F_1, and f_{e2} is the distance between P_2 and F_2.

Then the vergence of the object light at P_1 is $L_{P1} = n_o/\ell_{P1}$, where ℓ_{P1} is the distance from P_1 to the object. The vergence of the image light at P_2 is $L_{P2}' = n_i/\ell_{P2}'$, where ℓ_{P2}' is the distance from P_2 to the image. Figure 1.22 shows this on a diagram.

With L_{P1} and F_e defined, the Gauss equation can be used to find image distances from P_2 for various object distances from P_1.

$$L_{P1} + F_e = L_{P2}', \quad \ell_{P2}' = n_i/L_{P2}'$$

and the magnification becomes

$$M_T = L_{P1}/L_{P2}'$$

As drawn in Figure 1.22, P_1A is negative and P_2B is positive. Then

$$\ell_{P1} = \ell_1 + P_1A$$

and

$$\ell_{P2}' = \ell_2' + P_2B$$

so

$$\ell_2' = \ell_{P2}' - P_2B$$

The problem, then, becomes how to calculate F_e and how to find the locations of P_1 and P_2 relative to the physical front (A) and back (B) surfaces of the original optical system (dashed outline in Figure 1.22).

Some optical systems contain many lenses. In such cases, it would be laborious to trace rays through the real system each time the object distance was changed. However, once the equivalent lens model is determined, much time can be saved because only one refraction must be calculated to find an image. The following procedure is illustrated in Figure 1.23:

$$\ell_{P1} = \ell_1 + P_1A$$
$$L_{P1} = n_o/\ell_{P1}$$
$$L_{P1} + F_e = L_{P2}'$$
$$\ell_{P2} = n_i/L_{P2}'$$
$$\ell_n' = \ell_{P2}' - P_2B$$

where n (in ℓ_n') is the number of surfaces.

Principal Planes of Thick Lenses
(Two Refracting Surfaces)

If the system being modeled is a *single thick lens*, then F_e can be calculated by

$$F_e = F_1 + F_2 - (d/n_2)(F_1)(F_2)$$

where *d must be in meters*.

Then:

$$f_{e1} = -n_o/F_e, f_{e2} = n_i/F_e$$

where f_{e1} and f_{e2} are the distances between P_1 and F_1 and P_2 and F_2, respectively (*not* f_f and f_b).

Then, if the thick lens is in air ($n_o = n_i = 1.00$) the distance of P_1 from the front vertex (A) is:

$$P_1A = -\frac{F_2 \dfrac{d}{n_2}}{F_e} (n_o)$$

and the distance of B (the back vertex) from P_2 is

$$P_2B = +\frac{F_1 \dfrac{d}{n_2}}{F_e} (n_i)$$

In the equations for P_1A and P_2B, d may be in any unit since the meter units in F_1 and F_2 cancel with the meter units in F_e.

The same equations can be used for two thin lenses separated by air by setting $n_2 = 1.00$. Then

$$F_e = F_1 + F_2 - dF_1F_2, P_1A = -F_2d/F_e$$

and $P_2B = +F_1d/F_e$

For *thick* lenses, the *shape* of the lens helps to determine the positions of P_1 and P_2. Either P_1 or P_2 or both can be outside the lens.

For a single thick lens,

1. P_1 is always more upstream than P_2 to incoming object light.

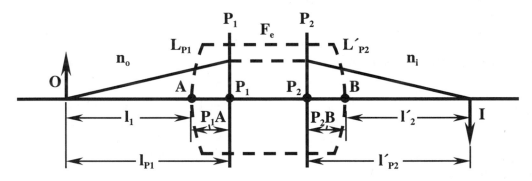

Figure 1.22. The distances, powers, and refractive indices used in the equations to determine the placement of P_1 and P_2.

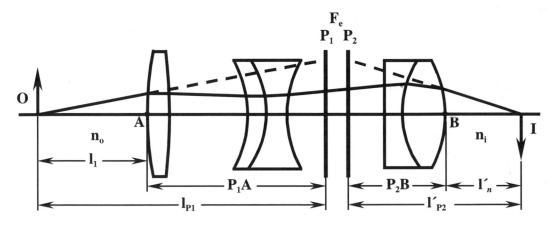

Figure 1.23. This diagram illustrates how the equivalent system can greatly simplify the calculations involved in raytracing between objects and images.

2. P_1 and P_2 are shifted in the direction of the surface with the greater curvature.
3. If one surface is plano ($F = 0$), P_1 or P_2 is at the surface that has curvature.

Example: Thick Lens

$F_1 = +10$ D, $F_2 = +5$ D, $n_2 = 1.50$, $n_1 = n_3 = 1.00$, $d = 10$ cm, $\ell_1 = -50$ cm.

Find ℓ_2' and m_T (Figure 1.24A).

By Full Raytrace

$\ell_1 = -50$ cm, $L_1 = n_1/\ell_1 = (1.00/-50)(100) = -2$ D $= L_1$

$L_1 + F_1 = L_1', -2 + (+10) = +8$ D $= L_1'$

$\ell_1' = n_2/L_1' = (1.50/+8)(100) = +18.75$ cm $= \ell_1'$

$\ell_2 = \ell_1' - d = +18.75 - 10 = +8.75$ cm $= \ell_2$

$L_2 = n_2/\ell_2 = (1.50/+8.75)(100) = +17.14$ D $= L_2$

$L_2 + F_2 = L_2', +17.14 + (+5) = +22.14$ D $= L_2'$

$\ell_2' = n_3/L_2' = (1.00/+22.14)(100) = +4.52$ cm $= \ell_2'$

$m_T = (L_1/L_1')(L_2/L_2')$
$= (-2/+8)(+17.14/+22.14) = -0.19x = M_T$

By Equivalent Lens

$F_e = F_1 + F_2 - (d/n_2)F_1F_2$ ($d = 10$ cm $= 0.1$ meters)

$= (+10) + (+5) - (0.1 \text{ m}/1.50)(+10)(+5)$
$= +11.67$ D $= F_e$

$P_1A = -[F_2(d/n_2)]/F_e$
$= -[(+5)(10 \text{ cm}/1.50)]/(+11.67) = -2.86$ cm

$P_2B = +[F_1(d/n_2)]/F_e$
$= +[(+10)(10 \text{ cm}/1.50)]/(+11.67) = +5.72$ cm

Figure 1.24B shows how this is done for the system in Figure 1.24A.

$\ell_{P1} = \ell_1 + P_1A = -50 + (-2.86)$
$= -52.86$ cm $= \ell_{P1}$

$L_{P1} = n_1/\ell_{P1} = (1.00/-52.86)(100) = -1.89$ D $= L_{P1}$

$L_{P1} + F_e = L_{P2}', -1.89 + (+11.67) = +9.78$ D $= L_{P2}'$

$\ell_{P2}' = n_3/L_{P2}' = (1.00/+9.78)(100) = +10.22$ cm (distance from P_2 to image)

$\ell_2' = \ell_{P2}' - P_2B = 10.22 - (+5.72)$
$= +4.51$ cm $= \ell_2'$ (distance from back vertex to image)

$m = (L_{P1})/(L_{P2}') = (-1.89)/(+9.78)$
$= -0.19x = m$

which agrees with the full raytrace.

It doesn't seem to be less work in this case to use cardinal points since F_e and the positions of P_1 and P_2 had to be calculated. However, if you need to locate the images for numerous object distances it would save time.

Nodal Points

In tracing rays through a *thin lens* the nodal ray passes through the center of the lens undeviated, so $\omega = \omega'$ (Figure 1.25A).

In a *thick lens* no ray passes through undeviated (unless it is coincident with the optical axis). However, a ray *can* be found that leaves the lens at the same angle to the axis as the angle at which it enters the lens ($\omega = \omega'$, that is, the object and image rays are parallel) (Figure 1.25B).

If the parallel entering and exiting rays are extended to the axis, the points at which they hit the axis defines the *nodal points* (N_1 and N_2) for a thick lens. The object ray is associated with the first nodal point (N_1) and the image ray is associated with the second nodal point (N_2).

To locate the nodal points:

1. If $n_o = n_i$, as happens when a lens is in air, then $f_{e1} = -f_{e2}$ and the nodal points have the same location as the principal points (P_1 and P_2). Then a ray directed toward P_1N_1 will exit the lens parallel to the object ray as if it were coming from P_2N_2. We have already encountered this ray in Figure 1.21 as the third predictable ray (nodal ray) in graphical raytracing through equivalent systems (Figure 1.26A).
2. If $n_o \neq n_i$, then $f_{e1} \neq -f_{e2}$ and the nodal points shift away from their corresponding principal points in the direction of the higher refractive

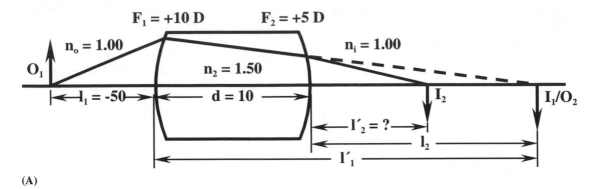

(A)

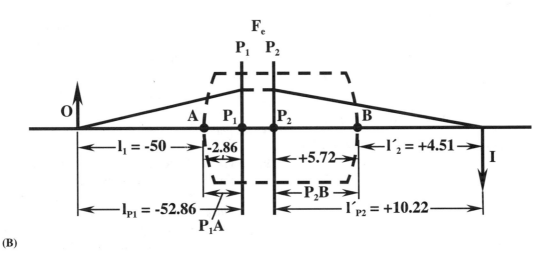

(B)

Figure 1.24. (A) The distances and powers required for a full raytrace through a single thick lens. (B) The equivalent system for a raytrace through the thick lens.

index side. When this happens, the distance from N_1 to N_2 still equals the distance from P_1 to P_2 ($N_1N_2 = P_1P_2$). But $F_1P_1 \neq P_2F_2$. Instead, the distance from F_1 to P_1 equals the distance from N_2 to F_2 ($F_1P_1 = N_2F_2$) (Figure 1.26B).

To locate the nodal points given P_1, P_2, F_e, and n_i:

1. $f_{e1} = -n_o/F_e$ and $f_{e2} = n_i/F_e$.
2. Distance $N_2F_2 = f_{e1}$.
3. N_1 is the same distance from N_2 as P_1 is from P_2.

A single refracting surface is the simplest example of how the nodal points can be separated from the principal points. In this case, P_1 coincides with P_2 and is located at the interface. N_1 coincides with N_2 and is located at the center of curvature (C) of the interface a distance r from P in the direction of the higher index where $r = f_{e1} + f_{e2}$ (Figure 1.27).

$$F_e = (n_i - n_o)/r, f_{e1} = -n_o/F_e, f_{e2} = n_i/F_e$$
$$[\text{or } f_{e2} = -(n_i/n_o)f_{e1}]$$

$$P_1N_1 \equiv P_2N_2 = r = f_{e2} + f_{e1}$$

STOPS

Until now we have not considered the sizes of lenses. However, real lenses have limited diameters and hence will limit the sizes of the bundles of rays going through the system.

Lenses are made of different sizes for a number of reasons including:

1. To determine the brightness of the image.
2. To determine the amount of detail in the image.
3. To determine the size of the field of view.

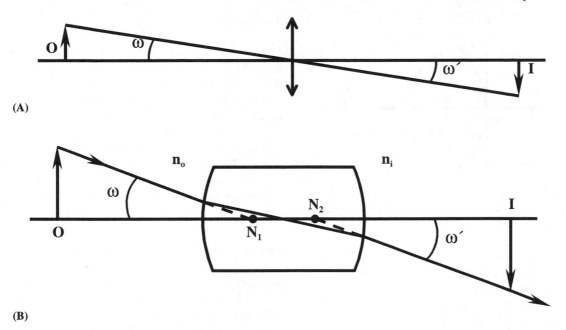

(A)

(B)

Figure 1.25. (**A**) The nodal ray passes through the center of a thin lens undeviated. (**B**) For a thick lens, no nonaxial ray passes through the lens undeviated. However, if the ray enters in the direction of N_1, the ray will exit parallel to the ray entering from the direction of N_2.

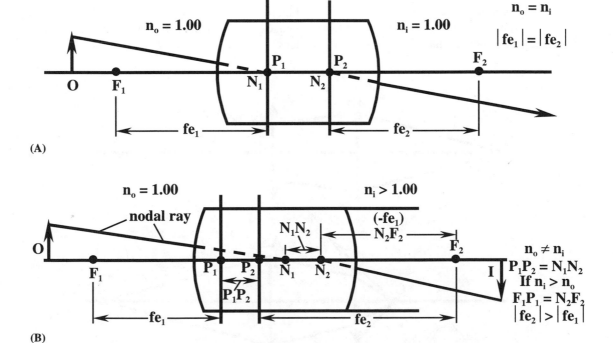

(A)

(B)

Figure 1.26. (**A**) If the object and image rays are in the same refractive index (e.g., a lens in air), then N_1 is located at P_1 and N_2 is located at P_2. (**B**) If the object and image rays are in a different refractive index, then N_1 and N_2 are shifted away from P_1 and P_2 in the direction of the higher index.

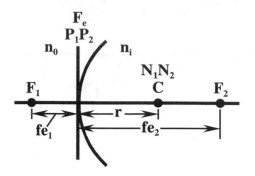

Figure 1.27. For a single refractive surface P_1 and P_2 are located at the surface and N_1 and N_2 are located at the center of curvature for the surface.

4. To determine the depth of field and depth of focus.
5. To reduce aberrations.
6. To eliminate stray light.
7. To improve economy.
8. To improve aesthetic appearance (e.g., spectacle lenses).

It is also common to use lensless apertures (usually circular holes) in an optical system for some of the same reasons. All of the *elements* (lenses or lensless apertures) that limit the passage of rays in an optical system are called *stops*. Two stops, the *aperture stop* and the *field stop*, serve special functions, after which they are named.

Aperture Stop

The aperture stop (AS) is the element in a system that limits the amount of light from an *axial object point* that reaches the image and, thus, it controls axial image brightness. For example, a simple lens can be its own aperture stop. A separate lensless aperture may also limit the bundle of rays and be the AS.

The AS may be one of the lenses in a compound system. Figure 1.28 illustrates that the particular element that becomes the AS may depend on the distance from the object to the system. Also, note that the smallest lens is not necessarily the AS.

Identification of the Aperture Stop

To determine which element is the aperture stop (AS), place your eye at the intended axial object point and look into the optical system in reverse. You will see the first element directly, as well as the *images* of all of the internal lenses and apertures formed by the lenses in front of them. The *image* that looks smallest is called the *entrance pupil* (*EP*) and the *lens or aperture* whose image it is, is the *aperture stop* (*AS*).

You can locate the EP and AS in a system (as in Figure 1.29) by finding the location and size of the image of every element as viewed through the front lens:

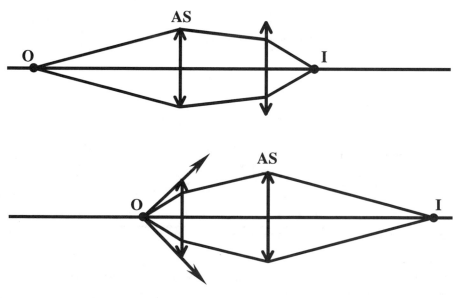

Figure 1.28. Which lens in a system is the aperture stop can depend on the distance of the object from the system.

1. *A* has no lens in front of it so it is its own image (*A'*).
2. The image of *B* through *A* is *B'*.
3. The image of *C* through *A* and *B* is *C'*.

Determine the angles the axial object point makes with the edges of all of the images. Then, the *image* that forms the smallest angle with the axial object point is the entrance pupil (EP) and the *element* whose image it is, is the aperture stop (AS).

Lens *A* has no lenses in front of it so its "image" *A'* is the lens itself. Lens *B* is imaged by lens *A* at *B'*. Lens *C* is imaged by lenses *B* and *A* at *C'*. The image diameters can then be calculated as the physical lens diameters multiplied by each respective magnification. In the above case, *C'* is the image that subtends the smallest angle with the eye at the intended axial object point so *C'* is the entrance pupil (EP) and lens *C* is the aperture stop (AS).

If a ray goes through the edge of object (*C*), it must also go through the edge of its image (*C'*).

The opposite is also true; by reversibility of rays, a ray directed toward the edge of image (*C'*) must come from the edge of object (*C*). Since the EP is an image of the AS, the cone of rays from the axial object point that is limited by the edge of the EP will, after all refractions, skim the edge of the AS. Thus, the size of the cone of light entering the system is limited by the outer rays that are directed toward the edge of the EP (Figure 1.30).

If you place your eye at the intended axial *image* (*I*) position and look through the system from behind, you will see the last element directly, as well as the images of all of the internal lenses and apertures. The image of the AS seen in this way is called the *exit pupil* (*XP*). For the lens system shown in Figure 1.30, since there are no lenses to the right of the AS (lens *C*), the AS is also the XP. The cone of rays from the axial image point directed toward the edge of the XP until it intersects the rearmost element in the system defines the physical extent of image rays exiting the system.

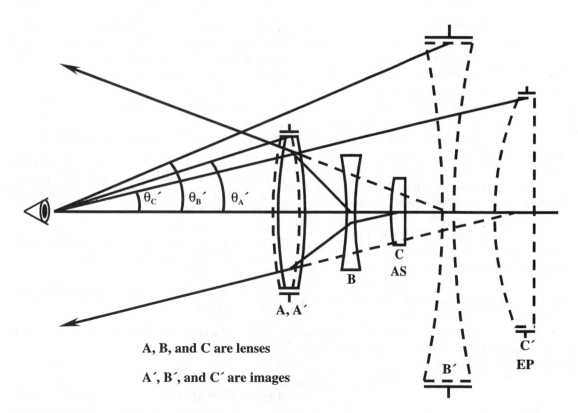

A, B, and C are lenses

A´, B´, and C´ are images

Figure 1.29. When you look through the front of a system of thin lenses, you see only the first lens with its actual location and size. You see each of the other lenses as an image formed by all of the lenses in front of it. When lines are drawn connecting the intended axial object point to the edge of each of the lens images, the edge that subtends the smallest angle belongs to the EP and the lens whose image it is, is the AS.

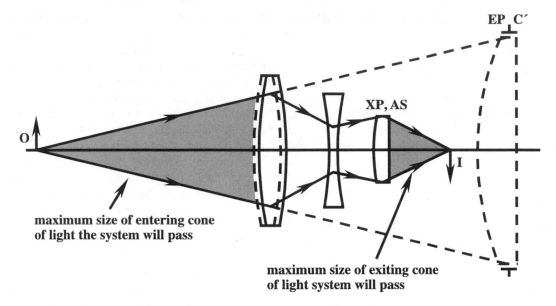

Figure 1.30. The largest cone of light impinging on the first lens from an axial object point that will make it through the entire system is limited by the size of the entrance pupil (EP). The largest cone of light that will leave the last lens to form an axial image is limited by the size of the exit pupil (XP).

You can see that the EP for object rays and the XP for image rays define the limits of the cones of light that can enter and exit the system.

So far our discussion of stops has been limited to *on-axis* objects and images. In order to understand how stops can affect the field of view of a system, we need to consider *off-axis* objects and images.

An *off-axis* object ray that is directed toward the center of the EP is called a *chief* or a *principal ray*. Since the EP is an image of the AS, the chief ray will also go through the center of the AS. Since the XP is also an image of the AS, the chief ray, after any further refractions, will exit the system as though coming from the center of the XP (Figure 1.31).

The importance of the chief ray is that it is the central ray of the bundle of rays that traverses the system. Thus, the center of a blur circle (a cross section of the cone of rays exiting the system) can be located by the chief ray, and the size of the blur circle can be determined by the intersection of an out-of-focus image plane (e.g., a screen) and the cone of light from the XP.

Field Stop

The field stop (FS) is the element in a system that, combined with the AS, limits the *off-axis* extent of

an object that can be imaged through the system. The FS is the element that if made larger would result in a greater field of view (more of the periphery of an off-axis object being imaged).

Identification of the Field Stop

To determine which element is the field stop:

1. Locate the images of all of the elements as seen through the front of the system. (The front element is its own image.) This has already been done as part of the procedure for finding the aperture stop (AS).
2. The element *image* whose edge forms the smallest angle with the center of the EP is the *entrance window*.
3. The element whose image is the entrance window is the FS.

This is illustrated in Figure 1.32 for the system in Figure 1.29.

Angular Field of View

The angular field of view is the angular extent of objects that can be imaged at the image plane. The entrance window is useful for finding the field of

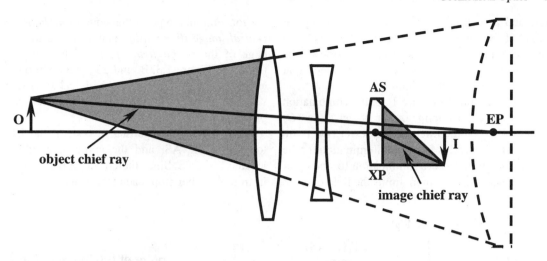

Figure 1.31. A ray from an off-axis object point that is directed into the system toward the center of the EP is called the chief ray. As this ray traverses the system, it stays in the center of the ray bundle and defines the image location even when the image is out of focus.

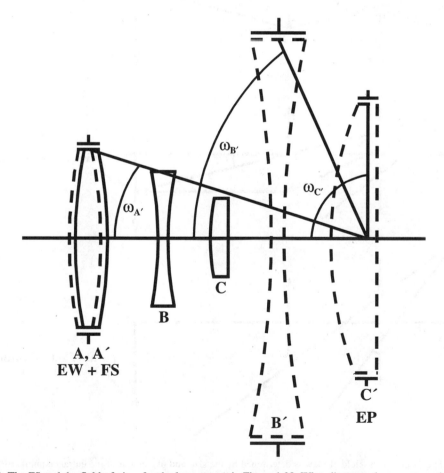

Figure 1.32. The FS and the field of view for the lens system in Figure 1.29. When lines are drawn connecting the center of the EP to the edge of each of the lens images, the edge that subtends the smallest angle belongs to the EW and the lens whose image it is, is the FS. The angle between the center of the EP and the edges of the EW is the field of view.

view and is well named. If you place your eye at the EP of the system, the entrance window is like a physical window (of the size and position of the image of the FS) that limits the size of objects that can be seen beyond the window.

In the diagrams in Figure 1.33, the combination of two stops causes points on the object arrow (O) farther off axis to be imaged with fewer rays (with less light). This varies from full illumination for the axial image point to zero illumination for the tip of the image arrow. This, then, limits the field of view.

By convention, the point that equals *one-half of the central image illumination* is considered to be the edge of the *useful field of view*. This gives $\omega_{A'}$ (= ω_e) in Figure 1.33B, and $2\omega_e$ (which allows an equal amount of field below the optical axis) agrees with the definition for angular field of view given previously.

Note that in this particular system, the EP is located at the AS, and the entrance window is located at the FS. Since there is no refractive power in front of either stop, each stop is its own image.

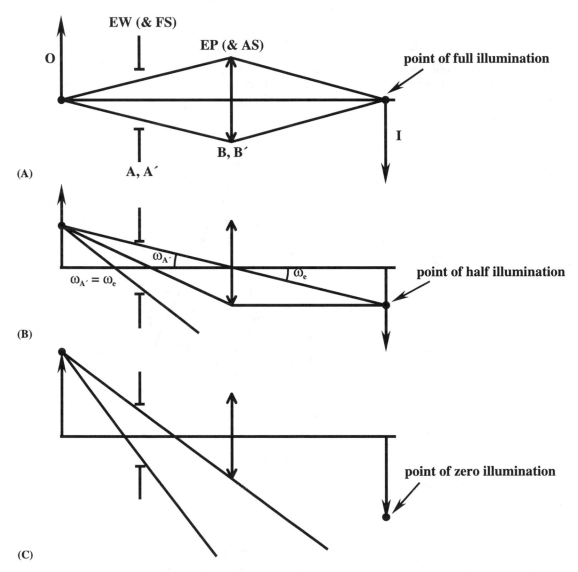

Figure 1.33. The extent of the field of view is determined by the size and placement of the entrance pupil (EP) and the entrance window (EW). The image illumination drops off gradually as object points become more off-axis (going from A to C), and field of view ($2\omega_e$) can be defined by that object point that results in a peripheral image half as bright as the central image.

DEPTH OF FIELD AND FOCUS

For a given distance ℓ of a point object from a lens, there is a definite distance ℓ' of the image point from the lens. If the object is moved closer to or farther from the lens (ℓ_2 or ℓ_1), then the image will move as well (ℓ_2' or ℓ_1'). If the image is still examined at ℓ' when the clearest image is at ℓ_2' or ℓ_1', a blur circle results rather than a sharp image point (Figure 1.34).

In all optical systems there is a critical blur circle size below which a smaller blur circle either cannot or need not be discriminated from a perfect point image. This may be due to the "grain" of film, the spacing of photoreceptors in the retina, or the ultimate limit to the image size of a point object due to diffraction. (Diffraction is discussed in Chapter 2.)

The range of object distances ($\ell_2 - \ell_1$) giving the largest tolerable blur circle diameter is the *depth of field*. The corresponding range of image distances ($\ell_2' - \ell_1'$) giving the same blur circle is the *depth of focus*.

Depth of field and focus can also be given as dioptric ranges:

Depth of field in diopters: $L_2 - L_1 = \dfrac{n_o}{\ell_2} - \dfrac{n_o}{\ell_1}$

Depth of focus in diopters: $L_2' - L_1' = \dfrac{n_i}{\ell_2'} - \dfrac{n_i}{\ell_1'}$

(Where n_o is the index the object is in and n_i is the index the image is in.)

The *dioptric* depth of field equals the *dioptric* depth of focus:

$$L_2 - L_1 = L_2' - L_1'$$

However,

$$\ell_2 - \ell_1 \neq \ell_2' - \ell_1'!$$

Example: A +7 D lens with a diameter (D) of 2.5 cm focuses an object 50 cm in front of the lens onto a screen behind the lens. If the greatest tolerable blur circle diameter in the image is 0.1 cm (Figure 1.35):

a. What is the total linear and dioptric depth of focus?

$F = +7$ D, $L + F = L'$, $(-2) + (+7) = +5$ D, $\ell' = 100/+5 = +20$ cm

$$\frac{x}{b} = \frac{1' + x}{D}, \frac{y}{b} = \frac{1' - y}{D}$$

If x and y are $\ll \ell'$, x or $y \approx b(\ell'/D) = 0.8$ cm in this case.

$$\frac{x}{0.1} = \frac{20 + x}{2.5}, 2.5x = 2 + 0.1x, 2.4x = 2,$$

$x = 0.833$ cm,

$$\frac{y}{0.1} = \frac{20 - y}{2.5}, 2.5y = 2 - 0.1y,$$

$2.6y = 2, y = 0.769$ cm

Therefore, linear depth of focus from $\ell' + x$ to $\ell' - y$ is 20.83 to 19.23 cm.

Range $= 20.83 - 19.23 = 1.60$ cm. (Equals $x + y$. Note that $x > y$, but for an approximation we have used $x = y$.)

b. What is the linear depth of field? That is, how far are the nearest and farthest extremes of the depth of field from the lens?

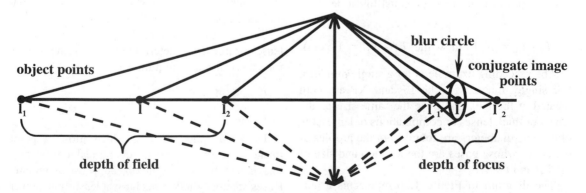

Figure 1.34. While an axial point object theoretically forms an image point in focus at one axial location, a range of object distances is tolerable if the resultant blur at the image plane is small enough.

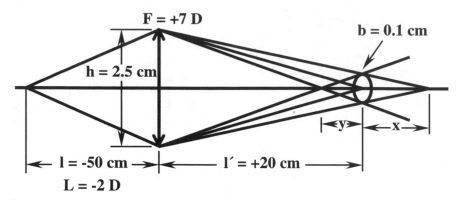

Figure 1.35. An example of depth of focus for a thin lens when a certain blur circle diameter (*b*) is tolerable.

The dioptric depth of field equals the dioptric depth of focus.

$$L_x' = 1/\ell_x' = 100/20.83 = +4.80 \text{ D}$$

$$L_y' = 1/\ell_y' = 100/19.23 = +5.20 \text{ D}$$

$$L_y' - L_x' = 5.20 - 4.80 = 0.40 \text{ D (or } \pm 0.20 \text{ D)}$$
depth of focus *and* depth of field.

Linear depth of field:

$$-2 \pm 0.2 \text{ D} \Rightarrow L_1 = -1.8 \text{ to } L_2 = -2.2 \text{ D}$$

$$L_1 = -1.8, \ell_1 = 100/-1.8 = -55.55 \text{ cm} = \ell_1$$

$$L_2 = -2.2, \ell_2 = 100/-2.2 = -45.45 \text{ cm} = \ell_2$$

Everything between ℓ_1 and ℓ_2 is "clear" (has an image blur circle ≤ 0.1 cm).

Note that while dioptric depth of field equals dioptric depth of focus,

$$(L_2 - L_1 = L_2' - L_1' = 0.40 \text{ D})$$

linear depth of field does not equal linear depth of focus,

$$(\ell_2 - \ell_1 = 10.1 \text{ cm} \quad \text{while} \quad \ell_2' - \ell_1' = 1.6 \text{ cm})$$

The preceding example is for a single thin lens. For single thin lenses, the EP and XP are both located at the lens and have the same size as the lens. For thick lenses or combinations of lenses, the blur circle diameters are found from the profiles of the cones whose bases are the location and size of the EP and the XP.

The diagram in Figure 1.36 represents a lens system where the front and back of the box represent the first and last lens surfaces in the system.

For a single thin lens, $\ell_{XP}' = \ell_{LENS}'$ and $D_{XP} = D_{LENS}$. But for a thick lens or a system of lenses, we require the EP and XP, which are a different size and location from the front and back lens surfaces.

AXIAL ASTIGMATISM

So far we have discussed spherical optical surfaces whose powers are the same for all *meridians* (diameters). It is also possible to make *astigmatic* lenses or mirrors whose powers vary along different meridians. There are few applications for optical elements that are deliberately made astigmatic, but the cornea and lens of most eyes have at least some astigmatism, so the topic is important for the correction of refractive error.

The most extreme case of an astigmatic lens is a cylinder where the power along one diameter is zero (called the *axis* of the cylinder) and the power along the diameter perpendicular to the axis is maximal (called the *power meridian*) (Figure 1.37).

The dioptric power in the power meridian for lenses or mirrors is determined in the same way as for spherical lenses and mirrors:

$$F_{lens} = (n_2 - n_1)/r$$

$$F_{mirror} = n/(r/2)$$

Unlike a spherical lens, which forms a point image from a point object, a cylindrical lens forms a line image from a point object. Most astigmatic lenses are not cylinders but have at least some power along all of their meridians. If the astigmatism is *regular,* then the meridians of greatest and least

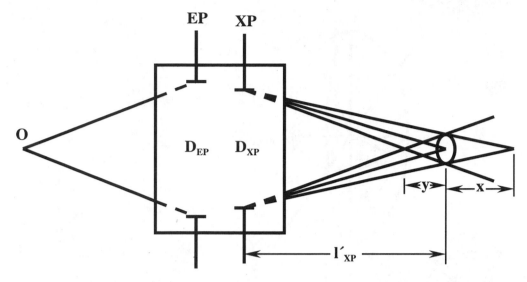

Figure 1.36. Depth of focus may be found for an optical system if the size and locations of the EP and XP are known. The object rays are traced to the edge of the EP and the image rays are traced from the edge of the XP.

power (called *principal meridians*) are at right angles to each other (Figure 1.38). The powers differ because the most powerful meridian has a shorter radius of curvature than the least powerful meridian. Such a surface is called *toric* because it is part of the surface of a toroid (a doughnut-shaped solid).

When an astigmatic lens has power in both meridians, point objects are still imaged as lines but there will be *two* line images, one for each power meridian. The line image in each case is perpendicular to the power meridian that forms it (Figures 1.39A).

The distance between the two line images is called the *interval of Sturm*. The envelope of the light beam between the two line foci is called the *conoid of Sturm*. Cross sections of the total envelope from the lens outward are shown in Figure 1.39B. A "point" focus does not exist in the envelope. The best focus is a blur circle between the two line images, which is called the *circle of least confusion*.

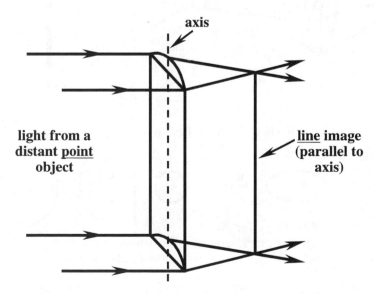

Figure 1.37. The power meridian of a pure cylinder is perpendicular to its axis. The line image that results from a point object is parallel to the cylinder's axis.

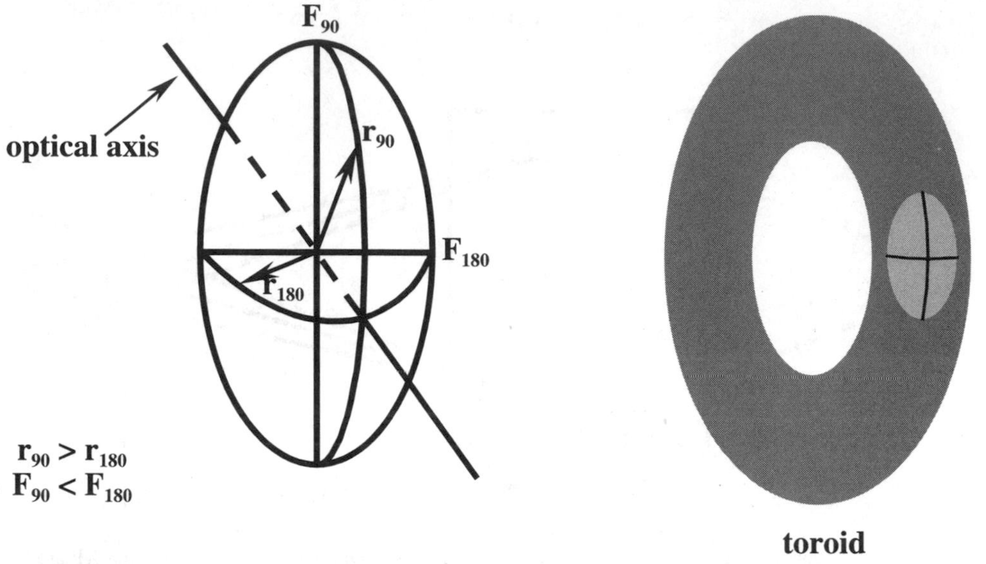

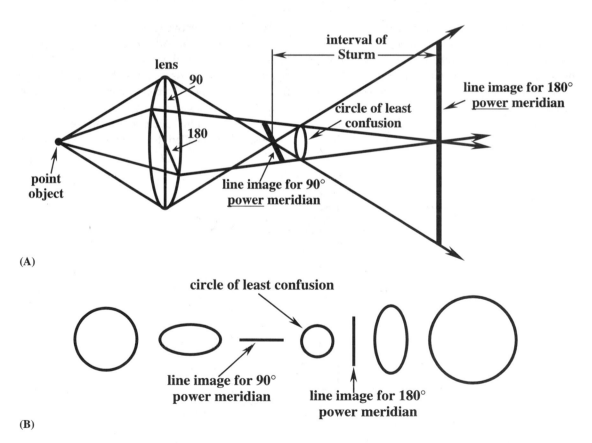

Figure 1.38. If a surface has regular astigmatism, the two power meridia are perpendicular. Such surfaces are referred to as toric because they can be described by a tangential section of a toroid (a doughnut-shaped solid).

Figure 1.39. (A) Since a toric surface has two power meridia, a point object will form two line images separated by a distance referred to as the interval of Sturm. (B) Cross sections of the envelope of rays formed by a toric surface progress from circular, to line, to circle of least confusion, to line, to circular again.

ABERRATIONS

So far we have assumed that if lenses and mirrors have perfectly spherical surfaces they will reproduce point objects located on a flat object plane as geometrically projected point images located on a flat image plane. This is only true to an approximation. To the extent that it is not true, an optical system is said to suffer from *aberrations*. This chapter discusses aberrations as the deviation of rays from their ideal location at the image plane. In Chapter 2 the concept of aberrations will be extended to wavefront error.

Chromatic Aberration

For the purpose of raytracing, we have used helium *d* light (yellow) to determine the refractive index (*n*). However, *n* will vary a small amount depending on the wavelength (λ) of the light being used. For the common materials used for lenses, short wavelength light (e.g., blue) has a greater *n* and is refracted more strongly than longer wavelength light (e.g., red). This is the reason why prisms break white light, which contains many wavelengths, into a spectrum of colors. The separation of light into its component colors is referred to as *dispersion*.

The three wavelengths in the visible spectrum that are commonly used to specify the refractive index (*n*) of optical materials are listed in Table 1.1. When we specify index of refraction for the media of the eye, the index for 555 nm is often used because that is the wavelength to which the eye is most sensitive when it is adapted to daytime illumination levels. Since this does not correspond to any practical spectral line, the 546 nm (green) mercury *e* line is frequently used as an approximation to 555 nm giving the index n_e.

Materials also differ in their *range* of *n*s ($n_F - n_C$). This range is called the *mean dispersion* and it

Table 1.1. Wavelengths Used to Specify *n* of Various Materials

	Spectral Sources
656 nm (red) called *C* light $\Rightarrow n_C$	hydrogen
587 nm (yellow) called *d* light $\Rightarrow n_d$	helium
486 nm (blue) called *F* light $\Rightarrow n_F$	hydrogen

can differ for different materials even if their n_d is the same. However, materials with a higher n_d *tend* to have a larger mean dispersion. Dispersive power is calculated as

$$V = \frac{n_d - 1}{n_F - n_C}$$

This is called the *V-value* or *number* (also *Abbe number* or *v-value*). If, for example, $V = 58.8$, this value means that, for 58.8 degrees of refraction of *d* light, we will get 1 degree of dispersion (separation) between *C* and *F* light. Note that the lower the *V*-value, the greater the dispersion (Figure 1.40).

Tables of n_d and *V* can be found for virtually all optical materials. Some tables use a shorthand notation in which decimal points are omitted from *n* and *V* and the 1 is omitted from *n*. For example, water which has $n_d = 1.334$ and $V = 54.7$ could be written as 334547.

The prism model of lenses suggests that lenses as well as prisms disperse light. Thus, the power and focal length of a lens are wavelength dependent (e.g., there is an F_d, an F_C, and an F_F, and their corresponding f_d, f_C, and f_F). This effect is called *chromatic aberration* (*CA*) of the lens. The location of the primary focal length is defined by n_d (yellow) light (giving F_d and f_d).

Longitudinal CA is the axial distance between the focal points for blue and red light.

Transverse CA is the radius of the blur circle at the yellow light (n_d) image plane due to the other colors being out of focus (Figure 1.41).

If the lens is "stopped down" (reduced in diameter), transverse CA decreases but longitudinal CA

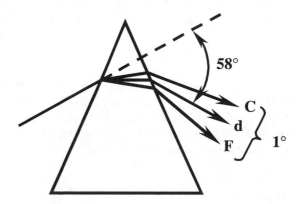

Figure 1.40. The *V*-value for a prism is the total angular deviation of a ray that results in one degree of difference in deviation between *C* (red) and *F* (blue) light.

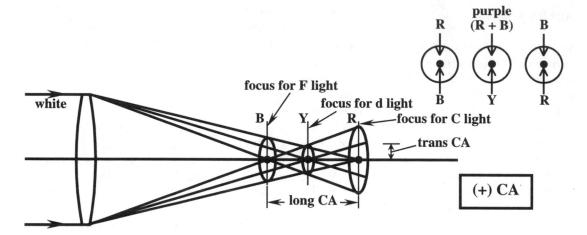

Figure 1.41. Transverse CA is the radius of the blur circle that results from *C* and *F* light being out of focus at the focal plane for *d* (yellow) light.

stays the same. Lenses can show longitudinal CA as a spread of either real or virtual image points.

A negative lens spreads the spectral order of colors in a direction opposite that of a positive lens whether the image is real *or* virtual. CA is (+) if *B* focuses before *R*. This is always the case with a plus lens. CA is (−) if *B* focuses after *R*. This is always the case with a minus lens. For this reason, a plus lens is said to have *positive CA* and a minus lens is said to have *negative CA*.

Longitudinal CA can also be expressed in diopters, usually based on the difference in *L′* for the wavelengths 486 nm (blue) and 656 nm (red) because these represent opposite sides of the visible spectrum (the *F* and *C* Fraunhofer lines, which are discussed in Chapter 2):

Dioptric CA $= L_F' - L_C'$

Dioptric CA for a distant object $= F_F - F_C$

$= \dfrac{F_d}{V}$, where $V = \dfrac{n_d - 1}{n_F - n_C}$

Example: A simple plus lens used as a camera lens will suffer from plus CA. Assume it has a 100 cm focal length and that it is made from crown glass ($n_d = 1.523$, $V = 58.6$). What is the longitudinal CA in diopters and in cm (Figure 1.42)?

$F_d = +1.0$ D

Then,

$$CA = F_F - F_C = \frac{F_d}{V} = \frac{+1.0\ \text{D}}{58.6} = 0.017\ \text{D}$$

As an approximation, the dioptric range of red (*C*) and blue (*F*) foci would be $F_d \pm 0.017/2 = 1.0 \pm 0.0085 = 1.009$ to 0.991 D. (Actually, blue light is responsible for a disproportionate part of the range but this will still give an accurate linear range.) The linear image distances would then be from $100/1.009 = 99.11$ cm to $100/0.991 = 100.91$ cm. Then the longitudinal CA is $\ell_C' - \ell_F' = 100.91 - 99.11 = 1.8$ cm = CA and a simultaneous focus for all wavelengths would be impossible.

Monochromatic Aberrations

The Gauss equation ($L + F = L'$) is based on a small angle approximation of Snell's law in which $\sin\theta \approx \theta$ in radians. Then, $n_1 \sin i = n_2 \sin r$ becomes $n_1 i \approx n_2 r$. This is accurate only when the angles of incidence or refraction on a surface are very small. Thus, it is a good approximation only for small lens apertures and small fields of view where the rays form a narrow pencil at the center of the lens, the *paraxial region* (Figure 1.43).

The small angle approximation, $\sin\theta = \theta$, comes from the first term of the series

$$\sin\theta = \theta - \frac{\theta^3}{3!} + \frac{\theta^5}{5!} - \frac{\theta^7}{7!} + \ \dots\ \text{(where } \theta \text{ is in radians)}$$

Using additional terms in the series gives a closer approximation to $\sin\theta$. Fewer terms are needed for a good approximation if θ is small. For off-axis rays and peripheral parts of the lens, θ quickly becomes

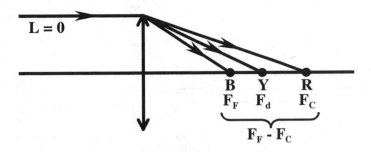

Figure 1.42. An example of longitudinal CA from a simple plus lens.

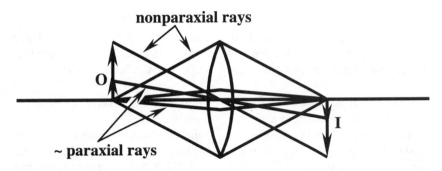

Figure 1.43. An illustration of nonparaxial and nearly paraxial rays for a single thin lens.

large enough that the next or "third-order" term is needed for a good approximation:

$$\sin \theta = \left(\theta - \frac{\theta^3}{3!} \right) \dots$$

Snell's law then is approximated by

$$n_1 \left(\theta - \frac{\theta_i^3}{3!} \right) \approx n_2 \left(\theta_r - \frac{\theta_r^3}{3!} \right)$$

The third-order approximation is adequate for modest angles outside the paraxial region. With a lot of algebra the third-order equation can be transformed into a power series expansion with five terms, which are referred to as the five *Seidel aberrations* (also known as *primary aberrations* or *third-order aberrations*). These are also called *monochromatic aberrations* to distinguish them from chromatic aberration. The five Seidel aberrations are (1) spherical aberration, (2) coma, (3) oblique (or radial) astigmatism, (4) curvature of field, and (5) distortion. Each Seidel aberration gives a transverse error, i.e., the difference in location between the paraxial (Gauss) image point and the point predicted by that third-order term.

If a system has significant aberrations, paraxial raytracing using the Gauss equation gives only a rough approximation of the location of image points. However, most optical systems are designed to correct aberrations, so paraxial raytracing usually finds the actual image locations and sizes. Also, Seidel aberrations are useful when designing optical systems because they give insight into which parameters in a system will be likely to reduce aberrations if they are varied.

Spherical Aberration

Spherical aberration is the only one of the five Seidel aberrations that affects on-axis objects. The rest occur only with off-axis objects. For a lens with spherical surfaces, the power of the lens varies for lens-ray intersections at different distances from the axis (annular zones). For plus lenses with spherical surfaces, the power of the peripheral zones is greater than the power for the central zones (a condition called *positive spherical aberration*). For minus lenses, the peripheral rays focus after the paraxial rays (called *negative spherical aberration*). Spherical aberration is illustrated in Figure 1.44.

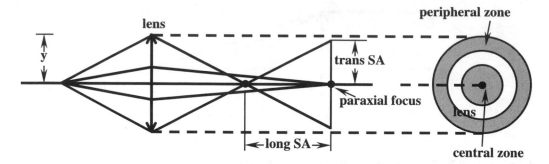

Figure 1.44. An illustration of positive SA from a plus thin lens. The peripheral rays focus closer to the lens than the central rays do.

The axial range of image points from the annular zones is called *longitudinal SA*. The radius of the blur circle at the paraxial image plane is called *transverse SA*.

Spherical aberration can be reduced in several ways, including stopping a lens down to a smaller diameter, changing the surface powers while keeping the total power the same (*bending* the lens), combining lenses with plus and minus aberrations so that the aberration cancels, or by using a gradient index material in which the *n* varies through or across the lens (a GRIN lens).

Comatic Aberration (Coma)

Coma is a Seidel aberration that occurs only for oblique rays (off-axis object points). On-axis object points result in good on-axis image points, but off-axis object points result in off-axis image points that are spread into a comet-shaped pattern (hence the name coma). The head of the comet always points either toward (positive coma) or away (negative coma) from the optical axis.

The degradation of a point object into a comet-shaped image is the result of a difference in lateral magnification for rays passing through different zones (annular rings) of the lens. Figure 1.45 shows positive coma in which the peripheral zones of a lens image object points as circles of image points. The length of the "comet" increases for object points farther off axis.

Unlike spherical aberration, plus or minus lenses can have *either* positive *or* negative coma. Coma can be corrected in several ways including stopping the lens down to a smaller diameter, bending the lens, reducing the field of view for the system, and combining lenses with plus and minus

coma so that the aberrations cancel. An optical system that is corrected for both spherical aberration and coma is called *aplanatic*.

Oblique (Radial) Astigmatism

Axial astigmatism results from toric lens surfaces (surfaces whose radii and power vary in different meridians). Spherical (nontoric) lenses also exhibit different powers in different meridians if the rays are *oblique* (from off-axis object points resulting in off-axis image points). This form of astigmatism, called *oblique* or *radial astigmatism,* results in each point object forming two mutually perpendicular line images separated by an interval of Sturm. There is no "point" image, but the smallest image of an object point is at the circle of least confusion where the bundle of rays becomes narrowest.

Of all the rays that traverse a lens to form an image, two types are of special interest, tangential rays and sagittal rays. *Tangential rays* are those that lie in the plane that contains both the rays and the optical axis (*tangential plane*) and form astigmatic line images perpendicular to that plane. This is the plane we have been using for drawing raytraces. *Sagittal rays* are those that lie in a plane that is perpendicular to the tangential plane (*sagittal plane*), and they form astigmatic line images perpendicular to the sagittal plane. Note that the orientations of the line images are perpendicular to the planes of the rays that form them (Figure 1.46).

Oblique astigmatism becomes a particularly bad problem when very large ray angles are encountered. This is especially true of spectacle lenses due to the wide field of view (widely off-axis object points). The correction is by lens bending. For each lens power (*Rx*), there is a front surface curvature

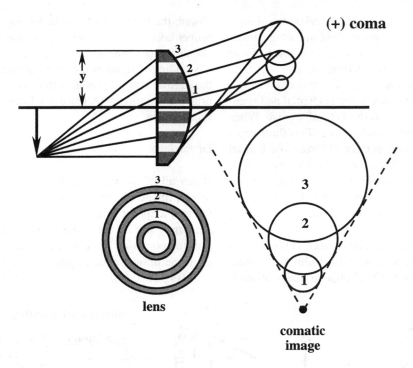

Figure 1.45. Coma in an off-axis image induced by a single plus lens. The peripheral zones of the lens introduce a greater lateral magnification than the central zones do.

(base curve), which minimizes oblique astigmatism. An optical system corrected for astigmatism is called *anastigmatic*.

Curvature of Field

If all of the above Seidel aberrations are eliminated, a point object will be imaged as a point whether it is on-axis *or* off-axis. However, the image points will usually fall on a curved rather than a flat surface so that if an extended image is projected onto a flat surface, not all of the points on the image can be in focus simultaneously.

In the absence of oblique astigmatism, this curved focal surface is called the *Petzval surface*. For plus lenses, the Petzval surface is concave toward the lens; for minus lenses, the Petzval surface is convex toward the lens.

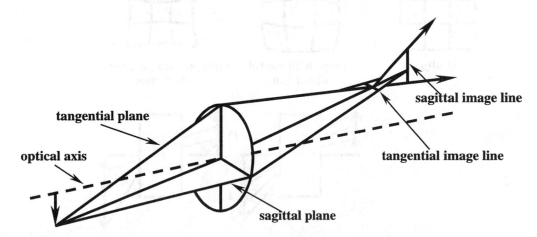

Figure 1.46. An illustration of oblique astigmatism induced by a single plus lens.

Curvature of field is intimately related to oblique astigmatism. In the absence of oblique astigmatism, tangential and sagittal rays from point objects focus together as points on the Petzval surface.

However, if oblique astigmatism is uncorrected, then the image surfaces of the tangential and sagittal lines will *not* fall on the Petzval surface. When this occurs, the tangential surface (*T*) is three times as far as the sagittal surface (*S*) from the Petzval surface (*P*). Therefore, the surface of best focus when oblique astigmatism *is* present is the surface between the *T* and *S* surfaces, which contains the circles of least confusion for all image points (Figure 1.47).

Curvature of field can be reduced (1) by using a curved focal surface (e.g., curved film or the naturally curved retina); (2) if oblique astigmatism is absent, the Petzval surface can be made flat by the proper combination of plus and minus lens powers and different refractive indices; or (3) by intentionally adding oblique astigmatism in such a way that the sagittal and tangential surfaces produce circles of least confusion that are all located on a flat image plane.

Distortion

When all of the other Seidel aberrations are corrected, image distortion remains. Point objects are focused as point images on a flat focal plane, but there may still be a difference in lateral magnification for points on the object at different distances from the optical axis. A grid as object shows this well (Figure 1.48).

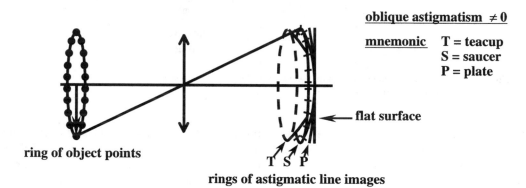

Figure 1.47. A 3-D representation of oblique astigmatism from a ring of point objects in front of a single thin lens.

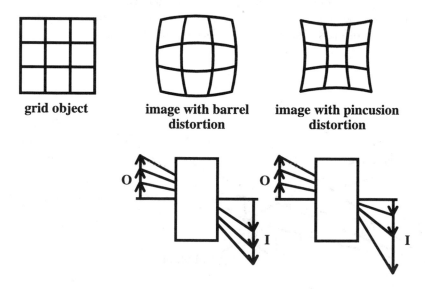

Figure 1.48. Lens systems (boxes) introducing barrel and pincushion distortion into the image from a grid object.

Distortion can be reduced by the proper selection of lens powers and stops but it is difficult to eliminate from wide field optical systems. This is why "fish-eye" camera lenses and door security peepholes have significant uncorrected distortion.

FURTHER READING

Fannin TE, Grosvenor T. *Clinical Optics*. Boston: Butterworth-Heinemann, 1987.

Freeman MH. *Optics*. 10th ed. Boston: Butterworth-Heinemann, 1990.

Keating MP. *Geometrical, Physical, and Visual Optics*. Boston: Butterworth-Heinemann, 1988.

Michaels DD. *Visual Optics and Refraction: A Clinical Approach*. 3rd ed. St. Louis: Mosby, 1985.

Meyer-Arendt JR. *Introduction to Classical and Modern Optics*. 2nd ed. Englewood Cliffs: Prentice-Hall, 1984.

Smith WJ. *Modern Optical Engineering*. 2nd ed. New York: McGraw-Hill, 1990.

Chapter 2
Physical Optics

Are not the Rays of Light very small Bodies emitted from shining Substances? For such Bodies will pass through uniform Mediums in right Lines without bending into the Shadow, which is the nature of Rays of Light. —Isaac Newton, 1730 (From Wade NJ. *A Natural History of Vision.* Cambridge, MA: MIT Press, 1998;23.)

Supposing the light of any given colour to consist of undulations, of a given breadth, or of a given frequency, it follows that these undulations must be liable to those effects which we have already examined in the case of waves of water, and pulses of sound. —Thomas Young, 1807 (From Wade NJ. *A Natural History of Vision.* Cambridge, MA: MIT Press, 1998;24.)

It is very important to know that light behaves like particles, especially for those of you who have gone to school, where you were probably told something about light behaving like waves. I'm telling you the way it *does* behave—like particles. —Richard Feynman, 1985 (From Feynman RP. *QED: The Strange Theory of Light and Matter.* Princeton: Princeton University Press, 1985;15.)

Some aspects of optics can only be understood through physical optics, which is the study of how light interacts with itself and with matter. The classical wave theory of light views light as a radiated electromagnetic field, which is often represented as waves, and the quantum theory of light views it as a stream of particles (photons). Even though intuition makes it difficult to conceive how light can have both a wave and a particle nature, quantum mechanics now gives a mathematically consistent and accurate description of light that includes both concepts.

CLASSICAL THEORY

Classical theory views light as electromagnetic radiation, in which for every point in its path an electric field periodically changes its strength in a direction 90 degrees to the direction in which the light travels. (There is also a magnetic field, but it is unimportant to most optical phenomena.) Although light waves are usually drawn as waves that might seem to represent something physically moving up and down, the height of the curve at each point actually represents the strength and direction in which the electric field would apply a force to positively charged particles (and the opposite direction for negative particles). The strength of the field at each point can also be shown by the lengths and directions of enclosed *E-vectors* (the arrows in Figure 2.1).

The highest and lowest points of the curve represent the *amplitude* (A) of the electric field (Figure 2.2). The *intensity* (I) of the field (energy per second) is proportional to the amplitude squared. *I* is roughly equivalent to *brightness*, but brightness is influenced by perceptual factors as well.

Electromagnetic magnetic radiation (EMR) is created by charges undergoing acceleration. This acceleration is commonly produced by charges moving back and forth along a line (as *oscillating dipoles*), either artificially within antennas or naturally as oscillating charges at the atomic level. This dipole oscillation creates a changing electric field, which oscillates at the same frequency as its source and travels away from the source at the speed of light (c). EMR is radiated most strongly in a direction perpendicular to the direction of charge oscillation (the dipole axis). Wavelength (λ), which is the distance over which the wave repeats itself, is inversely related to frequency (v) as $\lambda = c/v$, so higher frequency oscillations imply longer wavelengths.

The velocity of light differs depending on the medium it travels in, and is characterized by the *refractive index*, the ratio of the speed of light in a

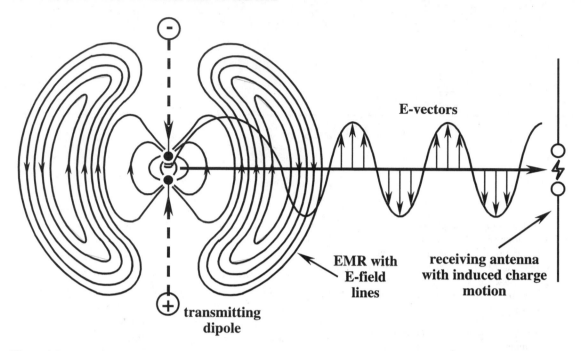

Figure 2.1. An oscillating dipole generates electric field lines like layers in an onion. This complex pattern is more commonly drawn as a sine wave, as shown to the right. The sine wave forms an envelope for the instantaneous strength and orientation of the E-field, which is shown as arrows perpendicular to the direction of travel.

vacuum to the speed of light in the medium. The type of medium does not affect v (the frequency), only V (velocity). For example, light has a lower V in a substance with a higher index of refraction (n), but v stays the same. This implies that as n increases, λ decreases; $\lambda_n = \lambda/n$ (where λ_n is the λ within medium of refractive index n). V for light in

a vacuum is symbolized by c. $c = 3.00 \times 10^8$ m/sec, which looks rounded but is fortuitously accurate to better than 0.1%.

Although the full EMR spectrum contains a continuous range of all frequencies and wavelengths, it is useful to partition it into bands according to the way its different regions are typically

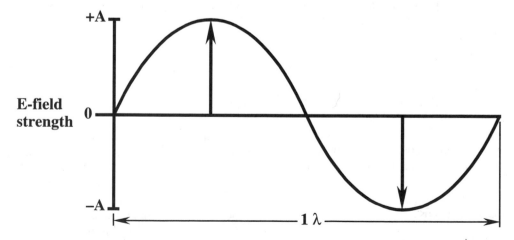

Figure 2.2. Graph of E-field strength over one cycle (one wavelength). The greatest electric field strength is the amplitude $+A$ and $-A$.

generated and detected. Also, these bands are characterized by frequency or wavelength depending on which is most directly known. *Microwaves* and *radio waves* are readily produced by electronic circuits in which the dipole consists of oscillating electrons in an antenna. They are characterized easily by frequency (v) because they have the same frequency as the circuits that produce them. The frequency of oscillation is slow enough that the electric field in the EMR can physically translate atoms or flip polar molecules in its path. Visible, IR (infrared), and UV (ultraviolet) radiation are usually produced by nature with an unknown v. They are usually characterized by wavelength (λ) because it is their wavelength that is most easily measured. *Infrared radiation (IR)* oscillates fast enough that atoms and molecules (collectively referred to as particles) in its path are not moved very far before the electric field reverses, so they merely vibrate. This produces heat through random collisions among the particles. *Visible light* has a still higher frequency, which can cause the outer (valence) electrons of atoms to jump to higher energy levels. EMR in the 400–700 nm wavelength range is "visible light" because photopigment molecules in the photoreceptor cells of the eye are triggered by these electron jumps, which triggering in turn initiates stimulation of the visual pathways to the brain. *Ultraviolet radiation (UV)* has a high enough frequency to remove all the outer electrons from atoms (ionization) and to break molecular bonds. Visible light will be central in our discussion of the optics of the eye, however, the nonvisible bands are also important because they are used in ophthalmic instruments and they can damage the eye (Table 2.1).

The wavelength of light is often measured variously in micrometers (μm, 10^{-6} m), nanometers (nm, 10^{-9} m), or angstroms (Å, 10^{-10} m). That is, 520 nm (green) is also 5200 Å and 0.520 μm. The average wavelengths of representative colors in the spectrum of visible light are given in Table 2.2.

Table 2.2. Average Wavelengths for Colors in the Visible Spectrum

Color	Wavelength
Red	650 nm
Orange	600 nm
Yellow	575 nm
Green	520 nm
Blue	460 nm
Violet	430 nm

Continuous Spectra

Although light produces the perception of single colors, most light is made up of a mixture of wavelengths. This can be demonstrated by passing light through a prism so that the component colors are spatially separated into a spectrum. A spectrum that contains all wavelengths without gaps is referred to as a *continuous spectrum*.

A heated solid emits EMR in a continuous spectrum as a result of the random thermal motion of its particles. As the temperature increases, a solid emits more total EMR so that it appears brighter, and the peak wavelength becomes shorter. Low heat produces EMR that is mostly in the IR range; it can't be seen but it can be felt as radiated heat. As the temperature increases, the peak output enters the visible spectrum and progresses from red to yellow to white, and finally to blue. When the spectral distribution peaks in the middle of the visible spectrum, the curve is flat enough that there is still a significant amount of radiation from the blue and red ends of the spectrum, so it appears white rather than green.

The continuous spectrum produced by a *black body radiator* can be used as a model for all thermal radiators. A black body radiator is one that absorbs all light incident on it, and any light it produces is a result of thermal emission. This ideal is approximated in the laboratory by an enclosed cavity that

Table 2.1. Characteristics of Infrared, Visible Light, and Ultraviolet

Band Name	Wavelength (λ)	Response of Atoms and Molecules
Infrared (IR)	100,000–700 nm	Molecular vibrations and heat
Visible light	700–400 nm	Orbital transitions in valence electrons
Ultraviolet (UV)	400–10 nm	Molecular bond breaking and ionization

has no internal source of light. Then, if the walls of the cavity are heated, they will fill the cavity with EMR. This can be observed if a small hole is placed in a wall of the cavity. The distribution of EMR power (energy per second) and wavelength depends only on the temperature of the cavity walls (Figure 2.3). Although a black body radiator is an idealized light source, its wavelength distribution can be used to approximate those of both natural and artificial sources of light produced by hot objects. It can also be used to approximate the color of light sources even if the color is not a result of thermal radiation. This is referred to as *color temperature,* which is useful for predicting the color rendition of objects illuminated by such a source. For example, the blue sky has a color temperature of about 20,000°K but the sky is, of course, cool.

The study of black body radiation was pivotal in establishing the quantum nature of light. In 1900 Planck discovered that the distribution of power versus wavelength radiated by a black body can be explained only if it is assumed that EMR energy is exchanged with the walls in quantum (packet) amounts. This implies that, unlike large mechanical systems such as guitar strings, which can be tuned over a continuous range of frequencies, atoms are capable of oscillating only at certain frequencies. This observation led Einstein to suggest that light itself is not a continuous flow of energy, but at a fine level it has a granularity in the form of particles (*photons*), each of which contains a set amount of energy.

THE QUANTUM NATURE OF LIGHT

A heated vapor of atoms at low pressure emits EMR, which is restricted to a set of very narrow ranges of wavelengths called *spectral lines*, rather than being a continuous spectrum. This is referred to as a *bright line spectrum*. Figure 2.4, for example, shows the line spectrum produced by heated hydrogen gas. Each element has a distinct pattern

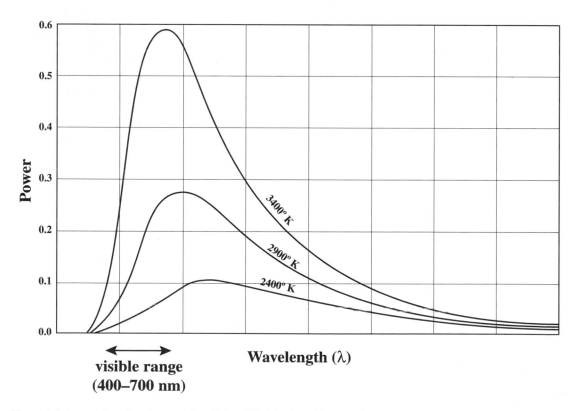

Figure 2.3. Power plotted against wavelength for a black body radiator. As the temperature of the black body rises, the total amount of radiant power increases and the power peaks at shorter wavelengths. (Modified from LeGrand Y. *Light, Color, and Vision.* 2nd ed. London: Chapman and Hall, 1968.)

Hydrogen Spectrum

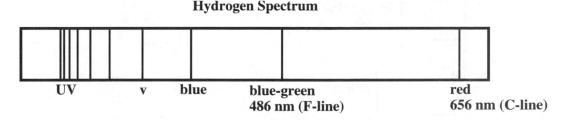

| UV | v | blue | blue-green
486 nm (F-line) | | red
656 nm (C-line) |

Figure 2.4. Line spectrum from a heated rarefied gas of hydrogen atoms. The dark lines in this drawing should be interpreted as bright lines against a dark background.

of spectral lines through which it can be identified, and the more prominent lines of some elements have their own letter designations.

A simplified explanation of bright line spectra is based on the quantization of electron orbits. For any given element, the electrons are restricted to a fixed set of orbits around the nucleus, and each of these orbits has a fixed amount of energy. An electron can move from one orbit to another only by giving up or receiving an amount of energy, which is the difference in energy between the two orbits. For example, an electron can jump to a higher orbit by absorbing energy from the random atomic collisions caused by heating the gas. This electron will then fall back to a lower energy orbit and create a photon whose energy equals the difference in energy between the two orbits ($E = E_{(outer)} - E_{(inner)}$) (Figure 2.5). The energy a photon possesses determines its frequency by $E = hv$ (where h is Planck's constant). Thus, higher frequency photons (shorter wavelengths) contain more energy than lower frequency photons (longer wavelengths).

Particularly strong spectral lines of certain elements are used to raytrace different colors of light through optical systems. Table 2.3 lists the spectral lines commonly used for this purpose.

If the light produced by a heated atomic gas is directly observed, the spectral lines appear bright, as described previously. However, if light with a continuous spectrum (white light) is passed through the same but cooler gas, the lines appear dark against the background of the continuous spectrum (Figure 2.6).

These dark lines correspond to wavelengths in the continuous spectrum that have been absorbed. When the gas is cool, its electrons are at their lowest energy levels and will absorb those photons that have just the right amount of energy to elevate them to higher energy levels. Although photons of

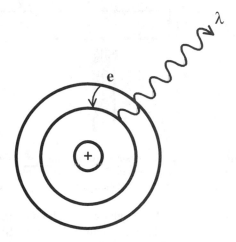

Figure 2.5. When electrons jump from a higher orbit to a lower orbit, the difference in energy can produce a photon whose wavelength is inversely proportional to the change in energy.

the same wavelength are reemitted when the electrons drop back to their original level, the photons are reradiated in all directions (scattered), so relatively few photons continue in the original direction. The spectrum of sunlight is an example of this. The Sun's surface produces a continuous spectrum because, even though it is a gas, gravity makes it dense enough to approximate the radiation of a heated solid. The Sun's atmosphere, which is between Earth and the Sun's surface, is cooler than the surface, so its constituent atoms absorb and

Table 2.3. Spectral Lines Used in Raytracing

	Color	Source	Wavelength
C	red	hydrogen	656 nm
d	yellow	helium	588 nm
e	green	mercury	546 nm
F	blue	hydrogen	486 nm

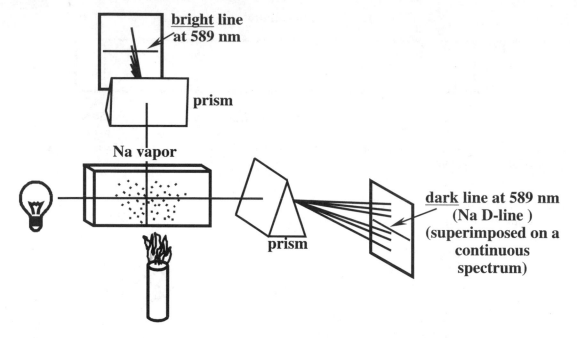

Figure 2.6. White light passing through a vapor of sodium atoms will have its 589-nm component (yellow-orange) strongly absorbed and reemitted (scattered). In the forward light direction this leaves a dark line in an otherwise complete continuous spectrum. Light scattered to the side produces a bright 589-nm line against a dark background.

reradiate those wavelengths whose photons match the energy level differences in their orbits. Since the reradiation is in random directions, their absence produces *dark* lines in the otherwise continuous spectrum of the Sun.

A gas made up of molecules (as opposed to atoms) produces a *banded* or *fluted* spectrum in which the lines are so close together in some areas of the spectrum that groups of lines appear to be continuous. This proliferation of lines results from the interaction of the bonds among the constituent atoms in the molecules.

Heated liquids and solids, as mentioned, emit *continuous* spectra. In this case the otherwise discrete electron energies are spread as a result of thermal motion and interactions among close neighboring atoms and molecules.

TRANSMISSION OF LIGHT BY MATTER

When EMR encounters atoms or molecules, it induces a dipole oscillation in the particles in the same direction and at the same frequency as its electric field. Since the particles have in turn become oscillating dipoles, they will reemit EMR of the same frequency as the absorbed EMR. EMR is absorbed most effectively if its frequency matches one of the frequencies at which the oscillating particles naturally resonate (called a *resonant frequency*). The closer the EMR's frequency is to a resonant frequency, the more effectively the EMR will be absorbed. This is another way of explaining why rarefied gases produce bright and dark line spectra. The spectral lines correspond to resonant frequencies that are absorbed very effectively and then reemitted. Since the reemission can be in any direction, the light does not necessarily continue in its original direction but is *scattered*.

Molecules in the atmosphere (N_2 and O_2) have resonant frequencies in the UV range. Therefore, the higher frequency (short wavelength) components of visible light are more effectively scattered than the lower frequency (long wavelength) components. This is why the atmosphere scatters blue light much more effectively than red. This is referred to as *Rayleigh scattering* or the *Tyndall effect* and follows the relationship that the intensity of scatter (I_s) is inversely proportional to the fourth power of the wavelength (λ) ($I_s \propto 1/\lambda^4$). However, this relationship between wavelength and effectiveness of scatter holds only if the scattering particles are much smaller than the wavelength of the passing light.

The atmosphere scatters violet light about seven times as effectively as red light, which explains why the sky is blue and sunsets are red. Sunlight passing through air molecules in the sky has its shorter wavelengths strongly scattered in all directions, so the sky looks blue. With the setting Sun, the light goes through a greater length of atmosphere and the shorter wavelengths are scattered so effectively that the remaining light that reaches us directly from the Sun looks red. Rayleigh scattering is responsible for the blue appearance of veins beneath the skin. Their blue color is *not* due to low oxygenation in venous blood. Veins are closer to the surface than arteries, so they are easier to see, and the blue component of light on the skin is scattered by the molecules in the walls of the veins. Rayleigh scattering from the molecules in irises, in the absence of the brown pigment melanin, gives them a blue color. Also, protein leaking out of the blood vessels into the aqueous of an inflamed eye produces Rayleigh scattering. A beam of white light in the aqueous is made visible by *flare* caused by the scatter of predominantly blue light.

If the scattering particles are large relative to the wavelength of the passing light, the amount of scattering no longer depends on the specific wavelength, and all component colors are scattered equally. This is referred to as *Mie scattering*. Clouds are white rather than blue because the water particles they consist of are large compared to the wavelength of light.

The previous discussion applies to rarefied gases. The interaction of light and *condensed matter* (solids and liquids) is complicated by the interactions among neighboring particles. The particles in condensed matter also have resonant frequencies and they also absorb best EMR whose frequency is close to a resonant frequency. However, the particles are close enough that before the EMR can be reemitted, the particles "bump into" each other and the EMR energy is converted to heat. As a result, condensed matter is opaque to EMR whose frequency is close to one of its resonant frequencies.

If in condensed matter the frequency of the EMR is *not* close to a resonant frequency, it is not strongly absorbed. Dipole oscillations will still be induced in the particles, but the oscillations will not be great enough to be dissipated as kinetic motion among adjacent particles. Instead, scattered EMR

of the same frequency will be emitted. Although the light is scattered, because the particles are close together, interference among the scattered waves will cause the light to continue in the same direction as the prescattered light. Thus, condensed matter is transparent to wavelengths that fall between the resonant frequencies. Glass is an example of a substance that has no resonant frequency in the visible spectrum. This makes glass transparent to visible light, and, therefore, a useful material for lenses. (However, if substances are added that *do* have resonant frequencies in the visible spectrum, the glass will appear colored.)

Metals are opaque for a different reason than that given above. They reflect, as well as absorb, an appreciable part of the light. Passing EMR causes the outer electrons, which in metals are only loosely tied to individual atoms (free electrons), to oscillate and produce dipole radiation. However, the interference among the scattered waves causes the reemission of light to be reinforced in the backward direction, so the light is reflected.

COMMON SOURCES OF LIGHT

Sunlight

The Sun is made of gas, but because the gas is very dense, its surface has the continuous spectrum of an incandescent solid and approximates that of a black body radiator.[1] By the time sunlight reaches ground level, however, it approximates the wavelength distribution of a black body radiator less well:

1. Sunlight is modified in a minor way by the dark lines in the solar spectrum.
2. On traversing Earth's atmosphere, air molecules, including water vapor, absorb broad bands of wavelengths mainly in the infrared ranges.
3. In the visible spectrum, the atmosphere scatters blue light so that at ground level the Sun appears less blue than it does from space and has a relatively flat distribution of its energy across the visible wavelengths, which makes it appear white.

It is sometimes argued that our eyes evolved to be most sensitive to light in the middle of the visible spectrum because the Sun's output peaks in this range. Soffer and Lynch[2] have published an interesting refutation of this claim.

About one-half of the energy of the sunlight reaching Earth is in the visible region of the spectrum. The other half is mostly IR, and only about 3% is UV radiation. Although UV radiation accounts for only a small proportion of sunlight, it is exceptionally energetic and can have disproportionately large effects.

Incandescent Lamps (Thermal Radiation)

Aside from sunlight our most common source of illumination is incandescent lamps, which include the common light bulb.[3] In incandescent lamps a current heats up a high resistance filament, and as a result the filament glows in a continuous spectrum. Its brightness and color (from the spectral distribution of its energy) depend on its temperature. Tungsten filaments are heated to about 2800°K and radiate a distribution of wavelengths that appears yellow (°K = °C + 273). Therefore, an object illuminated by an incandescent light bulb appears yellower than it would if it were illuminated by sunlight.

Incandescent lights do not have very high efficiency (light output per watt) because much of the electrical energy is wasted in producing IR radiation and heat. Tungsten filament lights can be made more efficient by raising the filament temperature to 3200–3400°K (which shifts more of the peak output into the visible range); but tungsten then evaporates and deposits on the walls of the globe, making it less transparent. Halogen lamps use a halogen gas in the globe to redeposit tungsten onto the filament. The globe can then be made smaller. In order to withstand the higher operating temperature, the globe is made of quartz rather than glass, hence the name *quartz-halide lamp*. The result is not only greater efficiency but also a whiter light, which gives a better color rendition of what is being illuminated. Modern ophthalmoscopes, for example, use quartz-halide lamps.

Gas Discharge Lamps

Some light sources have a wavelength distribution that is very different from incandescent sources. Gas discharge lamps emit a line spectrum when a rarefied atomic gas is excited by the passage of an electric current. The light produced is restricted to narrow spectral lines, the particular lines depending on the type of gas atoms used. However, the human eye is unable to detect the component lines and perceives the light as one color. As with incandescent lighting, objects illuminated by these unusual wavelength distributions can give color impressions that are significantly different from what they would be if illuminated by sunlight. There are several common gas discharge lamps[3]:

Neon: Neon tubing is used in advertising signs. When the tube is filled with neon it emits red light. However, the name *neon light* is sometimes used for tubes that produce other colors as well, by the addition of other gases, phosphors, or tinted glass.

Mercury vapor: These lamps are greenish with a strong component of UV, which is filtered out by the globe. Since mercury is a liquid, it must first be vaporized. This type of lighting is used for street and yard lights.

Sodium vapor: These lamps are yellow. They are used for street and yard lights. Sodium vapor lamps have been replacing mercury vapor lamps because they are more efficient; they produce more light per watt and are thus less expensive to run.

Low-pressure sodium: Most of output of these lamps is overwhelmingly in one spectral line at 589 nm, so colors are not seen and objects look yellow and unattractive.

High-pressure sodium: In these lamps, the spectral lines are broadened by an increase in pressure so a component of a continuous spectrum is present.

Fluorescent Lights

Fluorescent lights produce a continuous spectrum, but one that is quite unlike a black body in its distribution of power across wavelength. In fluorescent lights a current is run through a closed tube that contains a drop of mercury. When the mercury is vaporized, it emits a line spectrum with about 50% of its energy at 253.7 nm in the UV (which, of course, is invisible). The UV photons then strike a phosphor coating on the inside of the tube, which causes the phosphor to fluoresce as a continuous spectrum in the visible range. The particular color appearance depends on the type of phosphor. Some of the bright line spectrum from the excited mercury atoms "leaks" by the phosphor and can be seen against the continuous spectrum—although this output, including UV, is minimal. The older-style fluorescent lights tended to produce a bluish "cold" light, but the addition of different phosphors and gases can give a "warmer" (more yellow) or a whiter light. Fluorescent lights are more efficient than incandescent lights because they waste less energy as IR radiation and heat.[3]

Laser Light

Laser light has several characteristics that make it extremely useful. The beam can be highly directional, highly coherent, and highly monochromatic. No other light source possesses all of these qualities. Lasers have become pervasive in both diagnostic and therapeutic eyecare.

Lasers commonly use rarefied atomic gases or certain solids to produce line spectra. Usually only one of these lines is amplified into a laser beam, which is why lasers can produce very monochromatic light. Energy, through a process called pumping, is added to the lasing substance in order to excite electrons to higher energy levels. Pumping can be done in a number of ways, but the two most important are bombarding the atoms with photons if the laser medium is a solid or liquid and bombarding the atoms with electrons by running an electric current through the laser medium if it is a gas.

The excited electrons then drop to a lower orbit and emit a photon in one of two ways. In *spontaneous emission* electrons spontaneously drop to a lower energy level. The photons produced are emitted in random directions and are not in phase with each other—they are not coherent. In *stimulated emission*, an electron at an elevated energy level encounters a photon of the same wavelength as the photon it would emit if it were to fall to a lower level. This causes the electron to immediately jump to the lower orbit and emit a new photon of the same wavelength, phase, direction, and polarization as the stimulating photon. Thus, *one* photon encounters the atom but *two* coherent photons leave. These two photons can then encounter other elevated electrons, and so on, and a cascade of coherent photons is produced.

Stimulated emission under normal conditions accounts for minimal photon emission because most electrons are in their lowest energy orbit (*ground state*). This results in more light being absorbed than emitted. The electrons elevated through absorption quickly return to a lower orbit and reemit photons spontaneously (and incoherently) before other photons can trigger stimulated emission. However, certain energy levels, called *metastable states*, hold the elevated electrons for a considerably longer time than normal before the electrons return to a lower energy level. Due to the added delay, the pump elevates more electrons to the higher energy states than are at ground level—a condition referred to as a *population inversion*. Then, photons initially emitted spontaneously produce stimulated cascades of coherent photons going in their direction. The coherent cascades are made to go along the length of the laser axis by capping the length with two parallel mirrors to form a closed cavity. This causes those photons that by chance are traveling in the direction of the cavity's axis to reflect back and forth along what becomes a virtually infinite path, and all of the energy in the laser cavity is quickly recruited into the direction of the laser's axis. Then, if one of the mirrors is partially transmitting, a portion of the light will escape the cavity as a laser beam. (The word *LASER* is an acronym for **L**ight **A**mplification by **S**timulated **E**mission of **R**adiation.)

Most lasers emit far less power (watts) than a standard light bulb, but they can still be vision hazards due to the high collimation (directionality) of their beams. The degree to which a laser beam spreads is due, in part, to diffraction at the exit aperture and the spread is usually in the range of one milliradian (1 mm of spread per 1000 mm of travel).

A standard incandescent bulb rated as 100 watts might emit 20 watts of visible power, but it is emitted in all directions so that only 0.0016 milliwatts would fall on a 1-mm^2 area 1 meter away. On the other hand, a 1-milliwatt laser with a 1-mm^2 beam area directs *all* of its power onto a 1-mm^2 area 1 meter away. All of this light could easily fit through the pupil of an eye. A 5-milliwatt laser requires longer than one minute to cause retinal damage.[4] Since lid closure or eye aversion can reflexively protect the eye, lasers with powers up to 5 mW (the legal limit for laser pointers) are unlikely to cause accidental retinal damage.

A beam of light is said to be *coherent* when all of its light waves are *in phase* crest-to-crest and trough-to-trough. Most light sources do not produce coherent light. An example of an incoherent source is a frosted light bulb. In Figure 2.7, rays 1 and 3 are not coherent because, even though they have the same wavelength, they do not line up; that is, they are out of phase. Rays 1 and 2 are not coherent because they are a different wavelength. Lasers are capable of producing extremely coherent beams that are highly monochromatic and in lock step.

Filtered Light

The distribution of power across the spectrum of a light source can be altered by selective absorption so that its intensity or even its perceived color is changed.

The intensity (I) of transmitted light will not be as great when it leaves a material as when it entered it. This is due to absorption, reflection, and scattering. (In this section we are concerned only with absorption.) The fraction of the light incident on an optical system that is not absorbed is the *transmittance* (T). Thus, if 10% of the light energy is absorbed, the transmittance is 90% ($T = 0.9$). T is related to I_O, the intensity of the incident light, and I_T, the intensity of the transmitted light by:

$$T = \frac{I_T}{I_O} \quad \text{or} \quad I_T = I_O T$$

Optical density (D) is often used as a measure of transmission rather than transmittance (T) where:

$$D = \log_{10} \frac{1}{T} = -\log T$$

Example: If a filter transmits 0.1 of the incident light (I_O), then

$$D = \log (1/0.1) = \log 10 = 1.0$$

If

$$T = 0.01$$

then

$$D = \log (1/0.01) = \log 100 = 2.0$$

Optical density is easy to calculate because, if light passes successively through a number of filters:

$$D_{TOTAL} = D_1 + D_2 + D_3 + \dots + D_n$$

Thus,

$$T_T = (T_1)(T_2)(T_3) \dots (T_n)$$

is equivalent to

$$D_T = D_1 + D_2 + D_3 + \dots + D_n$$

Since the transmittance of optical materials depends on wavelength, optical density must be determined for each wavelength separately. If the transmittance is relatively uniform across wavelengths, the filter is referred to as a *neutral density* (*ND*) filter and it can be described by one number, the optical density. Neutral density filters reduce the amount of transmitted light with little change in perceived color. Filters that are more transparent to some wavelengths than to others are called *color filters* because they change the perceived color of transmitted light. Since their spectral transmittance differs for different wavelengths, they can't be described by one number and are usually characterized graphically as a plot of transmittance against wavelength.

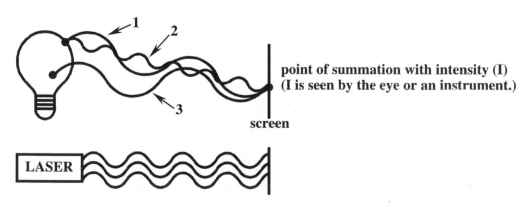

point of summation with intensity (I)
(I is seen by the eye or an instrument.)

screen

Figure 2.7. A comparison between incoherent light from a light bulb and coherent light from a laser.

Color filters are based on either selective absorption or interference from thin reflective films. Interference filters are usually used when a very narrow band of wavelengths is required, but these filters are expensive. For less stringent requirements, gelatin absorption filters are often adequate and are cheaper. Kodak produces a series of gelatin color filters, which are identified nominally by *Wratten numbers*.

POLARIZATION

In EMR the strength and direction of the electric field for each point in space can be represented by arrows (vectors) contained in the waveform. These will be referred to as *electric field vectors,* or simply as *E-vectors*. Looking along the direction of a light beam, the E-vector can be oriented in any direction and in most light sources it will randomly change its orientation from moment to moment so

all directions are usually represented[5] (Figure 2.8).

If all of the E-vectors are lined up in one plane, the light is said to be *plane polarized*. For example, a dipole oscillator in a radio transmitter would produce a plane-polarized wave whose E-vectors are aligned parallel to the dipole axis (along the length of the antenna) (Figure 2.9).

Most natural light is not polarized because the individual axes of the many particles acting as light-emitting dipoles are randomly oriented. The moment-to-moment E-vector size and orientation is the result of the contribution of all the individual E-vectors produced by those dipoles at each instant.

Polaroid filters are commonly used to produce linearly polarized light. If unpolarized light passes through a Polaroid filter, it becomes polarized in a plane that matches the filter's pass axis. Then if the light continues on to a second Polaroid filter, it will be able to pass or not to pass depending on the orientation of the second filter. The first filter is a

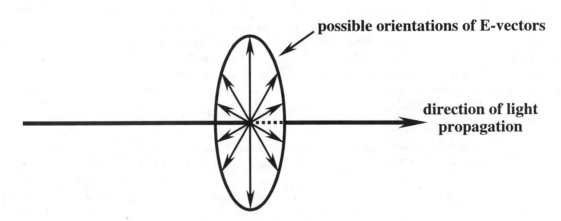

Figure 2.8. Electric field lines are oriented perpendicular to the direction of light travel, but their orientation about the direction axis is usually random. Such light is referred to as unpolarized.

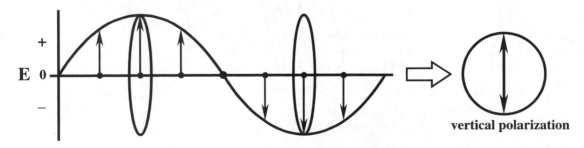

Figure 2.9. Light is said to be linearly or plane polarized when all of the electric field lines are oriented in a single plane. The plane of polarization is often illustrated by a diameter of a circle as seen against the direction of the light.

polarizer and the second filter is an *analyzer*. If the analyzer's pass axis is parallel to the polarizer's pass axis, all of the light from the polarizer will pass (neglecting reflection and nonpolarizing absorption). However, if the pass axis of the analyzer is rotated 90° to that of the polarizer, they are referred to as *crossed polarizers*, and no light will pass. If the pass axis of the analyzer is rotated to some angle between parallel and perpendicular to the pass axis of the polarizer, then the component of the E-vector amplitude (A) that can be projected onto the analyzer pass axis will get through.

Plane-polarized light can be broken down into E-vector projections along an x-axis and a y-axis. Thus, plane-polarized light at an oblique orientation can be represented by two perpendicular E-vectors of different amplitudes A_x and A_y along the x- and y-axes, whose vector sum gives the amplitude (A) and orientation (θ) of polarization. In Figure 2.10 the component A_x will get through the analyzer since it is parallel to the pass axis of the analyzer. However, A_y will not get through since it is perpendicular to the pass axis of the analyzer. It can be seen that $A_x = A_p \cos \theta$ where θ is the angle by which the pass axis of the analyzer differs from the axis of the polarizer.

It must be noted, however, that *intensity* (I) is proportional to A^2. Then, I_x is proportional to $A_x^2 = (A_p \cos \theta)^2 = A_p^2 \cos^2 \theta$. Therefore, $I_x = I_p \cos^2 \theta$. This is known as the *Law of Malus*.

Example: If the axis of an analyzer is set at $\theta = 45°$ to the axis of a polarizer, then

$$I_x = I_p \cos^2 45° = 0.5 \, I_P$$

Polarization by Reflection

If a beam of nonpolarized light is incident on the surface of a smooth, transparent, nonconductor such as glass, the fraction of the beam that is reflected will be polarized with the reflected E-vector perpendicular to the plane in which the ray travels (the plane of the drawing in Figure 2.11).

The reflected beam will be totally polarized for only one angle of incidence (i_B) called *Brewster's angle*. This angle will differ for substances depending on their refractive index (n) and is found by $\tan i_B = n_2/n_1$ which simplifies to $\tan i_B = n$ if n_1 equals 1.00 (air).

At other angles of incidence (i), the reflected beam will be only partially polarized.

Figure 2.12 shows that for $n = 1.50$, light at $i = 0°$ incidence is about 4% reflected independent of E-vector orientation. However, at $i_B = 56°$, about 15% of the light with perpendicular E-vector is reflected and *none* of the light with the parallel E-vector is reflected. At grazing angles of incidence (i nearly 90°), there is almost 100% reflectance independent of E-vector orientation. Note that, even at Brewster's angle, most of the light with a perpendicular E-vector orientation is transmitted rather than reflected.

Polarization by Scatter

Rayleigh scattering, but not Mie scattering, produces polarized light. The polarization is most complete for light scattered at right angles to the initial direction of a beam, and greater for shorter

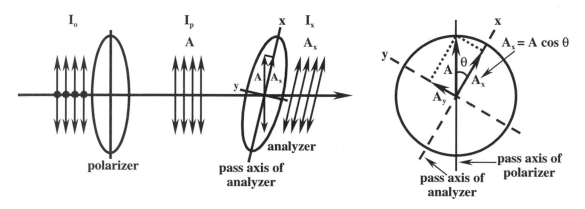

Figure 2.10. When light goes through two polarizing filters whose pass axes are not aligned, only the vector component of the light following the first filter that is projected onto the pass axis of the second filter will get through the second filter.

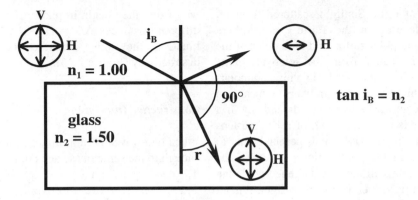

Figure 2.11. When unpolarized light strikes a transparent plate at an angle of incidence *i*, a percentage of it is reflected. When *i* equals Brewster's angle, all of the reflected light is linearly polarized with its E-vector perpendicular to the plane in which the light ray is drawn.

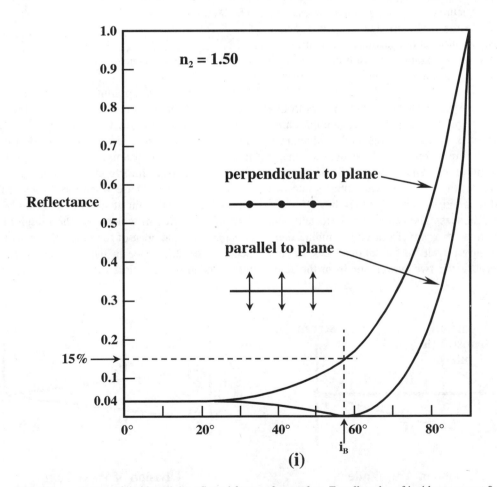

Figure 2.12. The percentage of incident light reflected from a glass surface. For all angles of incidence except 0 and 90, the reflected light is at least partially polarized. At Brewster's angle the reflected light is totally polarized.

wavelengths of light. Sunlight scattered from N_2 and O_2 molecules in the Earth's atmosphere accounts for the polarization and blue color of the sky. However, scatter from the relatively large water particles in clouds results in white, nonpolarized light. This gives photographers a means to increase the contrast between clouds and sky. If a Polaroid filter is placed in front of a camera lens and rotated so that its pass axis is perpendicular to the orientation of the polarization of the sky, the polarized skylight will become darkened while the clouds, which do not emit polarized light, remain relatively bright.

INTERFERENCE

If two or more waves overlap, the resultant instantaneous electric field strength at a given location is equal to the sum of all of the superimposed E-vectors. Since the E-vectors that are summed may be pointed in different directions (have different phases), the superposition can result in dim as well as bright light at that location—a phenomenon called *interference*.[5–7]

Interference can occur when light waves from a single source are divided and then recombined after having traveled through separate paths, which may have had different lengths. There are two major ways to achieve this. One way is to divide *one part* of a *wavefront* (a surface of equal phase) into two parts and recombine them after they have traveled different distances. The other way is to take two *different parts* of a wavefront and combine them after they have traveled different distances. In both cases, because the two waves are from the same wavefront, they begin in phase. If they then travel different distances $\Delta D = D_2 - D_1$ before recombination, they may interfere constructively or destructively (Figure 2.13).

Constructive Interference

When two waves of amplitudes a_1 and a_2 are close enough to the same phase at a point in space so that A_{1+2} is larger than a_1 and a_2, they are said to undergo *constructive interference*. For complete constructive interference, the total amplitude $A_{1+2} = a_1 + a_2$. Complete constructive interference occurs for two sources initially in phase when the distances from the sources to the point of summation are equal $(D_2 - D_1 = 0)$. But it also occurs if the difference in the distance each wave travels is an integer number (m) of λs. $D_2 - D_1 = m\lambda$ ($= 0\lambda$, 1λ, 2λ, etc.).

Destructive Interference

When two waves of amplitudes a_1 and a_2 are sufficiently out of phase at a point in space so that A_{1+2} is smaller than a_1 or a_2, they are said to undergo *destructive interference*. For complete destructive interference, the total amplitude $A_{1+2} = 0$. Complete destructive interference occurs for two sources initially in phase when the distances from the sources to the point of summation differ by $^1/_2\lambda$ $(D_2 - D_1 = {}^1/_2\lambda)$, in which case the trough of one wave cancels the crest of the other. But it will also occur if the difference in the distance each wave travels is an *odd* multiple of $^1/_2\lambda$s. $D_2 - D_1 = m\lambda$

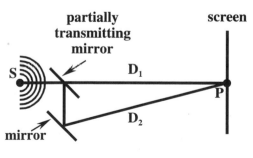

Division of Amplitude

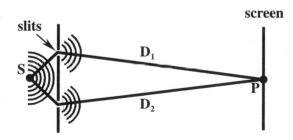

Division of Wavefront

Figure 2.13. Examples of the two major ways to produce interference experimentally.

$+ \frac{1}{2}\lambda = (m + \frac{1}{2})\lambda \ (=\frac{1}{2}\lambda, 1\frac{1}{2}\lambda, 2\frac{1}{2}\lambda, \text{etc.})$.

If the two waves combine (interfere) at a screen, film, retina, and so on, the intensity (I) at that point will be proportional to the resultant amplitude squared (A^2). For interference between two waves of equal amplitude (a), depending on the fractional λ path difference, the resultant amplitude A will be between $2a$ and 0 and the intensity I_T will be between $4I$ and 0.

Antireflection Coatings

All transmitting optical surfaces, no matter how well polished, will reflect a portion of the incident light (referred to as *Fresnel reflection*). The fraction of the incident intensity (I_I) that is reflected (I_R) off an optical interface is:

$$\frac{I_R}{I_I} = \left(\frac{n_2 - n_1}{n_2 + n_1}\right)^2, \ (I_I = \text{incident } I;$$

$I_R = $ reflected I).

Example: If n_1 is air and $n_2 = 1.523$, then:

$$\frac{I_R}{I_I} = \left(\frac{1.523 - 1.00}{1.523 + 1.00}\right)^2 = 0.04 \text{ or}$$

$I_R = 0.04 \ I_I \approx 4\% \text{ of } I_I$.

Thin films are often deposited on lenses in order to reduce reflections and increase transmission[7] (Figure 2.14). Then, the path difference between light reflected from the upper and the lower surface of the antireflective coating is $\Delta D = 2t = m(\lambda/n_2) + \frac{1}{2}(\lambda/n_2)$ (*destructive* interference), where t is the thickness and n_2 is the index of the coating. For the smallest t, $m = 0$, so, $2t = \frac{1}{2}(\lambda/n_2)$ and $t = \frac{1}{4}(\lambda/n_2)$. These films are sometimes called *quarter-wave coatings* for obvious reasons; however, the wavelength being referred to is in the medium of index n and is shorter than the wavelength in air ($\lambda_n = \lambda/n$).

For complete destructive interference by a quarter-wave coating, the amplitudes (a_1 and a_2) of the two reflected waves must be equal, as well as $\frac{1}{2}\lambda$ out of phase. Otherwise, $a_1 - a_2 \neq 0$.

$a_1 = a_2$ when $n_2 = \sqrt{n_3 n_1}$ ($= \sqrt{n_3}$ when n_1 is air). For optical crown glass of $n_3 = 1.523$, the coating material must have an $n_2 = \sqrt{1.523} = 1.23$. However, the closest practical coating material with an n near this is *magnesium fluoride* with an $n = 1.38$. Thus, $a_1 \neq a_2$ and the destructive interference is not perfect.

The $\frac{1}{4}(\lambda/n_2)$ coating thickness is best for the particular wavelength (color) chosen for destructive interference. This wavelength is usually chosen to be 555 nm (yellow-green) because the eye is most sensitive to this wavelength.

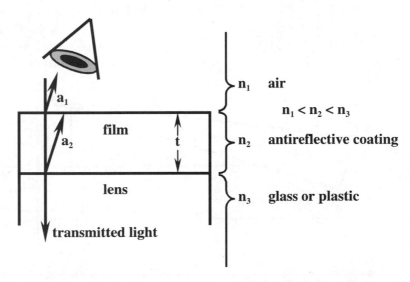

Figure 2.14. Reflection from glass or plastic with an antireflective coat. Reflected light from the outer and inner sides of the coating will recombine constructively or destructively depending on the thickness of the coating.

Example: For magnesium fluoride ($n = 1.38$), $t = \frac{1}{4}(\lambda/n_2) = \frac{1}{4}$ (555 nm/1.38) = 100.5 nm.

The destructive interference of reflected light is less effective for colors whose wavelengths differ from 555 nm and about 1.2% of the incident light is still reflected. Thus, with white light, red and blue are reflected more than yellow-green and the reflected mixture of red and blue light makes the reflection off coated lenses look purple. Even better results can be obtained by using multiple coatings of different materials and thicknesses. The reflection off such coatings often looks green.

Antireflection coatings are most necessary for optical systems with many lenses. For example, a camera lens with six air-spaced lenses has 12 surfaces. If each surface reflects 4% of the incident light, then 96% of the light incident on each surface is transmitted, and the total *transmitted* light = $(0.96)^{12} = 0.61 = 61\%$. This is a rather large light loss. Perhaps more important is the 39% of the light that is reflected, because this would produce ghost images and scattered light that would reduce image contrast. If all the surfaces have a magnesium fluoride antireflection coating, then each surface transmits $100 - 1.2\% = 98.8\%$ of the incident

light and all 12 surfaces would collectively transmit $(0.988)^{12} = 0.87 = 87\%$ of the light.

Double-Slit Interference

Young's double-slit experiment (in 1801) did more than any other demonstration to convince scientists for the next century that light was a wave (Figure 2.15).

A monochromatic (one λ) light source illuminates slit s_0. Slits s_1 and s_2 then become secondary wave sources, which start out in phase since they are both illuminated by the same wavefront. Where two crests meet in space, constructive interference results. This occurs where the waves differ in phase by integer multiples of λ (1λ, 2λ, 3λ, . . . $m\lambda$). When the crests meet troughs, destructive interference results. This occurs where the waves differ in phase by *odd* multiples of $\frac{1}{2}\lambda$ ($\frac{1}{2}\lambda$, $1\frac{1}{2}\lambda$, $2\frac{1}{2}\lambda$, . . . $m\lambda + \frac{1}{2}\lambda$). A screen set in front of the two slits will show alternate bright and dark bands (*fringes*), where the difference in distance between the wave paths from the two slits is right for constructive or destructive interference, respectively. (Young

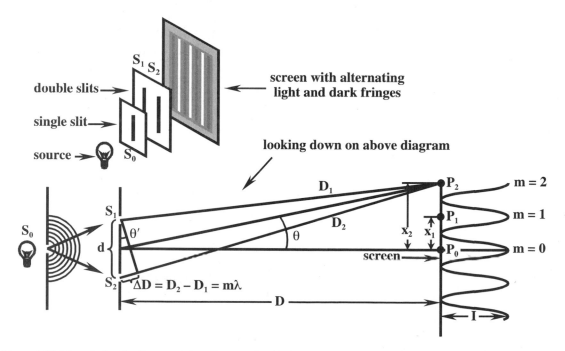

Figure 2.15. Young's double-slit setup. Two slits, s_1 and s_2, isolate separate wavelets from one wavefront. After traveling different distances to reach each point on a screen, the wavelets arrive in phase and produce a locally bright area, or arrive out of phase and produce a locally dark area.

originally used pinholes. The use of slits gives cylindrical rather than spherical wavefronts, but the principle is the same.)

Note in Figure 2.15 that the positions of the bright fringes ($P_1, P_2, \ldots P_m$) on the screen can be specified either as a distance x from P_0 (straight ahead where $\Delta D = 0$), or as an angle θ from P_0. The two waves arrive at each P_m having gone a difference in distance $\Delta D = m\lambda$ (where m, the number of whole λ shifts, is the order of the fringe). Since θ' is similar to θ (if $D \gg x$), the two triangles containing θ' and θ are similar triangles and $m\lambda/d = x/D$. Then, for bright fringes:

$$\theta_{rad} = x/D = m\lambda/d \text{ (bright fringes)}$$

and

$$x = m\lambda D/d \text{ where } m = 0, 1, 2, \text{ etc.}$$

The distance between adjacent fringes is nearly constant for small θ.

If the interfering waves are completely coherent and $a_1 = a_2$, then A_{1+2} varies between $2a$ and 0, and I varies between $4I$ and 0 (I_{max} is four times as great as the I for each separate wave). It should be noted that the conservation of energy is not violated. The extra energy in the bright fringes is accounted for exactly by the loss of energy from the dark fringes.

For waves of intermediate coherence, the difference in intensity between the bright and dark fringes becomes less. The fringes are still present but they lose their contrast since their peaks are not fully bright and their troughs are not completely dark. Then, fringe contrast (M) can be used as an indicator of how coherent the interfering waves are that have created the fringes. Michelson quantified this as *modulation* (M):

$$M = \frac{I_{max} - I_{min}}{I_{max} + I_{min}}$$

If the waves are fully coherent, $I_{min} = 0$ and regardless of what I_{max} is, $M = 1.0$. If the waves are completely incoherent, $I_{max} = I_{min}$ and $M = 0$.

DIFFRACTION

Interference fringes can be produced by a single slit as well as by two slits. In fact, double-slit interference is possible because each slit spreads its

light into a fringe pattern that is wide enough to overlap at the screen with the fringe pattern from the other slit.

This can be explained by *Huygen's principle,* which states that each point on a wavefront, even in the absence of matter, can be considered to be a point source of new waves (*wavelets*). The combined effect of the wavelets is to create a new wavefront farther along, which in turn advances the wavefront. However, if a pinhole or narrow slit is placed at a wavefront, only one wavelet is allowed to advance and the light acts as though it originated at the pinhole or slit (Figure 2.16).

According to Huygen's principle, a single *wide* slit can be thought of as made up of a large number of adjacent smaller *subslits*, each of which can be regarded as a new source of small *wavelets*. The wavelets from each subslit will then independently illuminate the entire image plane. Depending on the location of each subslit across the single-wide slit, the wavelets will travel different distances to combine at each point on the image plane. This produces phase differences, which produce an interference pattern of straight parallel fringes. Although it is an interference effect, in the case of a single opening, the interference is referred to as *diffraction.*[5,6]

Most optical systems have *circular apertures* (e.g., round lenses) rather than rectangular apertures (slits). This results in a diffraction pattern of con-

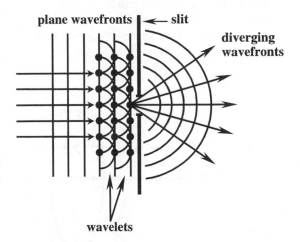

Figure 2.16. A wavefront may be conceived of as emitting a series of small wavelets whose combined effect is to advance the wavefront. A narrow slit or pinhole will allow only a small set of these wavelets to pass and act as a new source.

centric *circular* fringes. In Chapter 1 we use the refraction of rays to show how a lens produces a point image from a point object. A more realistic approach takes the wave nature of light and diffraction into consideration. If the lens is broken into *subareas*, each of which produces wavelets, the brightest area on the image plane will occur where the wavelets arrive most in phase, having traveled the same number of wavelengths (m) from the object point to the image point. Figure 2.17 shows two representative paths taken by light waves going from the object point to the image point. It can be seen that, for a suitably shaped lens, the number of wavelengths (m) can be made equal for all paths.

$$\frac{\ell_1}{\lambda} + \frac{t_1}{\lambda/n} + \frac{\ell_1'}{\lambda} = m \text{ and}$$

$$\frac{\ell_2}{\lambda} + \frac{t_2}{\lambda/n} + \frac{\ell_2'}{\lambda} = m$$

In Figure 2.17, path 2 has a greater length, but path 1 allows the wave to pass through a greater thickness (t) of lens where λ is shorter ($\lambda_n = \lambda/n$) so that both paths contain the same number (m) of λs.

An aberration-free optical system produces a diffraction pattern in the image plane that has a specific bull's-eye shape. Its center is a bright spot called the *Airy disk,* which contains about 84% of the light energy in the image. The remaining 16% of the energy is distributed around the Airy disk as a series of concentric rings, which rapidly become fainter and more closely spaced the farther they are

from the center of the pattern (Figure 2.18). The Airy disk has special significance because its size will place an irreducible limit on the fineness of detail in the image.

For small object distances such as occur with a microscope, the radius (h) of the Airy disk at the image plane is found by:

$$h = \frac{0.61\lambda}{NA}$$

where NA is the *numerical aperture*, which is usually marked on the side of the microscope objective.

For large object distances such as occur with a telescope objective, a camera lens, or the eye, the radius (h) of the Airy disk at the image plane (e.g., the retina) is found by:

$$h = 1.22 \frac{\lambda/n}{a} f$$

where a is the diameter of the entrance pupil (EP), f is the focal length, and n is the refractive index of the medium through which the image rays travel (this would be air for a telescope or camera lens, but vitreous for the eye). Recall that the entrance pupil is the image of the aperture stop as seen through all of the lenses and apertures in front of it. Thus, the EP for a telescope has the same size and location as the objective lens. For a camera lens, it is the image of the iris diaphragm as seen through the lens surfaces in front of it. And for the eye, the EP is the image of the anatomical pupil as seen through the cornea (i.e., the clinically measured pupil).

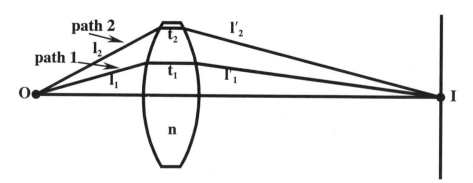

Figure 2.17. Two representative rays are drawn through a lens from an object point to the corresponding image point. Each path contains the same number of wavelengths so that they arrive in phase at the image plane and combine constructively to form the central spot of a diffraction pattern.

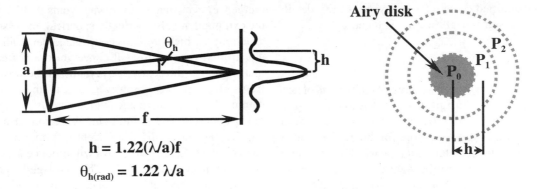

$$h = 1.22(\lambda/a)f$$

$$\theta_{h(rad)} = 1.22\ \lambda/a$$

Figure 2.18. Graphical profile of the light-intensity distribution produced by a single circular opening. The pattern is circular with a relatively large, bright central circular fringe (the Airy disk), which is flanked by successively dimmer, narrower circular fringes.

The radius of the Airy disk can also be given as an angle (θ) as pivoted at the center of the entrance pupil and projected into object space. In this case:

$$\theta_{radians} = 1.22\ \frac{\lambda}{a}$$

Resolving Power

Resolving power is a measure of how close together two image points can be and still be seen as two separate points. Even in the absence of aberrations, the resolving power of an optical system would be limited by the size of the Airy disk. For this reason, an aberration-free system is said to be *diffraction limited*.

Rayleigh's criterion is often used to calculate the resolving power of a diffraction-limited optical system. It states that two point images will just be resolved when the separation between the centers of their two Airy disks equals the radius (h) of the Airy disks. Thus, *linear resolving power* is h and *angular resolving power* is θ. From the preceding equations, it can be seen that an increase in the diameter of the entrance pupil results in a smaller Airy disk and a greater resolving power (Figures 2.18 and 2.19).

The amount of visual detail offered by a telescope's resolving power may not be useable unless

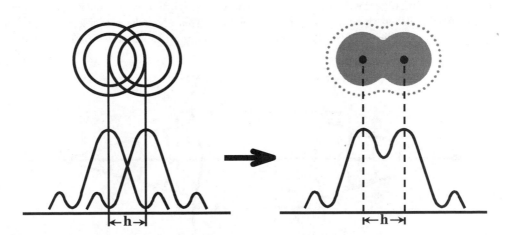

Figure 2.19. Graphical profile of the Airy disks from two adjacent image points. When the centers of the two Airy disks are separated by the radius of the disks, they are assumed to be as close as they can be and still be recognized as two image points (Rayleigh's criterion).

it is magnified enough for the eye to see this detail. The necessary magnification is found by:

$$M_{necessary} = \frac{RP_{eye}}{RP_{tel}}$$

Since the eye can resolve about 1 min of arc ($\approx 20/20$), the image from a telescope with a resolving power of 0.01 min of arc would have to be magnified $100\times$ or more for the eye to be able to appreciate the detail in the image. This is simply a matter of selecting the right focal length for the eyepiece to give this power, where $M_{telescope} = -f_{objective}/f_{eyepiece}$. A somewhat higher magnification might be used to make it easier for the eye to see the detail, but too great a magnification would reveal no additional detail and is referred to as *empty magnification*.

WAVEFRONT ABERRATION

Because it does not consider the effect of diffraction, exact raytracing gives only an approximation of the true quality of the image produced by an optical system. Seidel aberrations (discussed in Chapter 1) do even worse because of their small angle limitations. A more accurate and complete way to describe the aberrations in an optical system is by wavefront error.[8,9] This can be explained as follows.

A *wavefront* is a surface along the light path that contains all points of equal phase. For example, a point source would produce spherical wavefronts whose curved lines might conveniently represent crests. Light from a point object will emit perfectly spherical wavefronts. When these wavefronts go through an optical system, the wavefront curvature (vergence) is changed. If the wavefronts that leave the exit pupil are also perfectly spherical, the associated rays, which are lines constructed perpendicular to the wavefronts, will converge to a perfect image point at the center of curvature of the wavefronts (Figure 2.20). However, due to the wave nature of light, the image will be an Airy disk rather than a perfect point. If the wavefronts leaving the exit pupil differ sufficiently from perfect spheres, the aggregation of rays will produce a spot larger than the Airy disk. This enlarged spot encompasses the transverse aberrations found by raytracing.

Figure 2.21A shows a perfectly spherical wavefront leaving the exit pupil of an optical system. This serves as a reference wavefront against which the imperfect wavefront of an aberrated system may be compared. Since it is spherical, it will collapse to an Airy disk at the paraxial focal point. The actual wavefront is also shown centered on the exit pupil, but since it is aberrated, it has areas that deviate from the reference wavefront. The amount of deviation, in units of wavelength, can be mapped across the entire exit pupil to give a description of the *wavefront error* for the system. This gives another way of assessing the image quality of an optical instrument.

If the transverse aberrations are much smaller than the Airy disk, they will not significantly degrade the point image. Rayleigh concluded that the resolving power of an optical system would not be significantly diminished if the greatest path difference between the ideal and actual wavefront did not exceed one-fourth (i.e., one-quarter) of a wavelength of light. This gives the arguable rule that "quarter-wave" optics are essentially diffraction limited.

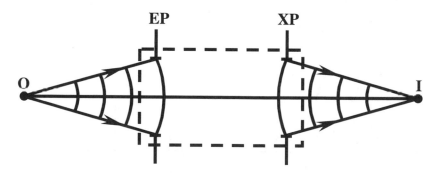

Figure 2.20. An object point sends a perfectly spherical wavefront toward the entrance pupil of an optical system. If the system has no aberrations, the wavefront that leaves the exit pupil will be perfectly spherical and collapse into an Airy disk pattern at its center of curvature.

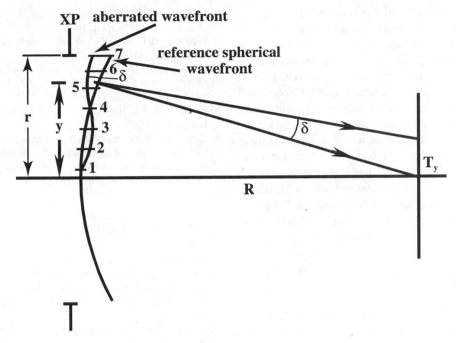

XP **aberrated wavefront**

reference spherical wavefront

(A)

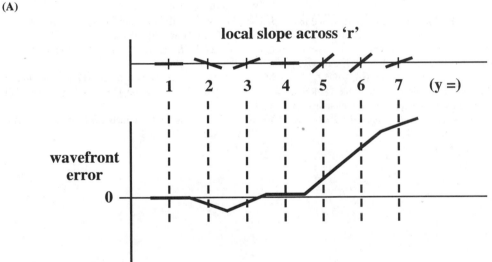

local slope across 'r'

1   2   3   4   5   6   7   (y =)

wavefront error   0

(B)

Figure 2.21. (**A**) The perfectly spherical image wavefront shown in Figure 2.20 is used as a reference wavefront against which to compare the true wavefront in an aberrated system. Any difference in slope between the reference and aberrated wavefronts at each location in the exit pupil will result in a transverse deviation T of the corresponding ray from the paraxial image point (transverse aberration). (**B**) Working backward, if the transverse aberration at the image plane is measured for rays from each location in the exit pupil, the slopes may be calculated and the aberrated wavefront reconstructed by the integration of those slopes.

Aberrated wavefronts may be compared directly to reference wavefronts by using *interferometers*. These are instruments that set up interference patterns between a reference wavefront and the wave- front to be tested. However, interferometers are usually very expensive, so it is often more practical to measure transverse aberrations, and, from them, *calculate* wavefront error. Figure 2.21B shows that there is a relationship between the difference in slope between the reference and aberrated wavefront and the resultant transverse error for rays at the image plane. Thus, if the transverse error is measured for rays going through different parts of the exit pupil, this measurement can be converted to a wavefront error slope at the exit pupil. Then, these slopes can be stitched together to reveal the true wavefront shape that would account for those slopes.[9] (For those versed in calculus, the wavefront is constructed by integrating its slopes.) We will return to the relationship between wavefront aberration and transverse aberration in Chapter 7 when we cover the measurement of refractive error by the use of wavefront sensors.

REFERENCES

1. Sliney D, Wolbarsht M. *Safety with Lasers and Other Optical Sources: A Comprehensive Handbook.* New York: Plenum, 1981.
2. Soffer BH, Lynch DK. Some paradoxes, errors, and resolutions concerning the spectral optimization of human vision. *Am J Phys.* 1999;67:946–953.
3. LaRocca A. Artificial Sources. In: Bass M. *Handbook of Optics, 1.* 2nd ed. New York: McGraw-Hill, 1995.
4. Robertson DM, Lim TH, Salomao DR, Link TP, Rowe RL, McLaren JW. Laser pointers and the human eye: A clinicopathologic study. *Arch Ophthal.* 2000;118: 1686–1691.
5. Jenkins FA, White HE. *Fundamentals of Optics.* 4th ed. New York: McGraw-Hill, 1976.
6. Freeman MH. *Optics.* 10th ed. Boston: Butterworth-Heinemann, 1990.
7. Meyer-Arendt JR. *Introduction to Classical and Modern Optics.* 2nd ed. Englewood Cliffs, NJ: Prentice-Hall, 1972.
8. Hecht E. *Optics.* 3rd ed. Reading, MA: Addison-Wesley Longman, 1998.
9. Geary JM. Catch a wave: wavefront sensors examine various parameters of light waves to produce accurate descriptions of how an optical system is performing. *Photonics Spectra.* March 1999;135–142.

FURTHER READING

Feinberg G. Light. *Sci Am.* 1968;219(3):50–59.
Feynman RP. *QED: The Strange Theory of Light and Matter.* Princeton: Princeton University Press, 1985.
Hecht E. *Optics.* 3rd ed. Reading: Addison-Wesley Longman, 1998.
Hecht J. *The Laser Guidebook.* 2nd ed. Blue Ridge Summit, PA: Tab Books, 1992.
Jenkins FA, White HE. *Fundamentals of Optics.* 4th ed. New York: McGraw-Hill, 1976.
Mauldin JH. *Light, Lasers and Optics.* Blue Ridge Summit, PA: Tab Books, 1988.
Meyer-Arendt JR. *Introduction to Classical and Modern Optics.* 2nd ed. Englewood Cliffs, NJ: Prentice-Hall, 1972.
Weisskopf VF. How light interacts with matter. *Sci Am.* 1968;219(3):60–71.

Chapter 3
Basic Optics of the Eye

[The cornea and sclera] is a rather hard and thick membrane which constitutes something like a round vessel in which all the eye's interior parts are contained. . . . [There] are three kinds of transparent glairs or humors which fill the entire space contained within these membranes . . . the one in the middle . . . which we call the crystalline humor, causes almost the same refraction as glass or crystal, and the other two . . . cause slightly less, about the same as ordinary water. —René Descartes (1637) (From Wade NJ. *A Natural History of Vision.* Cambridge, MA: MIT Press, 1998;81.)

GENERAL DESCRIPTION OF OCULAR OPTICS

Our exploration of the optics of the human eye begins in this chapter with the basic optical structure of the eye. Figure 3.1 shows a cross section of the human eye. Its *optical media* are the cornea, the aqueous humor, the crystalline lens, and the vitreous humor. The *aqueous humor* is the fluid between the cornea and the crystalline lens. It is a circulating fluid, produced by the ciliary body and eliminated in the angle between the posterior surface of the cornea and the anterior surface of the iris. A slight resistance to aqueous outflow inflates the eye with a pressure of about 15 mm Hg, which maintains its shape. The *vitreous humor* is a gel-like fluid located between the posterior surface of the crystalline lens and the retina. Unlike the aqueous, the vitreous is not circulated. The diameter of the eye from the anterior surface of the cornea to the retina varies considerably from one individual to another, but it is usually in the neighborhood of 24 mm (about the diameter of an American quarter).

Optically, the eye consists of a series of refractive surfaces defined by transitions between air, fluid, and solid tissues. As such, we could speak of a fluid aqueous lens and a fluid vitreous lens with as much right as a solid corneal lens and a solid crystalline lens. However, we traditionally think of the eye as consisting of two lenses, the cornea and the crystalline lens, whose surfaces are immersed in the fluids of the eye. The external surface of the cornea is covered with a tear film, but this layer is too thin to be refractively important.

The anterior surface of the *cornea* is convex and its posterior surface is concave. Because the concave surface has the shorter radius of curvature, the cornea, in isolation, would have a diverging, negative power. In the intact eye, however, the posterior surface is in contact with the aqueous, which weakens the negative power of this surface. The large change in index of refraction between air and the anterior cornea, on the other hand, gives a large positive power to the anterior surface that gives the cornea a net converging power that makes it the most powerful optical element in the eye.

The *crystalline lens* is biconvex, and, thus, also has a converging, plus power. Unlike the other optical media in the eye, the crystalline lens has an index of refraction that varies throughout its volume (it is a *gradient index,* or *GRIN,* lens). The analogy that is sometimes used is that the crystalline lens is layered like an onion with the highest index of refraction in the innermost layers and decreasing index going from the inner to the outer layers. The optical power of the crystalline lens is under motor control and can be increased for the viewing of near point objects, a process called *accommodation.*

The net converging power of the eye projects an image of objects in front of the eye onto the *retina,* a neurosensory layer on the back of the eye that

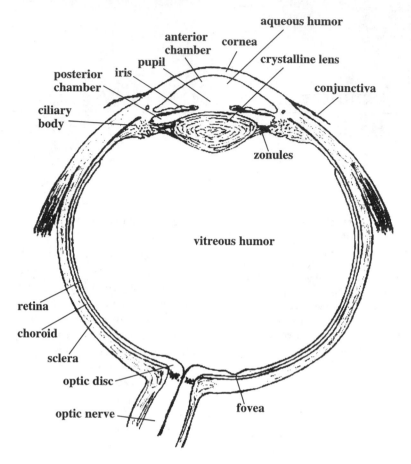

Figure 3.1. Cross section of the human eye.

initiates the neural processes of vision. The transduction of light energy into neuronal energy is accomplished by a layer of *photoreceptor cells* in the retina. The ability of the retina to detect light (*sensitivity*) and detail (*resolving power*) in projected images varies across its surface. This is due to differences across the retina in the types of photoreceptors and their densities, as well as to regional differences in the neuronal processing that takes place in the retina. The macula and its central portion, the *fovea*, are the parts of the retina most capable of processing fine detail. The fovea is the part of the retina we use to "look at something."

The *iris* of the eye is located just anterior to the crystalline lens, and is responsible for the eye's color. Although not itself a refractive surface, the iris is optically important because it forms the pupil of the eye. The iris is under motor control and can vary the diameter of the pupil between about 2 and 8 mm. Generally, the pupil constricts as object

luminance increases in order to control retinal illumination, but, as we shall see, its size has other optical consequences as well.

Although most commercial optical systems have spherical refracting surfaces, the eye has aspherical refracting surfaces. There is a great deal of variability in the asphericity of eyes, but the refractive surfaces are generally flatter peripherally than centrally. This peripheral flattening provides a better quality of retinal image than spherical surfaces would. Some commercial systems use aspherical optics to the same effect, but they are expensive to manufacture. Nature has no such economic concerns. Also, unlike commercial systems, the eye is not a centered system; the centers of curvature of the refractive surfaces do not all fall on one common optical axis. The crystalline lens is tilted with respect to the cornea, the pupil is slightly decentered, and the fovea is not on even the average optical axis. Nevertheless, the eye produces an adequate image in spite of this design flaw.

SCHEMATIC EYES

Because the optics of real eyes are very complex, schematic (model) eyes that are simpler than the real eye have been designed.[1] Schematic eyes are available with a range of complexity, but at a minimum, they include numerical values for radii of curvature, distances between refracting surfaces, and indices of refraction. The range of complexity allows the simplest schematic eye to be used, depending on the desired application. For instance, very simple schematic eyes can be used effectively to illustrate principles of visual optics such as power and refractive error, or to calculate roughly image size. More complex schematic eyes would be necessary to model aberrations in the retinal image or to calculate retinal image illuminance. For instance, to fully model aberrations a schematic eye might be required to include asphericity of surfaces, diameters of optical elements, and tilts and decentrations.

In this book we use primarily three schematic eyes: (1) the Gullstrand schematic eye No. 1, (2) the Gullstrand-Emsley schematic eye, and (3) the Emsley reduced eye. All three schematic eyes assume spherical refracting surfaces and a common optical axis. The Gullstrand schematic eye No. 1 has six refracting surfaces, the Gullstrand-Emsley schematic eye has three refracting surfaces, and the Emsley reduced eye has only one refracting surface.

Gullstrand Schematic Eye No. 1

The Gullstrand schematic eye No. 1 is also known as the Gullstrand exact schematic eye because it is the most comprehensive of the schematic eyes that Gullstrand described.[2] The numerical variables in the Gullstrand schematic eye No. 1 are given in Table 3.1, and it is illustrated in Figures 3.2 and 3.3. These values are based on the best data that were available at the time. The convergent refractive power of the anterior surface of the cornea is large because of the relatively large change in index of refraction from air to cornea. The power of the posterior surface of the cornea is negative, but small enough that the net corneal power accounts for

about two-thirds of the eye's power. The crystalline lens supplies the remainder of the power. The crystalline lens is modeled by an inner core surrounded by an outer cortex; thus, it has four refracting surfaces. The core of the crystalline lens has a higher index of refraction than the cortex. This was an attempt to model the gradient index nature of the crystalline lens.

The axial length of the Gullstrand schematic eye No. 1 is 24.0 mm, with most of this length consisting of the vitreous chamber. With refractive error referenced to the second principal plane, this eye has a refractive error of +1.00 D of hyperopia (farsightedness). According to Emsley, Gullstrand intended for this eye to be emmetropic and made it hyperopic to counteract the relative myopia

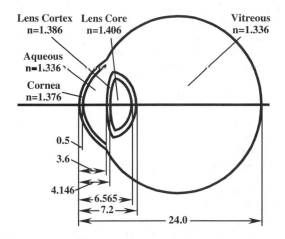

Figure 3.2. Index of refraction values and surface locations (in mm) in the Gullstrand schematic eye No. 1.

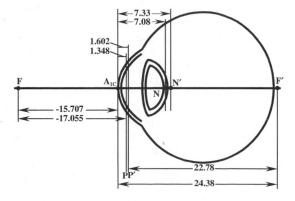

Figure 3.3. Locations of the principal planes, focal points, and nodal points (in mm from the anterior surface of the cornea) in the Gullstrand schematic eye No. 1.

Table 3.1. Gullstrand Schematic Eye No. 1

	Unaccommodated	Accommodated
Refractive Index		
Cornea	1.376	1.376
Aqueous humor and vitreous body	1.336	1.336
Lens cortex	1.386	1.386
Lens core	1.406	1.406
Position (mm)		
Anterior surface of cornea	0	0
Posterior surface of cornea	0.5	0.5
Anterior surface of lens	3.5	3.2
Anterior surface of equiv. core lens	4.146	3.8725
Posterior surface of equiv. core lens	6.565	6.5275
Posterior surface of lens	7.2	7.2
Radius of Curvature (mm)		
Anterior surface of cornea	7.7	7.7
Posterior surface of cornea	6.8	6.8
Anterior surface of lens	10.0	5.33
Anterior surface of equiv. core lens	7.911	2.655
Posterior surface of equiv. core lens	−5.76	−2.655
Posterior surface of lens	−6.0	−5.33
Refractive Power (D)		
Anterior surface of cornea	48.83	48.83
Posterior surface of cornea	−5.88	−5.88
Anterior surface of lens	5.0	9.375
Core lens	5.985	14.96
Posterior surface of lens	8.33	9.375
Corneal System		
Refractive power	43.05	43.05
Position of first principal point	−0.0496	−0.0496
Position of second principal point	−0.0506	−0.0506
First focal length	−23.227	−23.227
Second focal length	31.031	31.031
Lens System		
Refractive power	19.11	33.06
Position of first principal point	5.678	5.145
Position of second principal point	5.808	5.255
Focal length	69.908	40.416
Complete Optical System of Eye		
Refractive power	58.64	70.57
Position of first principal point	1.348	1.772
Position of second principal point	1.602	2.086
Position of first focal point	−15.707	−12.397
Position of second focal point	24.387	21.016
First focal length	−17.055	−14.169
Second focal length	22.785	18.930
Position of retina	24.0	24.0
Principal plane refractive error	+1.0	−9.6

induced by spherical aberration for rays going through the peripheral pupil.[3] Calculation of some of the variables in the Gullstrand schematic eye No. 1 are given in Appendix 3.1.

Gullstrand described both an unaccommodated state and a maximum accommodation state for the schematic eye No. 1 (see Table 3.1). The amount of accommodation exerted is 10.6 D, approximately the expected amplitude of accommodation for a young adult. The accommodated Gullstrand schematic eye models what happens in real eyes during accommodation. The only variables that change between the unaccommodated and accommodated eyes involve the crystalline lens. The anterior surface of the crystalline lens (and to a lesser extent the posterior surface) has a reduction in radius of curvature, and there is a decrease in the distance of the anterior surface of the crystalline lens from the anterior surface of the cornea.

Gullstrand-Emsley Schematic Eye

Gullstrand recognized that it was possible to use a simpler eye than the No. 1 to illustrate many optical principles. Therefore, he derived a schematic eye No. 2 in which the four surfaces of the crystalline lens in the schematic eye No. 1 were replaced by a single thin lens. However, for dealing with contributions of the ocular refractive components to the refractive error of the eye, it is necessary to have a thick crystalline lens. For this reason, Emsley[3] constructed what is now known as the Gullstrand-Emsley schematic eye. Emsley retained the thick crystalline lens of Gullstrand's schematic eye No. 1 but eliminated the core of the crystalline lens so that it had only two refractive surfaces, each with the same location and radius of curvature as in the Gullstrand No. 1 schematic eye. Also, he modeled the cornea with only one refractive surface. Thus, the Gullstrand-Emsley eye has three surfaces, as opposed to Gullstrand's eye No. 1, which had six surfaces. In addition, Emsley changed the index of refraction for the aqueous and vitreous to 4/3 in order to simplify calculations (an important consideration in the days before electronic calculators).

The Gullstrand-Emsley schematic eye is an emmetropic eye (i.e., its refractive error is zero; in other words, light from infinitely distant objects will focus on the retina). The variables in the

Table 3.2. Parameters in the Gullstrand-Emsley Schematic Eye (Unaccommodated)

Refractive Index	
Aqueous	1.333
Crystalline lens	1.416
Vitreous	1.333
Position (mm from cornea)	
Cornea	0
Anterior lens surface	3.6
Posterior lens surface	7.2
Retina	23.89
Radius of Curvature (mm)	
Cornea	+7.8
Anterior lens	+10.0
Posterior lens	−6.0
Refractive Power (D)	
Cornea	+42.735
Anterior lens	+8.27
Posterior lens	+13.778
Crystalline Lens System	
Equivalent power	+21.76
Position, 1st principal point	5.75
Position, 2nd principal point	5.91
Complete Optical System of the Eye	
Equivalent power	+60.49
Position, 1st principal point	1.55
Position, 2nd principal point	1.85
First focal length	−16.53
Second focal length	22.04
Position, 1st nodal point	7.06
Position, 2nd nodal point	7.36
Position, 1st focal point	−14.98
Position, 2nd focal point	23.89
Refractive error	0

Gullstrand-Emsley eye are listed in Table 3.2 and calculated in Appendix 3.2. This eye is illustrated in Figures 3.4 and 3.5.

Bennett and Rabbetts[4], and others have suggested minor modifications of the Gullstrand-Emsley schematic eye based on better estimates of the parameters of the average eye. However, the Gullstrand-Emsley eye has retained its popularity.

Emsley's Reduced Eye

The human eye can also be modeled as a single refracting surface, in which case it is referred to as a "reduced" eye. In this schematic eye the lens is eliminated, and its contribution to the total power is transferred to the cornea. Although this reduction

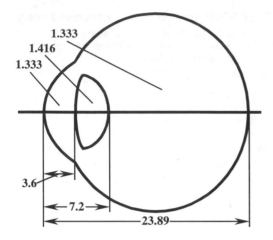

Figure 3.4. Index of refraction values and surface locations (in mm) in the Gullstrand-Emsley schematic eye.

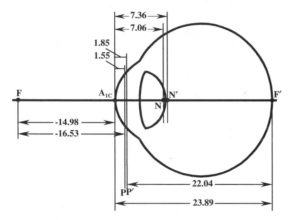

Figure 3.5. Locations of the principal planes, focal points, and nodal points (in mm from the anterior surface of the cornea) in the Gullstrand-Emsley schematic eye.

in complexity would appear to approach the absurd, there are some useful applications of the reduced eye, such as the calculation of retinal image size. A commonly used reduced eye is the Emsley reduced eye.[3] It has a total refractive power of +60 D, an index of refraction of 4/3, and it is given a length that makes it emmetropic. The radius of curvature of the "cornea" of the Emsley reduced eye is:

$$r = \frac{n' - n}{F} = \frac{1.333 - 1.000}{+60 \text{ D}} = +5.55 \text{ mm}$$

Note that this results in a corneal curvature that is much steeper than the approximately 7.7 mm for the average real human cornea.

Because the Emsley reduced eye has only one refracting surface, and it is emmetropic, the second focal point is on the retina. The second focal length and, consequently, the axial length of the Emsley reduced eye is:

$$f' = \frac{n'}{F} = \frac{1.333}{+60 \text{ D}}(1000) = +22.22 \text{ mm}$$

Note that this is somewhat shorter than the approximately 24 mm for the average human eye.

Since there is only one refracting surface, the first and second principal planes are both located at that surface, so the *equivalent* power (F_e) is the same as the corneal power (+60 D) and the *equivalent* second focal length (f_{e2}) is the same as f' (+22.22 mm).

All of these schematic eyes have spherical refracting surfaces, and, consequently, they do not model aberrations accurately. To fill this need, schematic eyes with aspheric surfaces have been developed. An example is the *Indiana eye*, which is a reduced eye modeled specifically to approximate the measured chromatic and spherical aberration of human eyes.[5] This schematic eye is identical to the Emsley reduced eye except that the single refracting surface has a specified asphericity and a pupil has been added.

With modern computers available there is no longer a need to limit a schematic eye to even the approximations used in Gullstrand's "exact" schematic eye. Attempts have been made to model the human eye as accurately as possible, including a gradient index crystalline lens.[6] Ironically, our computational abilities have now exceeded our knowledge of the exact parameters of the average eye. For example, we have only a crude knowledge of the aspheric nature of the anterior and posterior surfaces of the crystalline lens, but we could use that information to calculate the quality of a retinal image.

AXES AND ANGLES OF THE EYE

As mentioned earlier, the human eye is not a centered optical system. The optical axes of the cornea and lens are not coincident (i.e., the centers of curvature of their refracting surfaces do not all fall on one straight line). Nevertheless, we can define an approximation to the *optical axis* of the eye as the straight line that by best fit passes closest to all of the centers of curvature. Also, contrary to what one would expect if the eye were a precision optical system, the fovea of the retina is not on even the approximate optical axis of the eye. As a consequence, it is useful to define axes in addition to the optical axis, and to define the various angles formed at their intersections (Figure 3.6).

The *pupillary axis* is the line drawn through the center of the entrance pupil (the anatomical pupil as viewed through the cornea) at the angle that makes it perpendicular to the cornea. Unlike the optical axis, the location of the pupillary axis can be determined easily and it is close enough to the average optical axis that it is used clinically as an approximation to the optical axis. One method is for the examiner to place his eye directly adjacent to a flashlight while he directs the beam toward the eye being observed. When the location of the flashlight is set so that its reflection from the surface of the cornea appears to be centered in the entrance pupil, the pupillary axis is the line joining the flashlight to its reflected image.

The *line of sight* is the line that connects the object of regard (object being viewed) with the center of the entrance pupil. As such, the location of the line of sight can be determined easily. It is the ray directed from the object point to the cornea in the direction of the center of the entrance pupil. After refraction by the cornea and crystalline lens, the ray leaves the posterior crystalline lens surface along a line constructed from the center of the exit pupil to the fovea. Therefore, the line of sight is the

anterior segment of the chief ray that, after all refractions, intersects the fovea.

The *nodal axis* is a line from the object of regard to the first nodal point of the eye and then from the second nodal point of the eye to the fovea. Many authors refer to this line as the visual axis, although others argue that the visual axis should be defined differently.[7] To avoid confusion, we call this axis the nodal axis, and do not use the term *visual axis*.

The *achromatic axis* is a line from the object of regard directed toward the eye in a direction that minimizes lateral chromatic aberration. (This axis is discussed later in this chapter.)

Based on these axes, various angles of the eye have been defined as illustrated in Figure 3.6. *Angle alpha* is the angle formed at the first nodal point by the intersection of the optical axis and the nodal axis. *Angle kappa* is the angle formed at the first nodal point by the intersection of the pupillary axis and the nodal axis. *Angle lambda* is the angle subtended at the center of the entrance pupil by the intersection of the pupillary axis and the line of sight.

We would especially like to know for any particular eye how far the fovea is off the optical axis. This would require measurement of angle alpha. But, as we have noted, a true optical axis does not exist and, in any case, it would be hard to locate even an average optical axis. Thus, in a clinical examination of the eye, the pupillary axis is used as an estimate of the location of the optical axis and the angle lambda is used as an estimate of the angle

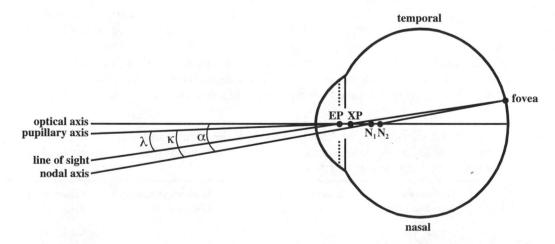

Figure 3.6. Angles of the eye in a right eye viewed from above. (EP = center of the entrance pupil of the eye; XP = center of the exit pupil of the eye; N$_1$ = first nodal point; N$_2$ = second nodal point; λ = angle lambda; κ = angle kappa; α = angle alpha.)

alpha. A point of confusion is that in a clinical setting angle lambda is often referred to as angle kappa. However, this cross use of terms is of little consequence because the line of sight is almost coincident with the nodal axis, so angles lambda and kappa are approximately equal.

The angles are considered positive in sign when the nodal axis or the line of sight in object space is nasal to the optical axis or the pupillary axis. All of the angles in Figure 3.6 are drawn as positive, which is typical of the majority of eyes. These angles are small, usually in the neighborhood of 5 degrees.

PURKINJE IMAGES

When light strikes a refracting surface, no matter how transparent or smooth, a small proportion of the incident light is reflected (known as *Fresnel reflection*). The images of a light source reflected from the refracting surfaces of the eye are known as Purkinje images, for the Czech physiologist Jan Evangelista Purkinje who first described them in detail in 1823.[8] Purkinje images have a number of clinical and research uses, such as measurement of the curvatures of the refracting surfaces of the eye (keratometry and phakometry), location of the axes of the eye, and estimation of the angle of deviation in strabismus (e.g., the Hirschberg test). (Some of these applications are described in detail later.)

The Purkinje images are numbered I, II, III, and IV, designating the order of the surface from which an external light source is reflected. Purkinje image I is formed by reflection from the anterior surface of the cornea. Purkinje image II is formed by reflection from the posterior surface of the cornea, Purkinje image III is formed by reflection from the anterior surface of the crystalline lens, and Purkinje image IV is formed by reflection from the posterior surface of the crystalline lens. Only Purkinje image I is formed by a simple reflection. To locate Purkinje images II, III, and IV by raytrace, the object rays must be traced into the eye through all of the refractive surfaces in front of the reflective surface, and after reflection they must be traced through the refractive surfaces in reverse order.

For an object about 1 m from the eye, Purkinje images I, II, and IV are located about 3 to 5 mm behind the anterior surface of the cornea and are close to the same size, with IV being a little smaller than the others. Purkinje image III is located about 10 to 11 mm behind the cornea and is considerably larger than the other Purkinje images. Purkinje images I, II, and III are erect images while Purkinje image IV is inverted. The locations and magnifications of the Purkinje images for the Gullstrand schematic eye No. 1 and the Gullstrand-Emsley schematic eye are given in Table 3.3. The tabulated results for the Gullstrand-Emsley schematic eye are calculated in Appendix 3.3. Because the Gullstrand-Emsley schematic eye has a single-surface cornea, Purkinje image II does not appear in the table for this eye. Note that the simplifications in going from the Gullstrand schematic eye No. 1 to the Gullstrand-Emsley schematic eye do not introduce large changes in the locations and magnifications of Purkinje images I, III, and IV. Figure 3.7 is a diagram showing the relative sizes, orientations, and locations of the Purkinje images. A triangular array of lights is used to illustrate which Purkinje images are erect or inverted.

Because the eye is not a coaxial (centered) optical system, the Purkinje images do not align perfectly on one line. The best approximation of the optical axis of the eye, then, is the line of best fit to these images. If an observer places his eye next to the light source, an estimate of the optical axis will

Table 3.3. Locations (Distances from the Anterior Surface of the Cornea) and Magnifications of the Purkinje Images for the Gullstrand Schematic Eye No. 1 and the Gullstrand-Emsley Schematic Eye (A negative magnification indicates an inverted image.)

Purkinje Image	Gullstrand Location (mm)	Schematic Eye No. 1 Magnification	Gullstrand-Emsley Location (mm)	Schematic Eye Magnification
I	3.84	+0.00384	3.88	+0.00388
II	3.75	+0.00337	—	—
III	10.54	+0.00746	10.51	+0.00744
IV	4.16	−0.00372	3.95	−0.00287

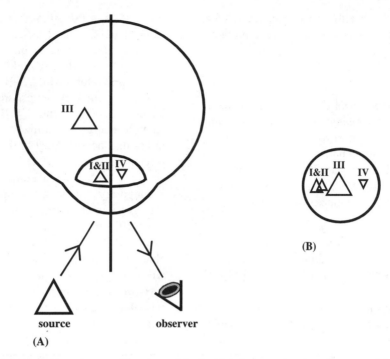

Figure 3.7. Relative sizes, orientations, and locations of the Purkinje images of a triangular array of lights; (**A**) in the eye, and (**B**) in the pupil as viewed by an observer.

be that line between the light source and Purkinje images that results in the Purkinje images being closest to superimposed.

During accommodation, the only easily noticeable change in the Purkinje images is that Purkinje image III moves forward and becomes smaller. Purkinje image IV may also become slightly smaller and move slightly deeper within the eye. Changes in Purkinje images III and IV have been used to study changes during accommodation in the radii of curvature and location of the surfaces of the crystalline lens. For instance, Gullstrand used such observations to determine parameters for his schematic eyes in the unaccommodated and the accommodated states.

The relative brightness of the Purkinje images may be calculated by using the equation for Fresnel reflection. Reflectance (R), the proportion of light incident on a refracting surface that is reflected from it, is given by:

$$R = \left(\frac{n_2 - n_1}{n_2 + n_1} \right)^2$$

Using the index of refraction values from the Gullstrand schematic eye No. 1, we calculate the following. For Purkinje image I, about 2% of the

light striking the cornea is reflected. This is based on the index of refraction for the tear film (1.334) rather than that for the cornea (1.376), because technically Purkinje image I is reflected from the tear film on the surface of the cornea. This is by far the brightest of the images because it is reflected at the surface with the largest change in index of refraction. About 0.02% of the light striking the posterior surface of the cornea is reflected, and about 0.03% of light is reflected at the anterior and posterior surfaces of the crystalline lens.

Purkinje image II is very difficult to distinguish because it is very close to Purkinje image I, whose much greater brightness obscures it. Viewed under high magnification Purkinje images I, II, and IV appear smooth, but Purkinje image III seems to have a diffuse orange peel-like appearance because the anterior surface of the crystalline lens is not as smooth as the other surfaces.

LIGHT AND THE EYE

The most important part of the electromagnetic spectrum for the eye is visible light because it is responsible for visual sensation. However, due to their effects on the health of the eye, ultraviolet (UV) and infrared (IR) radiation also are important.

Visible Light

The electromagnetic spectrum ranges from radio waves on the long wavelength side of the spectrum to gamma rays on the short wavelength side. However, the eye uses only a narrow band of this range to produce visual sensations. The sensory ineffectiveness of most of the electromagnetic spectrum is the result of a number of causes including

1. The limited power that a typical light source has in the extreme ranges of the spectrum.
2. Strong absorption of certain bands of the spectrum by the ocular media before it reaches the retina.
3. Insensitivity of the retinal photoreceptor cells to light on the long wavelength side of the visible spectrum.

Even within the visible spectrum, the retina has different sensitivities for different wavelengths. Under bright light (*photopic* conditions) the eye is maximally sensitive to 555 nm (yellow-green) light, but the sensitivity drops off to 20% of that value for wavelengths of about 489 nm (blue) and 637 nm (red). Under dim light (*scotopic* conditions) the eye is maximally sensitive to 510 nm light. Thus, under twilight conditions the eye becomes relatively more sensitive to blue light. This explains the phenomenon known as the *Purkinje shift* in which, if a red and a blue object appear equally bright under bright illumination, the blue object will appear brighter than the red object under dim illumination. (Transmission of visible light by the eye is discussed further in Chapter 4.)

UV Radiation

Most of the eye's UV light exposure is from the Sun; very little comes from artificial lighting. Although UV radiation is invisible, individual photons of UV light are energetic enough to break molecular bonds and damage tissues, including the eye. UV light is classified into three bands of wavelength, UV-C, UV-B, and UV-A.

UV-C (100–280 nm): The UV-C component of sunlight is almost completely absorbed by ozone (O_3) in the atmosphere. Chlorofluorocarbons (CFCs) used as coolants and spray can propellants released into the atmosphere destroy O_3 and allow more UV-C to reach the ground and (along with UV-B) can cause skin cancer. Germicidal lamps are effective due largely to UV-C (and UV-B), which have enough energy to ionize and thus break molecular bonds. Very little natural UV-C reaches the eye but UV-C from arc welding is absorbed by the corneal epithelium and causes a temporary but painful reduction in visual acuity. Refractive surgery using the excimer laser (193 nm) is an example of the controlled use of UV-C to reshape the cornea by surface ablation. Wavelengths shorter than 185 nm will not pass through air so are of little concern (this is referred to as "vacuum UV").

UV-B (280–315 nm): The UV-B band is readily transmitted through the atmosphere but it does not penetrate the eye very far. Most UV-B is absorbed by the corneal epithelium and is responsible for corneal flash burn from arc welding (along with UV-C) and snow blindness from reflected sunlight.

UV-A (315–400 nm): The cornea is transparent to UV-A, and most UV-A is absorbed by the lens, where it can cause cataracts. Because of absorption by the lens, little UV-A gets to the retina. As the lens ages, it becomes yellow (brunescent) so that it becomes an even more effective filter against UV-A. Most intraocular lens implants contain a dye that absorbs UV in order to protect the retina. Tanning lamps emit chiefly in the UV-A band.

Infrared Radiation

Infrared (IR) radiation is absorbed in the eye by causing vibration of water molecules so that its energy is converted to heat. A great deal of IR light is absorbed in the eye in the anterior chamber, but about half of IR light at 1000 nm is transmitted to the retina. The cutoff of visual sensitivity to IR is due to insensitivity of the retinal receptors rather than to lack of transmission to the receptors. Intense IR has been linked to cataracts due to heating of the lens, but such levels are usually found only in certain occupations such as working with molten glass.

ABERRATIONS OF THE EYE

Chromatic Aberration

Chromatic aberration occurs because all optical materials have slightly different refractive indexes for each wavelength. Thus the different wavelengths in object light are refracted by different amounts, and images in different colors may be axially blurred or laterally displaced. Most optical systems are designed to minimize this aberration. For example, optical designers often correct chromatic aberration by pairing plus and minus lenses that have opposite chromatic aberration so that chromatic aberration largely cancels. The eye does not directly correct for chromatic aberration by this means or any other; when polychromatic objects are observed, there is image blur on the retina for all colors except the one that is in focus.

We will use the Emsley reduced eye to illustrate the effect of *longitudinal chromatic aberration* (*LCA*) on the eye. If we add a pupil at its single refractive surface, the results from this model will not differ much from the real eye. In the Emsley eye all refraction is at a single corneal interface whose power F is $+60$ D. If the Emsley eye is filled with water (so that n equals 1.334 and dispersive power V equals 54.7), then:

$$LCA = F/V = +60/54.7 \approx +1.00 \text{ D}$$

This result is for the part of the spectrum between 486 nm (the blue hydrogen F-line) and 656 nm (the red hydrogen C-line). For the full visible spectrum (about 400–700 nm) the chromatic aberration is even greater ($\approx +1.75$ D). In the real eye, chromatic aberration has been measured to be about this amount and it is generated by the cornea and lens in approximate ratio to their powers. Unlike the Seidel aberrations, chromatic aberration varies little among different eyes.[9]

Longitudinal chromatic aberration is a measure of the axial distance between the images for two different wavelengths. Since it is relatively independent of the entrance pupil diameter, in itself, it is not a good indicator of the amount of blur induced by chromatic aberration. A measure that reflects retinal image blur better is *transverse axial chromatic aberration* (*TCA*). This is a measure of the blur circle diameter in one wavelength when another wavelength, usually spectrally central, is in

focus. In Figure 3.8, the blur circle size due to TCA is a function of both LCA and entrance pupil size.

The graph of chromatic aberration and wavelength isn't linear and much of the range of chromatic aberration is due to the blue end of the spectrum (Figure 3.9).

If a pinhole source of bright white light were viewed by an emmetropic eye so that yellow light were in focus on the retina, a yellow dot on the retina would be surrounded by a purple (red plus blue) halo. This difference in blur circle sizes for different colors allows cobalt filters to be used to directly perceive the effects of longitudinal chromatic aberration. A cobalt filter blocks the middle wavelengths of the spectrum while it passes the long and short wavelengths (red and blue). As shown in Figures 3.10A and B, an observer with the right amount of hyperopia looking through a cobalt filter at a bright white pinhole will see a blue pinhole with a red fringe, whereas an observer with the right amount of myopia will see a red pinhole with a blue fringe.

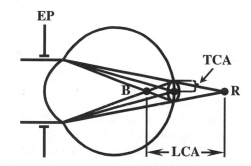

Figure 3.8. When the middle of the visible spectrum is in focus on the retina, blue light focuses in front of the retina and red light focuses behind the retina. This results in blur circles for blue and red light.

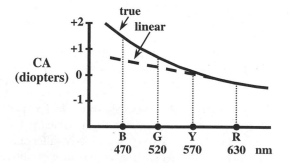

Figure 3.9. The graph of dioptric CA to wavelength is not linear. The blue end of the spectrum is responsible for a disproportionate amount of CA.

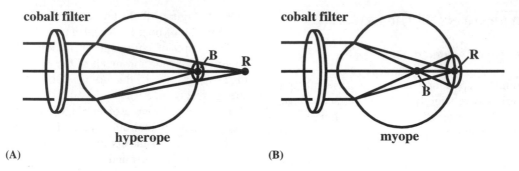

Figure 3.10. (**A**) Image formation in a hyperopic eye after transmission through a cobalt filter. (**B**) Image formation in a myopia eye after transmission through a cobalt filter.

One of a battery of tests that a doctor uses to determine a spectacle prescription (Rx) is the red-green (bichrome) test. This test uses ocular chromatic aberration to determine the Rx that results in focus of yellow light on the retina. If black letters against adjacent green and red backgrounds are made to look equally blurry, the letters on the green background will focus in front of the retina while the letters on the red background will focus behind the retina. The focus for yellow light will then be close to the retina.

Figure 3.8 suggests that chromatic aberration should produce considerable blur; even with uncorrected chromatic aberration, however, visual acuity is surprisingly good. Also, if chromatic aberration is reduced by using monochromatic light or achromatizing lenses (lenses that induce opposite chromatic aberration so that all wavelengths focus on the retina), visual acuity is not significantly improved. Thibos and colleagues[10] report from theoretical calculations that the effect of chromatic aberration on contrast for a 2.5-mm pupil is equivalent to only about 0.20 D of defocus. For high-contrast fine details, this amount of defocus might cause a Snellen acuity of 20/15 to be degraded to 20/20.

There are several reasons why visual acuity is not affected much by large amounts of chromatic aberration:

1. The lens turns yellow with age (brunescence) and filters out much of the blue light, which is the greatest offender. Sixty-year-olds may suffer only one-third as much blur from chromatic aberration as young people do[11] (however, this reported amount is controversial). Even the young lens filters out UV-A light, which otherwise would stim- ulate the retinal receptors and result in enormous amounts of chromatic aberration.

2. The retina contains a yellow pigment (xanthophyll) in the *macula* (an area that surrounds the fovea). This acts as a yellow filter, which filters out blue light (which is responsible for the greatest amount of chromatic aberration).

3. There are no "blue" receptors in the fovea (only "red" and "green" receptors). Thus, in this area, where the best retinal image is required, the receptors are relatively insensitive to the significantly blurred blue light. Without chromatic aberration, one would predict that blue light would produce better, not worse, visual acuity because shorter wavelength light produces a smaller Airy disk.

4. The luminous efficiency of the eye is greatest for 555-nm (yellow-green) light in the middle of the visible spectrum. Colors beyond blue-green on the short wavelength side and orange on the long wavelength side appear less than half as bright as yellow-green, so any blur is less noticeable for those wavelengths for which the blur is greatest.[12]

Even with all of the above ways that the eye minimizes the effects of chromatic aberration, its effects can be made very apparent under exceptional conditions, such as with the op-art posters that college students found so attractive in the 1960s. These often contain red and blue areas, which share common borders. The inability to focus simultaneously on both colors may cause accommodation of the lens to oscillate; the borders appear to vibrate and eyestrain is induced.

Another form of chromatic aberration is *chromatic difference of magnification*, often referred to as *lateral chromatic aberration*. In the eye this aberration causes the longer wavelengths in object light (e.g., red) to form larger images than the shorter wavelengths do (e.g., blue). The result is that for off-axis object points, the off-axis image points will be drawn out into radially oriented spectra that blur the image. Because the line of sight is aligned close to the achromatic axis (discussed later), lateral chromatic aberration is small and degrades the image much less than transverse chromatic aberration does. However, the stereoscopic mechanism in the visual cortex of the brain is remarkably sensitive to this color-dependent shift of the retinal image. This produces the false perception of stereopsis in flat objects, called chromatic stereopsis, whose explanation follows.

Chromatic Stereopsis

For most people, when red and blue objects are placed side by side against a black background, the red object appears to be closer than the blue object. Patients sometimes observe this effect when they are given the red-green test. The cause of this effect is the positive angle lambda of about 5° seen in most people, which gives a stereoscopic effect with binocular vision. Figures 3.11 and 3.12 show how this works. Each diagram in Figure 3.11 depicts the right eye seen from above. Figure 3.11B shows that

if the border between the red and blue fields is placed on the fovea, chromatic difference of magnification will form a blue image nasally and a red image temporally. Figure 3.12 shows that when the border is viewed with both eyes, the red images will project to a point closer than the blue images will. Disparity-detecting cells in the brain then interpret this as a difference in depth.

Figures 3.11 and 3.12 show the pupils centered on the optical axis. However, on average, pupils are decentered about 0.25-mm nasally (although there is quite a large variation among individuals).[1] The particular amount of decentration influences the depth effect induced by red or blue light. In Figure 3.13A the pupil is decentered enough to put the chief ray through the nodal point (decentered nasally > 0.25 mm). This eliminates chromatic difference of magnification and thus chromatic stereopsis is not seen. In Figure 3.13B further decentration causes the chromatic stereopsis effect to reverse so blue appears nearer than red. The line that goes through both the EP and the nodal point is called the *achromatic axis*. For most eyes the fovea is nearly on the achromatic axis so that lateral chromatic aberration is greatly reduced.

The specific stereo effect depends on the particular angle lambda (see Figure 3.6) and pupil decentration of the observer. A positive angle lambda

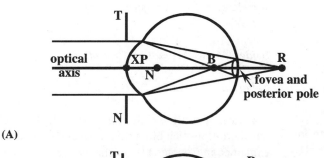

Fovea is on the optical axis, angle λ = 0.
R and B blur circles overlap with the Y point image.

(A)

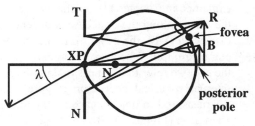

Fovea temporal to the optical axis (angle λ positive). Get <u>chromatic difference of magnification</u> where the R image is larger than the B image.

(B)

Figure 3.11. (A) Red and blue blur circles overlap with the yellow point image when the fovea is on the optical axis and angle λ = 0. (B) The fovea is temporal to the optical axis (angle λ is positive). This gives a chromatic difference of magnification in which the red image is more temporal than the blue image.

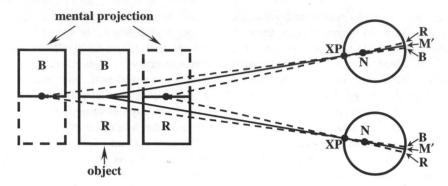

Figure 3.12. Two eyes are shown with the border between blue and red fields on the fovea (M′). The red chief ray projects temporally in both eyes, giving the perception that the red field is closer than the point of foveation; the blue ray projects nasally in both eyes, giving the perception that the blue field is farther than the point of foveation.

increases the effect where red appears closer than blue, whereas a nasal pupil decentration reduces this effect, or, if decentration is large enough, reverses it. The nasal pupil decentration seen in most people

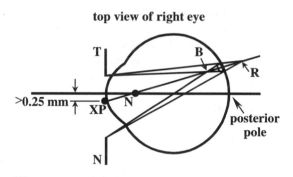

(A)

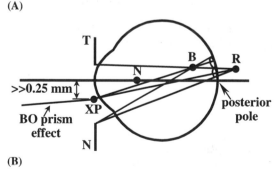

(B)

Figure 3.13. (A) If with a positive angle λ the entrance pupil is displaced nasally so that the chief ray passes through the nodal point as well as the center of the entrance pupil (EP), all wavelengths arrive at the same point on the retina and there is no chromatic stereopsis. (B) If the entrance pupil is displaced too far nasally, the blue chief ray will be displaced temporal to the red chief ray so that binocularly the blue field will appear to be closer than the red field.

functions to reduce chromatic difference of magnification and thus the chromatic stereopsis effect.

Although chromatic aberration results in blurred images, it may nevertheless have a beneficial use in the visual system. It has been demonstrated that some people require polychromatic light in order to accommodate accurately, so differential blur for colors may be a cue to the accommodative system as to the degree and direction that the crystalline lens power must be changed to regain focus.[13] Also, there is evidence that the eye uses the rather large dioptric range of chromatic aberration to increase the range of accommodation by focusing shorter wavelengths for near objects and longer wavelengths for far objects.

Seidel (Monochromatic) Aberrations

Spherical Aberration

Spherical aberration is the only one of the five Seidel aberrations that blurs axial images. Its effect, as explained in Chapter 1, is to change the location of the image along the optical axis depending on the distance (y) of the rays from the center of the entrance pupil. When restricting our discussion to the eye, we refer to SA measured in image space as internal spherical aberration (Figure 3.14A) and SA measured in object space as external spherical aberration (Figure 3.14B).

Internal spherical aberration (ISA) in diopters equals the difference in image vergence ($L' = n/\ell'$, where ℓ' is in meters) between peripheral rays (y_2) and paraxial (central) rays (y_1).

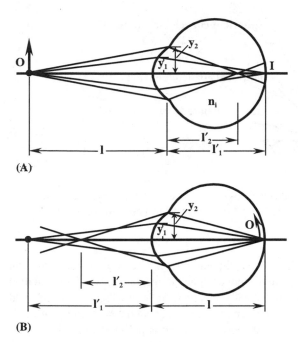

(A)

(B)

Figure 3.14 (**A**) For a given wavelength, in the typical eye the peripheral zones of the entrance pupil have a greater effective power than the central zones. This results in positive longitudinal spherical aberration. (**B**) When a point on the retina is used as an object, the external image also shows positive spherical aberration. This is how the spherical aberration can be measured clinically.

$$ISA = L_2' - L_1' = (n_i/\ell_2') - (n_i/\ell_1')$$

The corresponding longitudinal SA can be found by solving for the distances ℓ_2' and ℓ_1' so that linear $ISA = \ell_1' - \ell_2'$. (Then if $\ell_1' > \ell_2'$, the SA is plus in sign.) Transverse SA is the radius of the axial blur circle formed when the paraxial rays are in focus on the retina. It is a more direct indicator of retinal image blur than longitudinal SA is. (In the same way that transverse chromatic aberration is a more direct indicator of blur than longitudinal CA is.)

External SA (*ESA*) is found by placing an object at the fovea and finding the differences in image distance in front of the eye for different ys. ESA is more easily measured than ISA; for example, by retinoscopy through annular apertures of different radii (y). Once ESA is found, ISA is equal dioptrically.

A raytrace through the Emsley reduced eye reveals a large amount of plus spherical aberration (about +3.00 D for a 4-mm diameter pupil). In fact, for spherical surfaces, longitudinal spherical

aberration is proportional to y^2 and transverse spherical aberration is proportional to y^3. Thus, eyes with large pupils would be expected to form "blurred" images from point objects even when in best focus. Experimental measurements on the human eye show much less spherical aberration than predicted by raytracing through schematic eyes.[12] This is due to the fact that the cornea is not spherical but has a flatter curve (longer radius) peripherally than it has centrally. Actual corneal profiles differ greatly among individuals but they are generally described as elliptical (see Chapter 5). The aspheric surface of the typical cornea reduces the amount of spherical aberration from what a spherical cornea would have produced, but leaves a residual amount.

The preceding discussion is for the unaccommodated eye. When unaccommodated, the lens seems to contribute relatively little to the total amount of SA. However, when the lens accommodates, the anterior surface of the lens deforms to form a steeper center and a flatter periphery so that for the average person the SA for the entire eye may be further reduced and in some case may even become negative (Figure 3.15).

Spherical aberration varies considerably among eyes, presumably as a result of differences in the surface shapes of the cornea and lens. Also, spherical aberration is very asymmetric because spherical aberration in one power meridian may differ from that in another meridian.[13]

Diffraction theory predicts better visual acuity with larger pupils because larger pupils would result in a smaller Airy disk ($\theta_{rad} = 1.22 \lambda/a$, where a is the entrance pupil diameter). However, large pupils usually result in worse rather than better acuity.[14] This is due primarily to spherical aberration, which becomes large enough to offset the gain predicted by diffraction theory when, on average, the pupil diameter exceeds about 2.5 mm.

Coma

Coma does not affect on-axis object points but spreads off-axis image points into a comet-shaped blur (see Chapter 1). Because the fovea usually is not on the optical axis, coma may be a significant aberration at the fovea. Thus, the two major Seidel aberrations at the fovea are spherical aberration and coma.

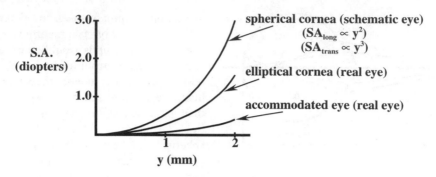

Figure 3.15. A graph of dioptric spherical aberration to the radii of entrance pupil zones in millimeters. An eye with all spherical refractive surfaces would have much more spherical aberration than the typical real eye with aspherical refractive surfaces.

Oblique (or Radial) Astigmatism

Even with well-centered spherical optics, oblique off-axis rays (from objects in the peripheral field) experience different lens powers depending on whether they go through the tangential or sagittal meridian of a lens (see Chapter 1). This produces oblique astigmatism, in which a point object is imaged as two line images aligned at right angles in different image planes. With a converging system, the tangential line focus is closer to the last lens than the sagittal line focus is. The smallest image that can be obtained is a circular spot (the circle of least confusion) between the two line images.

There are usually several diopters of oblique astigmatism in the peripheral field of the human eye, but this is still less astigmatism than if the eye had all spherical surfaces. Advantageously, the eye is curved enough that, on average, the retina is located between the two line foci so that the circle of least confusion remains close to the retina[15] (Figure 3.16).

Even though retinal circuitry in the peripheral field is not designed to respond to smaller detail than it typically receives, oblique astigmatism and field curvature can be great enough that they have an additional degrading effect on peripheral visual acuity.[16]

Curvature of Field

In the absence of oblique astigmatism, the focal "plane" is a specific curved surface called the Petzval surface. In the presence of oblique astigmatism, the actual best focal surface is that of the circles of least confusion. This best focal surface for the eye is close to the retina, as mentioned, and is significantly in front of the Petzval surface.

Distortion

Off-axis images on the retina suffer from significant distortion, but this is relatively unimportant because the brain can correct for this defect perceptually, possibly in the same way that it adapts to

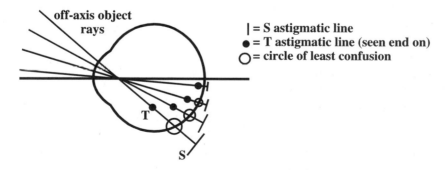

Figure 3.16. The eye suffers from both field curvature and oblique astigmatism. The curvature of the retina compensates for this, at least in part, by having a curvature that places the retina at the image surface for the circles of least confusion.

distortion induced by a new spectacle Rx. Also distortion does not blur point images, it simply shifts them from their geometrically projected positions.

In designing spectacle lenses, oblique astigmatism, curvature of field, and distortion produced by the spectacle lens are the more important of the five Seidel aberrations. Spherical aberration and coma are relatively unimportant because the pupil of the eye becomes the aperture stop for the system and restricts the size of the beam of light from any given object point that passes through the spectacle lens. The front and back surface powers of the spectacle lens are selected to reduce oblique astigmatism and match the curvature of field to the retina. Distortion is usually not corrected.

APPENDIX 3.1

CALCULATION OF SOME OF THE VARIABLES IN THE GULLSTRAND SCHEMATIC EYE NO. 1 (UNACCOMMODATED)

Given the radius of curvature of the anterior surface of the cornea of +7.7 mm, and the index of refraction of the cornea of 1.376, the power of the anterior surface of the cornea is +48.83 D:

$$F_{1C} = \frac{n_2 - n_1}{r} = \frac{1.376 - 100}{+0.0077 \text{ m}}$$

$$F_{1C} = +48.83 \text{ D}$$

The power of the posterior surface of the cornea is –5.88 D:

$$F_{2C} = \frac{n_3 - n_2}{r} = \frac{1.336 - 1.376}{+0.0068 \text{ m}}$$

$$F_{2C} = -5.88 \text{ D}$$

Given these surface powers and the thickness of the cornea of 0.5 mm, the equivalent power can be calculated:

$$F_{ec} = F_{1C} + F_{2C} - \left(\frac{d}{n_2}\right)(F_{1C})(F_{2C})$$

$$F_{ec} = +48.83 \text{ D} + (-5.88 \text{ D}) - \left(\frac{0.005 \text{ m}}{1.376}\right)$$

$$(+48.83\text{D})(-5.88 \text{ D})$$

$$F_{ec} = 43.05 \text{ D}$$

The equivalent power of the cornea is +43.05 D. The cornea is thus a high power converging lens. The following is the calculation of the location of the first principal plane of the cornea:

$$\overline{A_{1C}P_C} = \frac{n_1 \cdot d \cdot F_{2C}}{n_2 \cdot F_{ec}}$$

$$\overline{A_{1C}P_C} = \frac{(1.0)(0.0005 \text{ m})(-5.88 \text{ D})}{(1.376)(+43.05 \text{ D})}$$

$$\overline{A_{1C}P_C} = -0.0496 \text{ mm}$$

The minus sign indicates that the first principal plane of the cornea (P_C) is to the left of anterior to the anterior surface of the cornea (A_{1C}).

The distance of the second principal of the cornea (P_C') from the posterior surface of the cornea can be calculated as follows:

$$\overline{A_{2C}P'} = -\frac{n_3 \cdot d \cdot F_1}{n_2 \cdot F_C}$$

$$\overline{A_{2C}P'} = -\frac{(1.336)(0.0005 \text{ m})(+48.83 \text{ D})}{1.376 + 43.05 \text{ D}}$$

$$\overline{A_{2C}P'} = -0.55 \text{ mm}$$

The second principal plane of the cornea is therefore 0.55 mm anterior to the posterior surface of the cornea. We can find the location of the second principal plane of the cornea with respect to the anterior surface of the cornea, as it is expressed in Table 3.1, by deducting the corneal thickness. When we do so, we find that the second principal plane of the cornea is 0.05 mm anterior to the anterior surface of the cornea:

$$\overline{A_{1C}P_C'} = \overline{A_{1C}A_{2C}} + \overline{A_{2C}P_C'}$$

$$\overline{A_{1C}P_C'} = +0.50 \text{ mm} + (-0.55 \text{ mm})$$

$$\overline{A_{1C}P_C'} = -0.05 \text{ mm}$$

By the previous calculations, we know that the equivalent power of the cornea in the Gullstrand schematic eye No. 1 is +43.05 D, and the principal planes of the cornea are slightly anterior to the anterior surface of the cornea.

The crystalline lens in the Gullstrand schematic eye No. 1 is a four-surface converging lens. The core of the crystalline lens has an index of refraction of 1.406. The surrounding cortex of the crystalline lens has an index of refraction of 1.386. The radii of curvature of each of the surfaces and their locations are given in Table 3.1. The equivalent power of the crystalline lens is +19.11 D. The anterior and posterior surfaces of the lens are 3.6 mm and 7.2 mm from the anterior surface of the cornea. The principal planes of the crystalline lens are 5.678 mm (P_L) and 5.808 mm (P_L') from the anterior surface of the cornea, and are therefore located in the crystalline lens.

The thick lens equation for equivalent power can be used to determine the equivalent power of a complex optical system consisting of two lenses, such as the eye. F_1 becomes the equivalent power of the first lens in the system (the cornea). F_2 becomes the equivalent power of the second lens (the crystalline lens). The value d in this formula is the distance from the second principal plane of the first lens (P_C') to the first principal plane of the second lens (P_L). The index of refraction used in the formula is the index of refraction of the substance between the two lenses in the system; this would be the aqueous in the eye. First of all, the distance from $P_c{}'$ to P_L would be:

$$\overline{P_C{}'P_L} = \overline{A_{1C}P_L} - \overline{A_{1C}P_C{}'}$$

$$\overline{P_C{}'P_L} = 5.678 \text{ mm} - (-0.0506 \text{ mm})$$

$$\overline{P_C{}'P_L} = 5.728 \text{ mm}$$

The calculation of the equivalent power of the eye is as follows:

$$F_e = F_1 + F_2 - \left(\frac{d}{n}\right)(F_1)(F_2)$$

$$F_{eeye} = F_{ec} + F_{eL} - \left(\frac{\overline{P_C{}'P_L}}{n}\right)(F_{ec})(F_{eL})$$

$$F_{eeye} = +43.05 \text{ D} + (+19.11 \text{ D})$$

$$- \left(\frac{0.005729 \text{ m}}{1.336}\right)(+43.05 \text{ D}) + (19.11 \text{ D})$$

$$F_{eeye} = +58.64 \text{ D}$$

The formula for the location of the first principal plane, when applied to a complex optical system, yields the distance from the first principal plane of the first lens in the system to the first principal plane of the complete system of two lenses. In the case of the eye, this would be the distance from the first principal plane of the cornea to the first principal plane of the eye. The variable d would be the same as in the preceding equivalent power calculation.

$$\overline{A_1 P} = \frac{(n_1)(d)(F_2)}{(n_2)(F_e)}$$

$$\overline{P_C P_{eye}} = \frac{(n_{air})(\overline{P_C{}'P_L})(F_{eL})}{(n_{aqueous})(F_{eeye})}$$

$$\overline{P_C P_{eye}} = \frac{(1.00)(0.005729 \text{ m})(+19.11 \text{ D})}{(1.336) + (58.64 \text{ D})}$$

$$\overline{P_C P_{eye}} = 1.3974 \text{ mm}$$

The distance from the anterior surface of the cornea to the first principal plane of the eye can then be found as follows:

$$\overline{A_{1C}P_{eye}} = \overline{A_{1C}P_L} + \overline{P_C P_{eye}}$$

$$\overline{A_{1C}P_{eye}} = (1.3974 \text{ mm}) + (-0.0496 \text{ mm})$$

$$\overline{A_{1C}P_{eye}} = 1.3478 \text{ mm}$$

When applied to a two-lens system, the formula for the location of the second principal plane yields the distance from the second principal plane of the second lens to the second principal plane of the complete system. In the case of the eye, this would be the distance from the second principal plane of the crystalline lens to the second principal plane of the eye.

$$\overline{A_2 P'} = -\frac{(n_3)(d)(F_1)}{(n_2)(F_e)}$$

$$\overline{P_L{}'P_{eye}{}'} = -\frac{(n_{vitreous})(\overline{P_C{}'P_L{}'})(F_{ec})}{(n_{aqueous})(F_{eeye})}$$

$$\overline{P_L{}'P_{eye}{}'} = \frac{(1.336)(0.005729 \text{ m}) + (43.05 \text{ D})}{(1.336) + (58.64 \text{ D})}$$

$$\overline{P_L{}'P_{eye}{}'} = -4.206 \text{ mm}$$

The distance from the anterior surface of the cornea to the second principal plane of the eye is 1.602 mm.

$$\overline{A_{1C}P_{eye}{}'} = \overline{A_{1C}P_L{}'} + \overline{P_L{}'P_{eye}{}'}$$

$$= 5.808 \text{ mm} + (-4.206 \text{ mm})$$

$$= 1.602 \text{ mm}$$

The first focal length of the eye can be calculated as follows:

$$f = -\frac{n_1}{F_e}$$

$$f_{eye} = -\frac{n_{air}}{F_{eeye}}$$

$$f_{eye} = \frac{1.00}{+58.64 \text{ D}}$$

$$f_{eye} = -17.05 \text{ mm}$$

The first focal point of the Gullstrand Schematic eye No. 1 is 15.7 mm in front of the anterior surface of the cornea:

$$\overline{A_{1C}F_{eye}} = \overline{A_{1C}P_{eye}} + \overline{P_{eye}F_{eye}{}'}$$

$$\overline{A_{1C}F_{eye}} = \overline{A_{1C}P_{eye}} + f_{eye}$$

$$\overline{A_{1C}F_{eye}} = 1.35 \text{ mm} + (-17.05 \text{ mm})$$

$$\overline{A_{1C}F_{eye}} = -15.70 \text{ mm}$$

The second focal length of the Gullstrand schematic eye No. 1 can be calculated as follows:

$$f' = \frac{n_3}{F_e}$$

$$f_{eye}' = \frac{n_{vitreous}}{F_{eeye}}$$

$$f_{eye}' = \frac{1.336}{+58.64 \text{ D}}$$

$$f_{eye}' = 22.78 \text{ mm}$$

The location of the second focal point of the eye with respect to the anterior surface of the cornea is:

$$\overline{A_{1C}F_{eye}'} = \overline{A_{1C}P_{eye}'} + \overline{P_{eye}'F_{eye}'}$$

$$\overline{A_{1C}F_{eye}'} = \overline{A_{1C}P_{eye}'} + f_{eye}'$$

$$\overline{A_{1C}F_{eye}'} = 1.60 \text{ mm} + (22.78 \text{ mm})$$

$$\overline{A_{1C}F_{eye}'} = 24.38 \text{ mm}$$

The locations of the nodal points can be determined using the relation that the distance from the first focal point to the first nodal point is equal to the second focal length, and the distance from the second focal point to the second nodal point is equal to the first focal length.

$$\overline{F_{eye}N_{eye}} = f_{eye}' = 22.78 \text{ mm}$$

$$\overline{A_{1C}N_{eye}} = \overline{A_{1C}F_{eye}} + \overline{F_{eye}N_{eye}}$$

$$\overline{A_{1C}N_{eye}} = -15.70 \text{ mm} + 22.78 \text{ mm}$$

$$\overline{A_{1C}N_{eye}} = 7.08 \text{ mm}$$

$$\overline{F_{eye}'N_{eye}'} = f_{eye} = -17.05 \text{ mm}$$

$$\overline{A_{1C}N_{eye}'} = \overline{A_{1C}F_{eye}'} + \overline{F_{eye}'N_{eye}'}$$

$$\overline{A_{1C}N_{eye}'} = 24.38 \text{ mm} + (-17.05 \text{ mm})$$

$$\overline{A_{1C}N_{eye}'} = 7.33 \text{ mm}$$

The locations of the principal planes, focal points, and nodal points in the Gullstrand schematic eye No. 1 are given in Figure 3.3. The principal planes are just behind the cornea. The nodal points are close to the posterior surface of the crystalline lens. The first focal point is 15.7 mm in front of the anterior surface of the cornea. The second focal point is 24.38 mm from the anterior surface of the cornea. Because the axial length of the Gullstrand schematic eye No. 1 is 24.0 mm, the second focal point is located 0.38 mm behind the retina.

Because the second focal point is behind the retina, the Gullstrand schematic eye No. 1 is a hyperopic eye. One way to calculate the refractive error of this eye is to compare the vergence of light leaving the second principal plane of the eye after parallel light strikes the eye to the vergence of light that would be necessary leaving the second principal plane in order to have a focused image on the retina. If parallel light strikes the eye, the vergence of light theoretically leaving the second principal plane is equal to the equivalent power of the eye, +58.64 D. An image would then be formed at the second focal point. To find the vergence of light theoretically leaving the second principal plane that would focus on the retina, the distance from second principal plane to the retina must first be known.

$$\overline{A_{1C}R} = \overline{A_{1C}P_{eye}'} + \overline{P_{eye}'R}$$

$$\overline{P_{eye}'R} = \overline{A_{1C}R} - \overline{A_{1C}P_{eye}'}$$

$$\overline{P_{eye}'R} = 24.00 \text{ mm} - 1.60 \text{ mm}$$

$$\overline{P_{eye}'R} = 22.40 \text{ mm}$$

The vergence of light necessary for focus on the retina is equal to the index of refraction in image space (vitreous) divided by the distance from the second principal plane to the retina.

$$L' = \frac{n'}{\ell_1}$$

$$L' = \frac{1.336}{0.0224 \text{ m}}$$

$$L' = +59.64 \text{ D}$$

Because the equivalent power of the eye is +58.64 D, an additional +1.00 D would need to be placed at the principal plane in order to have focus on the retina. Therefore, we can say that the principal plane refractive error of the Gullstrand schematic eye No. 1 is +1.00 D, or 1.00 D of hyperopia.

APPENDIX 3.2

CALCULATION OF VARIABLES IN THE GULLSTRAND-EMSLEY SCHEMATIC EYE

The Gullstrand-Emsley schematic eye has three refracting surfaces. The cornea is a single refracting surface with a radius of curvature of $+7.8$ mm. The index of refraction of the aqueous is 4/3 (see Table 3.2). The power of the cornea is $+42.735$ D:

$$F = \frac{n_2 - n_1}{r}$$

$$F = \frac{1.333 - 1.00}{+0.0078 \text{ m}}$$

$$F = +42.735 \text{ D}$$

The crystalline lens has two refracting surfaces and one index of refraction. The equivalent power of the crystalline lens is:

$$F_{el} = F_{1L} + F_{2L} - \left(\frac{d}{n}\right)(F_{1L})(F_{2L})$$

$$F_{el} = (+8.27 \text{ D}) + (13.778 \text{ D}) - \left(\frac{0.0036 \text{ m}}{1.416}\right)$$
$$(+8.27 \text{ D})(+13.778 \text{ D})$$

$$F_{el} = +21.76 \text{ D}$$

The locations of the principal points of the crystalline lens can then be determined.

$$\overline{A_{1L}P_L} = \frac{(n_1)(d)(F_2)}{(n_2)(F_e)}$$

$$\overline{A_{1L}P_L} = \frac{(1.333)(0.0036 \text{ m}) + (13.778 \text{ D})}{(1.416) + (21.76 \text{ D})}$$

$$\overline{A_{1L}P_L} = 2.147 \text{ mm}$$

The distance of the first principal point of the crystalline lens from the cornea would be:

$$\overline{A_C P_L} = \overline{A_C A_{1L}} + \overline{A_{1L} P_L}$$

$$\overline{A_C P_L} = 3.6 \text{ mm} + 2.147 \text{ mm}$$

$$\overline{A_C P_L} = 5.747 \text{ mm}$$

For the second principal point of the crystalline lens,

$$\overline{A_2 P_L'} = \frac{(n_3)(d)(F_1)}{(n_2)(F_e)}$$

$$\overline{A_2 P_L'} = \frac{(1.333)(0.0036 \text{ m})(+8.27 \text{ D})}{(1.416)(+21.76 \text{ D})}$$

$$\overline{A_2 P_L'} = -1.288 \text{ mm}$$

The distance of the second principal point of the crystalline lens from the cornea would be:

$$\overline{A_C P_L'} = \overline{A_C A_{2L}} + \overline{A_{2L} P_L'}$$

$$\overline{A_C P_L'} = 7.2 \text{ mm} + (-1.288 \text{ mm})$$

$$\overline{A_C P_L'} = 5.912 \text{ mm}$$

The equivalent power of the eye can now be calculated. The value of d in the equivalent power formula is the distance from the second principal point of the cornea to the first principal point of the crystalline lens. Since the cornea is a single refracting surface, the corneal vertex and the corneal principal points are all coincident. Therefore, d is the distance from the cornea to the first principal point of the crystalline lens.

$$F_e = F_1 + F_2 - \left(\frac{d}{n}\right)(F_1)(F_2)$$

$$F_{eeye} = (+42.735 \text{ D}) + (21.76 \text{ D}) - \left(\frac{0.005747 \text{ m}}{1.333}\right)$$
$$(+42.735 \text{ D}) + (21.76 \text{ D})$$

$$F_{eeye} = +60.49 \text{ D}$$

The position of the first principal point of the eye would be 1.55 mm from the cornea:

$$\overline{P_c P_{eye}} = \overline{A_c P_{eye}} = \frac{(n_1)(d)(F_2)}{(n_2)(F_e)}$$

$$\overline{A_c P_{eye}} = \frac{(1.00)(0.005747 \text{ m})(+21.76 \text{ D})}{(1.333)(+60.49 \text{ D})}$$

$$\overline{A_c P_{eye}} = 1.55 \text{ mm}$$

The location of the second principal point of the eye is 1.85 mm from the cornea:

$$\overline{P_L'P_{eye}'} = -\frac{(n_3)(d)(F_1)}{(n_2)(F_e)}$$

$$\overline{P_L'P_{eye}'} = -\frac{(1.333)(0.005747 \text{ mm})(+42.735 \text{ D})}{(1.333)(+60.49 \text{ D})}$$

$$\overline{P_L'P_{eye}'} = -4.06 \text{ mm}$$

$$\overline{A_C P_{eye}'} = \overline{A_C P_L'} + \overline{P_L'P_{eye}'}$$

$$\overline{A_C P_{eye}'} = 5.912 \text{ mm} + (-4.06 \text{ mm})$$

$$\overline{A_C P_{eye}'} = 1.852 \text{ mm}$$

The first focal length of the eye is:

$$f = -\frac{n_{air}}{F_{eeye}}$$

$$f = -\frac{1.00}{+60.49 \text{ D}}$$

$$f = -16.53 \text{ mm}$$

Therefore, the position of the first focal point is:

$$\overline{A_C F_{eye}} = \overline{A_C P_{eye}} + \overline{P_{eye} F_{eye}}$$

$$\overline{A_C F_{eye}} = 1.55 \text{ mm} + (-16.53 \text{ mm})$$

$$\overline{A_C F_{eye}} = -14.98 \text{ mm}$$

The second focal length of the Gullstrand-Emsley schematic eye is:

$$f' = \frac{n_{vitreous}}{F_{eeye}}$$

$$f' = \frac{1.333}{+60.49 \text{ D}}$$

$$f' = +22.04 \text{ mm}$$

The position of the second focal point of the eye is thus:

$$\overline{A_C F_{eye}'} = \overline{A_C P_{eye}'} + \overline{P_{eye}'F_{eye}'}$$

$$\overline{A_C F_{eye}'} = 1.85 \text{ mm} + 22.04 \text{ mm}$$

$$\overline{A_C F_{eye}'} = 23.89 \text{ mm}$$

Since the axial length of the Gullstrand-Emsley schematic eye is 23.89 mm, the second focal point is on the retina and the eye is emmetropic.

The location of the first nodal point of the eye can be found from the following relation:

$$\overline{FN} = \overline{P'F'}$$

The location of the first nodal point is therefore 7.06 mm behind the cornea:

$$\overline{A_C N} = \overline{A_C F} + \overline{FN}$$

$$\overline{A_C N} = \overline{A_C F} + \overline{P'F'}$$

$$\overline{A_C N} = -14.98 \text{ mm} + 22.04 \text{ mm}$$

$$\overline{A_C N} = +7.06 \text{ mm}$$

The location of the second nodal point can be derived using the following relation:

$$\overline{F'N'} = \overline{PF}$$

The second nodal point of the eye is therefore 7.36 mm behind the cornea:

$$\overline{A_C N'} = \overline{A_C F'} + \overline{F'N'}$$

$$\overline{A_C N'} = \overline{A_C F'} + \overline{PF}$$

$$\overline{A_C N'} = -23.89 \text{ mm} + (-16.53 \text{ mm})$$

$$\overline{A_C N'} = +7.36 \text{ mm}$$

APPENDIX 3.3

CALCULATION OF THE LOCATIONS AND MAGNIFICATIONS OF PURKINJE IMAGES I, III, AND IV IN THE GULLSTRAND-EMSLEY SCHEMATIC EYE

Note that this schematic eye would not have a Purkinje image II because it has a single surface cornea.

LOCATION AND MAGNIFICATION OF PURKINJE IMAGE I

The radius of curvature of the cornea in the Gullstrand-Emsley schematic eye is +7.8 mm, so the focal length of the cornea as a mirror is:

$$f = \frac{-r}{2} = \frac{-(0.0078 \text{ m})}{2}$$
$$= -0.0039 \text{ m}$$

The location of Purkinje image I is ℓ', as follows:

$$-\frac{1}{\ell'} = \frac{1}{\ell} + \frac{1}{f}$$
$$-\frac{1}{\ell'} = \frac{1}{-1 \text{ m}} + \frac{1}{-0.0039 \text{ m}}$$
$$\ell' = 0.003884 \text{ m}$$
$$\ell' = 3.88 \text{ mm}$$

Purkinje image I is located 3.88 mm behind the cornea. Its magnification is:

$$M = -\frac{\ell'}{\ell} = \frac{-0.0038848 \text{ m}}{-1 \text{ m}}$$
$$= +0.00388$$

LOCATION AND MAGNIFICATION OF PURKINJE IMAGE III

In the Gullstrand-Emsley schematic eye, Purkinje image III is formed by (1) refraction at the cornea, (2) reflection from the anterior surface of the crystalline lens, and (3) refraction at the cornea. For refraction at the cornea:

$$L_1 = \frac{1}{\ell_1} = \frac{1}{-1 \text{ m}} = -1.00 \text{ D}$$
$$L_1' = L_1 + F = -1.00 + 42.735$$
$$L_1' = +41.735 \text{ D}$$
$$\ell_1' = \frac{1.333}{+41.735 \text{ D}} = +0.03194 \text{ m}$$
$$\ell_1' = 31.94 \text{ mm}$$

The image formed by refraction at the cornea is 31.94 mm behind the cornea. Because the anterior surface of the crystalline lens is 3.6 mm behind the cornea, this image would be 28.34 mm behind the anterior surface of the crystalline lens:

$$\ell_2 = 31.94 \text{ mm} - 3.6 \text{ mm}$$
$$= 28.34 \text{ mm}$$

This (ℓ_2) is the object distance for reflection from the anterior surface of the crystalline lens. The focal length of the anterior surface of the lens is:

$$f = -\frac{r}{2} = \frac{-(+0.01 \text{ m})}{2}$$
$$= -0.005 \text{ m}$$

Therefore, for reflection from the anterior surface of the lens:

$$-\frac{1}{\ell_2'} = \frac{1}{\ell_2} + \frac{1}{f}$$
$$-\frac{1}{\ell_2'} = \frac{1}{+0.02834 \text{ m}} + \frac{1}{-0.005 \text{ m}}$$
$$\ell_2' = +0.00607 \text{ m}$$
$$\ell_2' = +6.07 \text{ mm}$$

The image formed by reflection from the anterior surface of the crystalline lens is 6.08 behind that surface. For the subsequent refraction at the cornea, the object distance is measured from the cornea, requiring the addition of the distance from the anterior lens surface to the cornea. If we "flip" the optical system to retain our convention of light going from left to right, the object distance for refraction at the cornea is:

$$\ell_3 = -6.07 \text{ mm} + (-3.6 \text{ mm})$$
$$= -9.67 \text{ mm}$$

Therefore, for refraction at the cornea:

$$L_3' = L_3 + F$$

$$= \frac{1.333}{-0.00967 \text{ m}} + 42.735 \text{ D}$$

$$L_3' = -95.15 \text{ D}$$

$$\ell_3' = \frac{100}{-95.15 \text{ D}}$$

$$\ell_3' = -0.01051 \text{ m}$$

Purkinje image III is thus 10.51 mm behind the cornea. The magnification of Purkinje image III in the Gullstrand-Emsley schematic eye is:

$$M = \frac{L_1}{L_1'} \times \left(\frac{\ell_2'}{-\ell_2} \right) \times \frac{L_3}{L_3'}$$

$$= \frac{-1.00}{41.735} \times \left(\frac{0.00607}{-0.02834} \right) \times \frac{-137.88}{-95.15}$$

$$= +0.00744$$

LOCATION AND MAGNIFICATION OF PURKINJE IMAGE IV

In the Gullstrand-Emsley schematic eye, Purkinje image IV is formed by (1) refraction at the cornea, (2) refraction at the anterior crystalline lens surface, (3) reflection from the posterior crystalline lens surface, (4) refraction at the anterior lens surface, and (5) refraction at the cornea.

As found above for Purkinje image III, refraction at the cornea will form an image 28.149 mm behind the anterior surface of the crystalline lens; therefore, for refraction at the anterior surface of the lens:

$$\ell_2 = +0.02834 \text{ m}$$

$$L_2' = L_2 + F$$

$$= \frac{1.333}{+0.02834 \text{ m}} + 8.27 \text{ D}$$

$$= +55.32 \text{ D}$$

$$\ell_2' = \frac{1.416}{+55.32 \text{ D}}$$

$$= +0.0256 \text{ m}$$

Refraction at the anterior lens surface forms an image 25.6 mm behind that surface. This image is 22.0 mm from the posterior lens surface, when the thickness of the lens is considered:

$$\ell_3 = 25.6 \text{ mm} - 3.6 \text{ mm}$$

$$= 22.0 \text{ mm}$$

This distance is the object distance for reflection from the posterior surface of the crystalline lens. The focal length of the posterior lens surface as a mirror is:

$$f = -\frac{r}{2} = -\frac{(-0.006 \text{ m})}{2}$$

$$= +0.003 \text{ m}$$

Therefore, for reflection at the posterior lens surface:

$$= -\frac{1}{\ell_3'} = \frac{1}{\ell_3} + \frac{1}{f}$$

$$\frac{1}{\ell_3'} = -\frac{1}{+0.003 \text{ m}} - \frac{1}{+0.022 \text{ m}}$$

$$\ell_3' = -0.00264 \text{ m}$$

The image is formed 2.64 mm in front of the posterior lens surface. This is 0.96 mm behind the anterior lens surface:

$$\ell_4 = 3.6 \text{ mm} - 2.64 \text{ mm}$$

$$= 0.96 \text{ mm}$$

If the optical system is reversed to retain the convention of light traveling from the left to right, the sign of the object distance for refraction at the anterior lens (ℓ_4) surface is reversed; therefore, for refraction at the anterior surface of the crystalline lens:

$$L_4' = L_4 + F$$

$$\frac{1.333}{\ell_4'} = \frac{1.416}{-0.00096 \text{ m}} + 8.27 \text{ D}$$

$$\ell_4' = -0.000909 \text{ m}$$

The image formed by refraction at the anterior lens surface is 0.909 mm behind that surface. It is 4.509 mm behind the cornea:

$$\ell_5 = -3.6 \text{ mm} + (-0.909 \text{ mm})$$

$$= -4.509 \text{ mm}$$

Therefore, for refraction at the cornea:

$$\frac{1}{\ell_5'} = \frac{1.333}{-0.004509 \text{ m}} + 42.735 \text{ D}$$

$$\ell' = -3.95 \text{ m}$$

Purkinje image IV for the Gullstrand-Emsley schematic eye is 3.95 mm behind the cornea. Its magnification is:

$$M = \frac{L_1}{L_1'} \times \frac{L_2}{L_2'} \times -\frac{\ell_5'}{\ell_3} \times \frac{L_4}{L_4'} \times \frac{L_5}{L_5'}$$

$$= \frac{-1.00}{41.735} \times \frac{47.05}{55.32} \times \frac{-0.00264}{0.0022}$$

$$\times \frac{-1475.00}{-1466.73} \times \frac{-295.70}{-252.97}$$

$$= -0.00287$$

REFERENCES

1. Thibos LN, Bradley A. Modeling the refractive and neurosensory systems of the eye. In: Mouroulis P, ed. *Visual Information: Optical Design and Engineering Principles.* New York: McGraw-Hill, 1999;101–159.
2. Gullstrand A. The optical system of the eye. In: Southall JPC, trans-ed. *Helmhotz's Treatise on Physiological Optics, 1.* 3rd ed. New York: Dover, original German ed. 1909, English trans. 1924, reprinted 1962;350–358.
3. Emsley HH. *Visual Optics, 1: Optics of Vision.* 5th ed. London: Butterworth-Heinemann, 1953;343–348.
4. Bennett AG, Rabbetts RB. *Clinical Visual Optics.* 2nd ed. London: Butterworth-Heinemann, 1989;252–255.
5. Thibos LN, Ye M, Zhang X, Bradley A. Spherical aberration of the reduced schematic eye with elliptical refracting surface. *Optom Vis Sci.* 1997;74:548–556.
6. Smith G, Pierscionek BK. The optical structure of the lens and its contribution to the refractive status of the eye. *Ophthal Physiol Opt.* 1998;18:21–29.
7. Bennett AG, Rabbetts RB. *Clinical Visual Optics.* 3rd ed. London: Butterworth-Heinemann, 1998;220–221.
8. Duke-Elder S, Abrams D. *System of Ophthalmology, 5: Ophthalmic Optics and Refraction.* Duke-Elder S, ed. St. Louis: Mosby, 1970;96–97.
9. Atchison DA. Visual optics in man. *Aust J Optom.* 1984;67:141–150.
10. Thibos LN, Bradley A, Zhang X. Effect of ocular chromatic aberration on monocular visual performance. *Optom Vis Sci.* 1991;68:599–607.
11. Millodot M. The influence of age on the chromatic aberration of the eye. *Albrecht v. Graefe's Arch Clin Exper Ophthalmol.* 1976;198:235–243.
12. Fry GA. The optical performance of the human eye. In: E Wolf, ed. *Progress in Optics, 8.* London: North-Holland, 1970;51–131.
13. Walsh G, Charman WN. Measurement of the axial wavefront aberration in the human eye. *Ophthal Physiol Opt.* 1985;5:23–31.
14. Leibowitz H. The effect of pupil size on visual acuity for photometrically equated test field at various levels of luminance. *J Opt Soc Am.* 1952;42:416–422.
15. Millodot M. Effect of the aberrations of the eye on visual perception. In: JC Armington, J Krauskopf, BR Wooten, eds. *Visual Psychophysics and Physiology.* New York: Academic, 1978;441–452.
16 Charman WN. Limits on visual acuity performance set by the eye's optics and the retinal cone mosaic. In: JJ Kulikowski, V Walsh, IJ Murray, eds. *Limits of Vision.* Vol. 5 of J Cronly-Dillon, ed. *Vision and Visual Dysfunction.* Boca Raton: CRC Press, 1991;81–96.

FURTHER READING

Atchison DA. Visual optics in man. *Aust J Optom.* 1984;67:141–150.
Freeman MH. *Optics.* 10th ed. Boston: Butterworth-Heinemann, 1990.
Smith G, Atchison DA. *The Eye and Visual Optical Instruments.* Cambridge: Cambridge University Press, 1997.
Walker BH. *Optical Engineering Fundamentals.* New York: McGraw-Hill, 1995;235–256.

Chapter 4
The Retinal Image

Thus vision is brought about by a picture of the thing seen being formed on the concave surface of the retina. That which is to the right outside is depicted on the left on the retina, that to the left on the right, that above below, and that below above. . . . The greater the acuity of vision of a given person, the finer will be the picture formed in his eye. —Johannes Kepler, 1604 (From Wade NJ. *A Natural History of Vision.* Cambridge, MA: MIT Press, 1998;9.)

If an optician should try to sell me an instrument possessing the faults mentioned above [of the eye], it seems to me without overstressing the matter that I should think myself wholly justified in using the most severe language with regard to the carelessness of his work and returning the instrument under protest. With regard to my eyes, however, I shall do no such thing but, on the contrary, I shall be glad to keep them as long as possible notwithstanding their shortcomings. . . . —Hermann von Helmholtz, 1903 (From Duke-Elder S, Abrams D. In: S Duke-Elder, ed. *System of Ophthalmology, 5. Ophthalmic Optics and Refraction.* St. Louis: Mosby, 1970;125.)

Chapter 3 introduced the basic optics of the eye, including surface powers, axes, and aberrations. In this chapter we use these concepts to examine the retinal image including its size, its illumination, and its quality. Finally, we cover the subject of entoptic images.

RETINAL IMAGE SIZE

The human eye has a relatively high dioptric power, so that for objects at any reasonable distance in front of the eye, the retinal image is inverted and tremendously minified. Our greatest interest is to determine the size and quality of the image formed on the *fovea* and the surrounding *macula*, the posterior area of the retina used to examine fine detail. Because this area is small relative to the curvature of the retina, it can be considered to approximate a flat surface. Given this qualification, the methods given in Chapter 1 to determine image size can be applied.

In any optical system, an object ray directed toward the first nodal point (N_1) at an angle θ degrees with the optical axis will enter image space as though coming from the second nodal point (N_2) at an equal angle θ with the optical axis. In the eye this nodal ray allows us to calculate both linear and angular image size (Figure 4.1.)

Note from Chapter 3 that N_1 and N_2 in the Gullstrand and the Gullstrand-Emsley schematic eyes are located near the posterior surface of the crystalline lens and are separated from each other by only about 0.25 mm. In the Emsley single surface eye, N_1 and N_2 combine into just one nodal point (N), which is located at the center of curvature of the cornea, and is separated from the retina by about the same distance as N_2 is in the other two

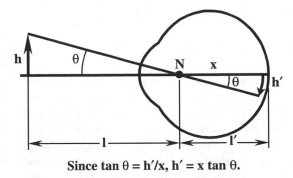

Since tan θ = h′/x, h′ = x tan θ.

Figure 4.1. The two nodal points in the eye are located near the posterior surface of the lens. These points are so close together that for an approximation a straight ray may be traced from an object point through the average nodal point to find the corresponding image point.

schematic eyes. Therefore, the Emsley reduced eye can be used to simplify calculations of retinal image size, at least in the central field, without introducing much error. An examination of Figure 4.1 shows by similar triangles that:

$$h/\ell = h'/\ell' \text{ and } h' = h(\ell'/\ell)$$

Example: A 20/20 letter 6 meters from a patient would be 8.73 mm tall. What is the image height of this letter on the patient's retina? If the object of height $h = 8.73$ mm is –6000 mm from the cornea, its distance from N is $\ell = -6005.55$ mm, and the distance from N to the retinal image is $\ell' = 22.22 - 5.55$ mm $= +16.67$ mm (neglecting a small shift in N due to 1/6 D of accommodation). Then, $h' = h(\ell'/\ell) = (8.73$ mm$)(16.67/-6005.55) = -0.024$ mm. The minus sign indicates that the image is inverted.

Object sizes are often given as the angle θ that the object makes with the nodal point N_1. The retinal image then makes the same angle θ with N_2. An examination of Figure 4.1 shows that:

$$\tan \theta = h'/x$$

so

$$h' = x \tan \theta$$

Example: A 20/20 letter subtends an overall angle of $\theta = 5$ minutes of arc (= 0.0833 degrees) as viewed by a patient. Then, $h' = -x \tan \theta = (16.67$ mm$)(\tan - 0.0833°) = -0.024$ mm (in agreement with the previous example).

RETINAL ILLUMINATION

Transmittance of the Eye

The fraction of the light incident on the cornea that the eye transmits to the retina varies with wavelength. As mentioned in Chapter 3, UV-C and UV-B are absorbed by the cornea, whereas UV-A is largely absorbed by the lens. UV radiation would be able to stimulate the photoreceptor cells and become part of the visible spectrum if it were not absorbed. Indeed, in the days before artificial lenses were used to replace a surgically removed crystalline lens, such patients could see by UV-A radiation. Different wavelengths in the IR spectrum

are variably transmitted to the retina but the photons are not energetic enough to cause the changes in the photoreceptor cell pigments necessary for visual sensation. Visible light is, of course, transmitted to the retina, although a surprisingly large part of it, especially the shorter wavelengths, is still absorbed and scattered by the ocular media. Figure 4.2 shows light transmission (T) through the young eye for various wavelengths in the visible spectrum. Surprisingly, T reaches a maximum of only 0.7 at the red end of the spectrum and falls off to as little as 0.1 at the violet end. As the eye ages, an even greater percentage of the visible light is absorbed, especially at the blue end of the spectrum, and an increase in scatter further prevents light from forming a useful image.[1]

Stops and the Eye

Although simple raytracing can be used to find the boundaries of a retinal image, it reveals little about the amount of light falling onto the image (its *illuminance*). In most optical systems, uniformly luminous extended objects do not produce a uniformly illuminated image. For most systems, the part of the image that is closest to the optical axis receives the greatest illumination and there is a progressive reduction in illumination for parts farther from the axis. At some distance off-axis, the illumination becomes low enough that we define this to be the edge of the "useful" field of view (e.g., when the illumination is half that of the axial illumination).

In order to analyze image illumination, it is necessary to review the concepts about stops introduced in Chapter 1. That chapter notes that one element in a system (either a lens or powerless aperture), called the aperture stop (AS), limits the bundle of rays from an axial object point that can pass unobstructed to the corresponding axial image point. Thus, the AS determines the illumination of the axial image point. If there are two or more elements, one of the other elements, called the field stop (FS), in combination with the AS, limits the bundles of rays from off-axis object points that can pass unobstructed to their corresponding off-axis image points. Thus, the FS determines the useful field of view.

The optical elements in the eye that can be the AS are the cornea, the anatomical pupil, and the

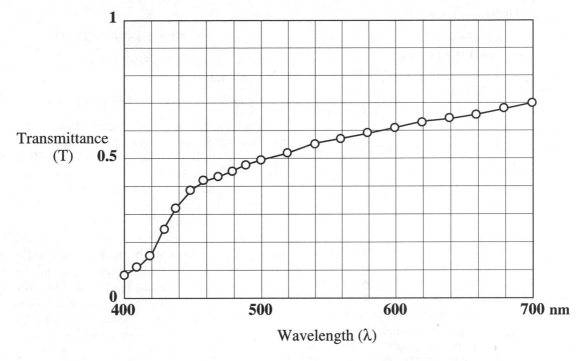

Figure 4.2. Percent transmittance of light through young eyes for wavelengths in the visible spectrum. (Modified from LeGrand Y. *Light, Colour and Vision.* New York: Wiley, 1957;89.)

lens. If we look into the eye from the intended axial object point, an image of each optical element is formed by all of the refractive elements in front of it. The *image* that appears angularly smallest as viewed from the axial object point is the entrance pupil (EP), and the *element* whose image it is, is the AS. In the eye the image that appears to be smallest is the pupil. Thus, the EP is the clinically measured pupil as viewed through the cornea, and the AS is the anatomical pupil. The EP identifies the boundaries of the cone of rays in

object space that will be included in the retinal image point.

Example: Find the location and size of the EP of the Gullstrand-Emsley schematic eye. The AS is the anatomical pupil so the EP would be the anatomical pupil as imaged by the cornea in front of it. Light now comes out of the eye from the pupil to you as an observer. In order to follow the convention of light traveling from left to right, the eye is drawn reversed in Figure 4.3.

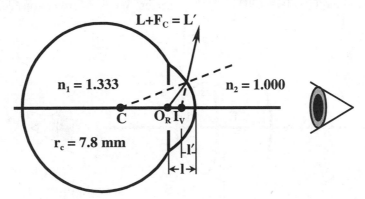

Figure 4.3. A Gauss raytrace to locate the entrance pupil for the eye.

For the Gullstrand-Emsley Eye:

$r_c = +7.80$ mm, $n_{aq} = 1.333$, ℓ (distance of iris from cornea) $= -3.6$ mm

$F_C = (n_2 - n_1)/r = (1.000 - 1.333)/-7.8$ mm
$(1000) = +42.73$ D

$\ell = -3.6$ mm, $L = n_1/\ell = (1.333/-3.6)(1000)$
$= -370.37$ D

$L + F_C = L' = -370.37 + (+42.37)$
$= -327.64$ D

$\ell' = n_2/L' = (1.000/-327.64)(1000)$
$= -3.05$ mm

$m = L/L' = -370.37/-327.64 = +1.13x$

Thus, the image of the pupil as seen from outside the eye is -3.05 mm behind the cornea (about 0.5 mm closer than the anatomical pupil), erect, and 13% larger than the anatomical pupil.

The image of the anatomical pupil (AS) as viewed from the image side through all of the elements behind it (i.e., the surfaces of the crystalline lens) is the exit pupil (XP). The XP identifies the boundaries of the cone of rays that will leave the posterior surface of the crystalline lens to make up the retinal image.

Example: Find the location and size of the XP of the Gullstrand-Emsley schematic eye. Since the AS (anatomical pupil) sits on the anterior lens surface, the anterior lens surface has no effect on the placement of the XP and only the posterior lens surface ($F_{2L} = +13.78$ D) needs to be considered (Figure 4.4).

ℓ (lens thickness) $= -3.6$ mm

$L = n_L/\ell = (1.416/-3.6)(1000) = -393.33$ D

$L + F_{2L} = L'$
$-393.33 + (+13.78) = -379.55$ D $= L'$

$\ell' = n_v/L' = (1.333/-379.55)(1000)$
$= -3.51$ mm $= \ell'$

$m = L/L' = -393.33/-379.55 = +1.036x$

Therefore, the XP is 3.51 mm in front of the posterior surface of the lens (or 0.09 mm behind the anterior surface of the lens) and the XP is approximately 3% larger than the anatomical pupil. We can use the anatomical pupil as the XP by approximation because there is very little difference in location or size.

The boundary of the cone of light from an axial object point that can make it through the eye to the corresponding retinal image point is found by drawing rays from the axial object point toward the cornea in the direction of the edge of the EP. Then at the cornea the rays are refracted toward the edge of the AS. And finally, after refraction by the lens, the rays leave the posterior lens surface coming from the direction of the XP (Figure 4.5).

The field stop (FS) is the element that when viewed through the front of the system forms the image that makes the smallest angle with respect to the center of the EP. This angle (ω) subtends half of the field of view. Figure 4.6 shows this for the eye.

Inspection of Figure 4.6 shows that rays from increasingly off-axis object points are able to pass through the center of the anatomical pupil until the rays directed toward the center of the EP become limited by the edge of the cornea. Since the edge of the cornea is behind the EP, when a ray enters the cornea in the direction of the center of the EP, that side of the field of view can be greater than 90 degrees! Without further consideration, this would

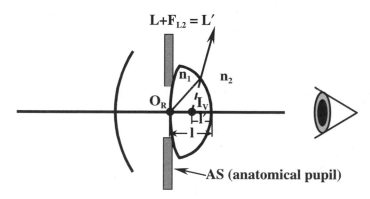

Figure 4.4. A Gauss raytrace to locate the exit pupil for the eye.

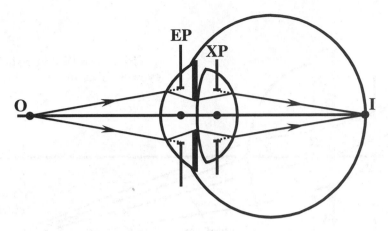

Figure 4.5. The limits of the bundle of rays from an on-axis object point that contribute to the corresponding on-axis retinal image point.

make the cornea the FS for the eye. However, the peripheral retina stops short of the corneal limit of the field of view and thus the retina becomes a *functional* field stop in the same way that the film frame in a camera limits the camera's field of view. For this reason, the retina is usually regarded as being *the* field stop for the eye. An example of this functional limit is a lack of viable retina in the extreme nasal field of view. Apparently, nature is conservative in not maintaining retina at a location where the only view would be that of the nose.

In Figure 4.7, if the eye is focused on the tip of the object arrow, then a bundle of rays from that object will reach the corresponding image point on the retina. Of all of the possible rays in that bundle, two are especially useful:

1. *Nodal ray:* By definition, the nodal ray is directed from the off-axis object point toward the first nodal point. After all refractions, it will exit the last refractive surface from the direction of the second nodal point in a direction that is parallel to the entering nodal ray. The nodal points in the human eye are located near the posterior surface of the crystalline lens. Because they are separated by only about 0.25 mm, they are drawn in Figure 4.7 as one point (*N*). This ray is then essentially undeviated and, thus, is the most convenient ray to trace.

2. *Chief ray:* By definition, the chief ray is directed from the off-axis object point toward the center of the EP. After refraction, it will physically pass through the center of the AS (the anatomical

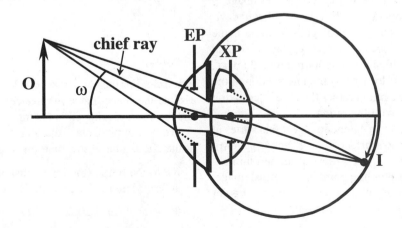

Figure 4.6. The limits of the bundle of rays from an off-axis object point that contribute to the corresponding off-axis image point.

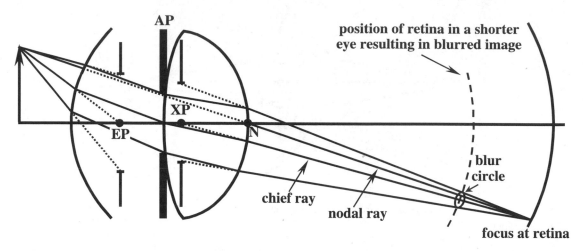

Figure 4.7. When the retinal image is in focus either the chief ray or the nodal ray can be traced to find an image point. However, when the retinal image is not in focus only the chief ray strikes the retina at the center of the blur circle.

pupil), and then emerge from the lens as though it came from the center of the XP. Although the chief ray is more difficult to trace, it is very useful because it locates the centers of the blur circle profiles when the image plane intersects the cone of image rays at various distances along the optical axis.

Figure 4.7 shows that the nodal ray and the chief ray will meet at the retina only if the image point is in focus at the retina. Since the chief ray remains in the center of the cone of light going through an optical system, it will also go through the center of any blur circle. Thus, it will define the location of an image point on the retina even if the image is blurred. The nodal ray, on the other hand, will deviate from the center of the image blur circle if the image is not in focus. For this reason, in finding the size or magnification of a blurred retinal image, the image point is located by the intersection of the chief ray with the retina rather than the intersection of the nodal ray with the retina.

If the eye views an extended object that varies in brightness over its surface (i.e., it has a pattern), each point on the object will result in an illumination of the corresponding point in the retinal image. The illumination E_0 at the axial retinal image point can be determined by the equation[2]:

$$E_0 = B\pi \sin^2\theta' \, (n_i/n_o)$$

where B = luminance ("brightness") of the part of the extended object being imaged. (If B is in candelas/m^2, E is in lumens/m^2),

θ' is the angle subtended by the radius of the XP at the image point,

where

$$\theta' = \tan^{-1}\left(\frac{D_{XP}/2}{\ell_{XP}}\right)$$

n_o = the index of the medium the object is in.

n_i = the index of the medium the image is in.

ℓ_{XP}' = the distance between the XP and the retina

Example: For the Gullstrand-Emsley schematic eye, assume the object has a luminance $B = 100$ *cd/m²* and the anatomical pupil is 6.0 mm in diameter.

We will approximate the location and diameter of the XP as that of the anatomical pupil.

XP to the retina (the image distance from the anterior lens) is 20.29 mm. Then,

$\theta' = \tan^{-1} (6/2)/20.29 = 8.41°$, and

$E = (100)(3.14)(\sin^2 8.41°) = 6.72$ lm/m²

The meaning of the preceding equation can be understood in terms of a photometric principle. The XP when viewed from the image plane appears to have the same luminance (less absorption) as the corresponding area of the object it is imaging. Then, $E = B\pi \sin^2\theta$, where E is the illumination of the image plane (e.g., lumens per square meter) and B is the luminance of the object (e.g., [lumens per steradian] per square meter). The term $\pi \sin^2\theta$ is the steradians (solid angle) into which the light is projected. Thus, the illuminance at the image plane can be treated as though the XP were a luminous disk of object luminance B. Looking out of the eye from a part of an extended retinal image, the XP would have the same luminance as the corresponding part of the extended object. This luminance would change over the separate areas that make up the variable illumination of the object pattern.

The astute reader may note that the transmittance (T) does not appear in the preceding equation. This is because the photometric unit of luminance (B) incorporates spectral transmittance and spectral sensitivity of the eye. If we were to apply this equation to a nonocular system, the luminance would be replaced by radiance, which is a purely physical term, and transmittance (T) would then have to be included.

This equation is an approximation. The XP is large compared to its distance from the retina, yet it treats all parts of the XP as being the same distance from the retinal point in question. Also, it neglects the Stiles-Crawford effect in which light going through the peripheral pupil is less effective in stimulating the cone receptors than light going through an equal area of the central pupil.

Once the relative illumination on axis is found, the following equation gives the relative illumination at an angle ϕ off-axis as measured from the center of the XP[2] (Figure 4.8).

$$E_\phi = E_0\left(\frac{d_0}{d_\phi}\right)\cos\phi\cos\omega$$

where, ϕ is the angle between the optical axis and the line from the center of the XP, which intersects the retina at the location where E is being evaluated, ω is the angle of incidence on the retinal location for E_ϕ of a line from the center of the exit pupil, and, d_0 and d_ϕ are the lengths of the lines from the center of the XP to the retinal surface at 0 and ϕ degrees, respectively.

It may seem intuitive that the retinal illumination should drop off for images farther off-axis due to the elliptical foreshortening of the pupil for peripheral objects. However, the drop-off is not as great as might be expected. The curvature of the retina shortens the peripheral paths so that the inverse square law predicts a brighter image. Also, the curved retina allows the retinal surface to remain more nearly perpendicular to the oncoming light than otherwise so that the surface itself does not appear excessively foreshortened to the oncoming light and more light is captured per surface area. The net effect is that there is very little drop-off of retinal illumination with increase in degrees off-axis. By contrast, the illumination of flat film by a single thin camera lens falls off by $\cos^4\theta$ so that at 60° the illumination is only 0.0625 times the central illumination.

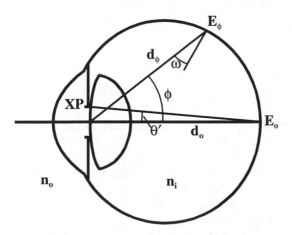

Figure 4.8. Diagram showing the meaning of the symbols used in the equation to determine retinal illumination.

RETINAL IMAGE QUALITY

Point Spread and Line Spread Functions

Because of optical limitations, point objects are not imaged as points on the image plane, but are spread out over an area. The graph of the illuminance across this image is called a *point spread function* (Figure 4.9). Similarly, a thin line object will form an image that has its width spread out over the image plane. A graph of the illuminance of a line image across its width is referred to as a *line spread function*.

Several factors are responsible for the width of the point or line spread function:

1. *Focus:* An out-of-focus image increases the width of the spread function.
2. *Aberrations:* Aberrations spread image light beyond the boundaries of its geometrically determined size even if the image is examined at its best focus. If the eye had a true optical axis and the fovea were on it, only the *axial* aberrations (i.e., chromatic aberration and spherical aberration) would affect the image at the fovea. However, the fovea on average is 5 degrees temporal to the "optical axis" and the refractive surfaces of eye include tilts and decentrations. Therefore, there is no true optical axis and coma may also degrade foveal images.
3. *Diffraction:* Due to the wave nature of light and to the limited size of the pupil (EP), diffraction spreads light from a point object into an extended pattern at the image plane.

When there are no aberrations and focus is perfect, the point spread function becomes a pure diffraction pattern in which light is concentrated in a central *Airy disk* surrounded by progressively fainter rings (Figure 4.10). When the central disk is produced by a distant point object, the Airy disk contains 84% of the light energy present in the entire pattern. The size of the Airy disk can be specified by its angular radius θ_A.

$$\theta_A = 1.22(\lambda/a)$$

where θ_A is the *radius* of the Airy disk in *radians*, λ equals the wavelength of light in the image, and *a* equals the entrance pupil (EP) diameter (diameter of the clinically measured pupil).

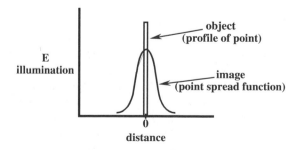

Figure 4.9. The illumination profile for a geometrically projected "point" image is actually spread out into a wider area as a point spread function.

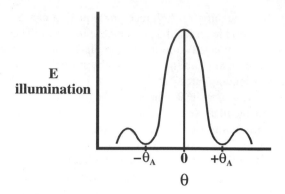

Figure 4.10. The illumination profile for a diffraction limited system is a diffraction pattern whose center is the Airy disk between $-\theta_A$ and $+\theta_A$.

In a *diffraction-limited system* (one whose spread function is due only to diffraction), the smaller the Airy disk is, the closer two image points can approach each other and still be recognizable as two separate points. Rayleigh considered that the closest that two image points could be and still be resolved as two separate points is the radius of the Airy disk (θ_A). In this case, the two Airy disks would overlap by an amount equal to their radii, so the edge of each disk would overlap to the center of the other. This rule is referred to as *Rayleigh's criterion*.

Example: For a 2.5-mm diameter EP and 555-nm light:

$\theta_{radians} = 1.22(0.000555$ mm$)/(2.5$ mm$)$
$= 0.000271$ radians $= 0.93$ min arc
(about 1 min arc, which is equivalent to 20/20 VA)

Figure 4.11 graphically shows how under one set of experimental conditions, pupil diameter relates to visual acuity.[3] For a 2.0- to 3.0-mm diameter pupil, diffraction effects contribute about as much to the spread function as spherical aberration does. Below about 1.5 mm, diffraction effects contribute much more to the spread function than spherical aberration does, so that for smaller pupils the spread function enlarges as a result of diffraction and follows Rayleigh's criterion. Visual acuity remains relatively constant for pupil diameters up to about 4.0 mm, after which the effect of spherical aberration increases to the point where visual acuity decreases again. (Such data are complicated by

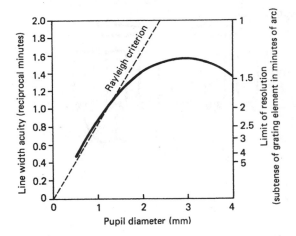

Figure 4.11. Resolving power of the eye on average is maximal for a 2.5-mm pupil. Smaller pupils do worse due to diffraction and larger pupils do worse due to increasing spherical aberration. (Reprinted with permission from Bennett AG, Rabbetts RB. *Clinical Visual Optics*. 2nd ed. London: Butterworth-Heinemann, 1989;28.)

the fact that smaller pupils produce fainter retinal images, which in itself can result in lower acuity.)

Anatomical Limits to the Resolving Power of the Eye

Even if the optical system of the eye could project a perfect image onto the retina, there are physiological limitations to how fine the retinal image detail can be and still be detected by the nervous system. Two main types of photoreceptor cells form a mosaic on the retina, the *cones* and the *rods*.

There are about six million cone cells in the retina. They are active in *photopic* (light-adapted) conditions and are capable of detecting color and fine image detail. The cone cells have their greatest concentration in the macula, and this concentration is especially great in the *fovea* at the center of the macula. This exceptional concentration of cones makes the fovea the part of the retina that is most capable of processing fine detail in the retinal image.

In the central fovea, each cone has a pathway to the visual cortex that is not shared by other cones. Since the centers of adjacent cone outer segments are about 2 μm apart, the least distance between two spots that could be separated and still be seen as two spots is about 4 μm (since two cones would be stimulated with one unstimulated cone between

them). Since 1 arc min (20/20) corresponds to about 5 μm, the angular separation of the two spots separated by 4 μm would correspond to about 0.8 min arc, which is close to 20/15 (which is considered good acuity for humans) (Figure 4.12). The fact that the image detail supplied by the optics of the eye and the retinal "grain" is about equal may be due to a conservatism on nature's part to not maintain a system's capability beyond what is necessary. Farther from the fovea the density of the cones decreases, as does photopic visual acuity.

There are about 120 million rod cells in the retina, so rods far outnumber cones. Rods are active under *scotopic* (dark-adapted) conditions and are capable of detecting dim stimuli, but do not detect color and fine detail. Rods are absent in the fovea but their density is greater than that of the cones even in the surrounding cone-rich macula, and their density increases up to about 10 to 20 degrees from the fovea where scotopic visual acuity is greatest. However, even though rods outnumber cones in the periphery, photopic visual acuity is always better than scotopic visual acuity because rods summate their signals onto ganglion cells so that sensitivity is gained by the sacrifice of acuity (Figure 4.13). The falloff of photopic visual acuity is shown on the graph in Figure 4.14.[4]

There is a close match between optical and anatomical limits to resolving power. However, in the young eye the foveal retina can discriminate finer detail than the optics supply. Also in the periphery, if oblique astigmatism is corrected, somewhat better acuity can usually be obtained.

Standard Visual Acuity

Standard visual acuity has several names—minimum resolvable, minimum separable, or minimum angle of resolution (MAR). It is generally 0.5 min to 1.0 min arc. There are other types of visual acuity not covered here, such as stereoacuity and vernier acuity.

As a subjective test, patterns are reduced in size until they can no longer be identified. This is not purely a test of resolving power since it requires pattern recognition and can be affected by intelligence, education, motivation, cortical disease, and so on even when MAR is otherwise normal. For example, an illiterate patient may not be able to read a Snellen chart even if there is a clear image on his retina.

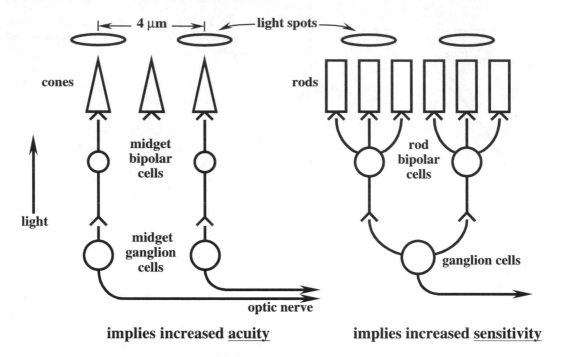

Figure 4.12. Schematic diagrams of cone and rod circuits in the retina. Private channels (cones) favor acuity and converging channels (rods) favor sensitivity.

1. *Snellen acuity (minimum legible acuity):* Standardized letters that are shown to patients have an overall size that is five times that of the individual line width used to construct the letters. Figure 4.15 shows this for the Snellen E.

   The Snellen fraction is the distance in feet the letter is from the patient over the distance in feet at which the letter subtends 5 min overall (finest detail is 1 min) (e.g., 20/40). In the metric system distances are measured in meters so 20/20 = 6/6, 20/40 = 6/12, and so on since 20 feet is approximately 6 meters. Decimal visual acuity

(or relative VA) is obtained by dividing through the Snellen fraction, for example, 20/20 = 1.0, 20/200 = 0.1, and so on.

The overall size of a 20/20 letter is 8.87 mm though it is easier and more accurate to measure a 20/200 letter, which is 88.7 mm or 8.87 cm. (This is based on a chart distance of 20 feet. It is 8.73 cm when based on a chart distance of 6 meters since 20 feet actually equals 6.096 meters.) To obtain the letter size for a shorter lane, change the letter size (y) in proportion to the change in distance.

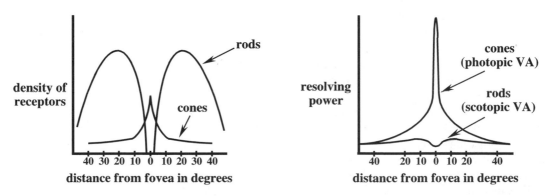

Figure 4.13. Resolving power of the eye from fovea to periphery roughly follows the density of the retinal receptors. It is maximal centrally for cones but about 20 degrees peripherally for rods.

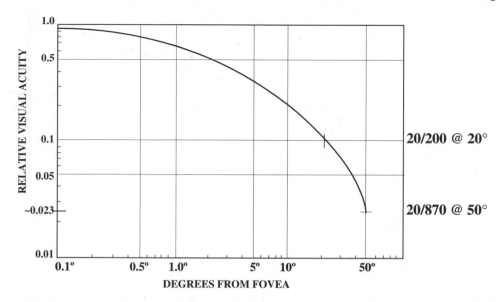

Figure 4.14. Graph of relative visual acuity versus field eccentricity. (Reprinted with permission from Smith WJ. *Modern Optical Engineering: The Design of Optical Systems.* 2nd ed. New York: McGraw-Hill, 1990:123.)

Example: At 15 ft, $y/15$ ft $= 8.87$ mm/20 ft, a 20/20 letter is 6.65 mm overall. Or, you could use $y = x \tan(5/60)°$, but if x is in feet you would then have to convert y from feet to millimeters (Figure 4.16).

In a 15-foot lane 20/20 VA would be recorded more accurately as 15/15 or a 20/400 letter as 15/300, but this is almost never done because the angular size is identical and the only difference is the slightly greater amount of accommodation that is required by the nearer chart. However, for very short viewing distances the numerator *is* changed.

Example: If a low-vision patient walks up to within 5 feet of a chart to read the 20/400 letter:

a. In a 20-foot lane, this is recorded as 5/400.
b. In a 15-foot lane, this is recorded as 5/(400 × (15/20)) = 5/300. (This latter calculation can be avoided by using handheld charts of 20-foot letters that are brought to the patient.

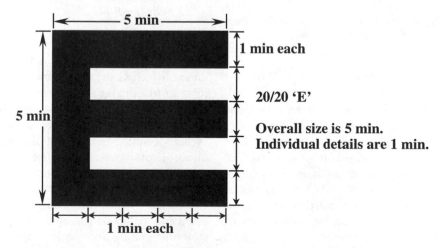

Figure 4.15. A standard Snellen letter is laid out on a square grid so that the line and spacing width are equal. For a 20/20 letter, the finest detail is 1 min arc and the overall size is 5 min arc.

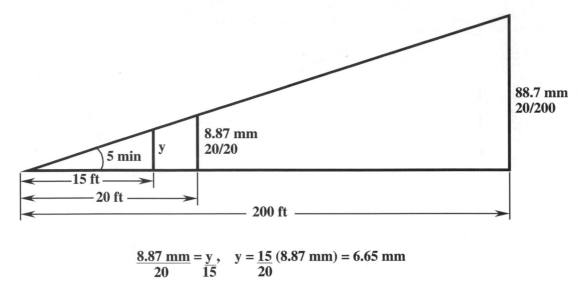

$$\frac{8.87 \text{ mm}}{20} = \frac{y}{15}, \quad y = \frac{15}{20}(8.87 \text{ mm}) = 6.65 \text{ mm}$$

Figure 4.16. Similar triangles can be used to determine the linear size of a Snellen letter when the distance is changed but the angular subtense is constant.

2. *Illiterate E (or tumbling E):* The patient determines the orientation of the prongs of an *E,* which are oriented up, down, left, or right.
3. *Landolt C:* The patient determines orientation of the break in what is essentially a rotated Snellen C. The Broken Wheel Test is a modification of this test for use with children. The child is asked which silhouetted cars in a sequence have gaps in their tires.
4. *Grating:* A grating is a series of light and dark bars whose luminance varies as a square wave, or more typically as a sine wave. The bar spacing is reduced until the observer can no longer detect the pattern. Gratings allow the direct use of the modulation transfer function.

Modulation Transfer Function

Resolving power for optical instruments or visual acuity for the visual system is only one way to assess the performance of an optical system. Another method is to assess the loss in contrast between object and image (as the ratio of image contrast to object contrast). When this is plotted against a range of detail, it is called the *modulation transfer function (MTF)* for the optical system. (The phase of the contrast may also change, in which case it is called the optical transfer function, but this is unimportant for the present discussion.)

The MTF is obtained by using gratings of various bar widths as targets to test optical systems. The bar spacing is usually described in terms of *spatial frequency*, the number of cycles ("line" pairs) per millimeter or degree. A line pair (one cycle) consists of one light and one dark line. Note that a higher spatial frequency implies greater detail.

The contrast of the gratings (called modulation in optical terms) is defined as (Figure 4.17):

$$M = \frac{B_{max} - B_{min}}{B_{max} + B_{min}}$$

This is the Michelson definition of contrast and it should be noted that it differs from Weber's definition, which is more common in psychophysics [$C = \Delta B/B$, or in the above terms $C = (B_{max} - B_{min})/B_{min}$]. Michelson's contrast is used for repetitive spatial changes in luminance such as gratings. Weber's contrast is used for differences in luminance across borders of isolated objects such as visual field targets.

Figure 4.18 shows that even in an aberration-free optical system, diffraction effects produce an inevitable reduction in contrast. Note that the closer the grating line spacing approaches the size of the diffraction pattern's spread function, the lower the contrast becomes.[4]

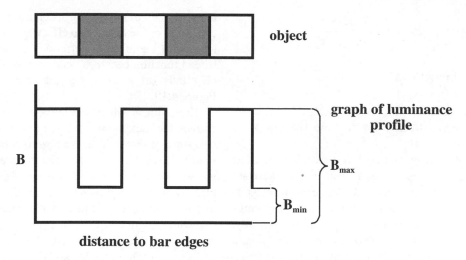

Figure 4.17. A square wave grating and its corresponding luminance profile.

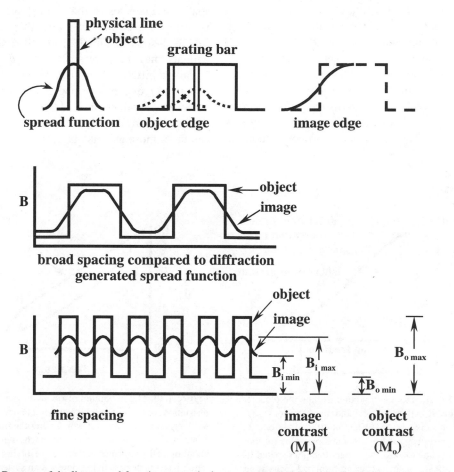

Figure 4.18. Because of the line spread function, an optical system spreads the image of a square wave grating so that light from the bright bars blurs into the dark bars. If the spread function is wide enough compared to the bar spacing, this causes a decrease in the image contrast of the grating.

$$B_i = \text{image } B, \quad M_i = \frac{B_{i(max)} - B_{i(min)}}{B_{i(max)} + B_{i(min)}}$$

$$B_o = \text{image } B, \quad M_o = \frac{B_{o(max)} - B_{o(min)}}{B_{o(max)} + B_{o(min)}}$$

Also note that with broad spacing M_i is approximately equal to M_o, but for fine spacing M_i is much less than M_o.

A grating may have its luminance distributed as a sine wave rather than as a square wave. These are referred to as sine wave gratings. Sine wave gratings have an advantage over square wave gratings in that they are easier to analyze mathematically. No matter what the shape of the spread function, a sine wave object grating is always imaged as a sine wave grating having the same frequency (but a different contrast). Sine wave gratings are usually used in preference to square wave grating in vision research and clinical practice.

The modulation transfer function is a plot of the reduction in modulation (contrast) (M_i/M_o) when going from object to image, against a range of grating spacings (spatial frequency) in line pairs per degree or millimeter. For a diffraction-limited (aberration-free) optical system, the spread function is relatively small since it is due only to the effects of diffraction. Thus, modulation is decreased in the image mainly as the grating spacing approaches the small size of the diffraction effects. For optical systems with significant aberrations or defocus, the spread function becomes wider and image contrast (M_i) falls off more sharply, as for example in Figure 4.19.

The point at which the curve meets the x-axis defines the maximum resolving power of the system since at that point there is zero contrast in the image. This is basically the point that we find when we assess the best resolving power of the eye with high contrast objects as with visual acuity. The fact that the best optical system is not necessarily the one with the greatest resolving power is illustrated by the example in Figure 4.20.

In this graph, optical system 2 has the greatest resolving power, but optical system 1 will produce images with far more contrast. In many cases, most of the useful information in an image is from lower spatial frequencies so that optical system 1 would be superior even though it doesn't reveal detail as fine as system 2. This helps explain why cataract patients may have reasonably good acuities but complain bitterly about their vision. Visual acuity, being only one point on the MTF, tells us little about the overall contrast of the image. Figure 4.21 shows an example of how lower spatial frequencies can be of more use than higher spatial frequencies.

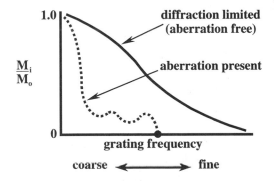

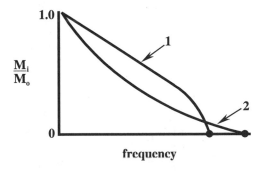

Figure 4.19. The modulation contrast function plots reduction in contrast between object and image for a range of spatial frequencies. For a diffraction-limited system, the image contrast changes from its maximal value for low spatial frequency to zero for a specific higher spatial frequency. Optical systems suffering from bad focus or aberrations give images with less contrast and they have a lower frequency cutoff for zero contrast.

Figure 4.20. The maximum resolving power of an optical instrument or the eye is the spatial frequency for which the MTF crosses the x-axis, at which point the image has zero contrast. The entire MTF contains much more information about optical performance than just resolving power. System 2 has a better resolving power than system 1, but system 1 gives better contrast over its range of spatial frequencies.

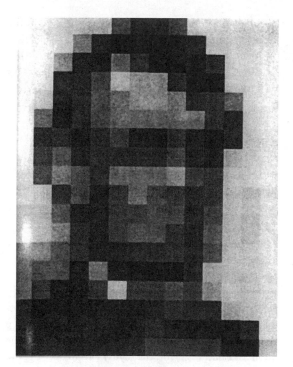

Figure 4.21. A pixilated image of Abraham Lincoln. The edges of the pixels have high spatial frequency components, which are unnecessary and make identification of the image difficult. Squinting the eyelids or using a plus blurring lens in front of the eye eliminates the high spatial frequencies. The lower spatial frequencies remain and the image looks more natural. (Reprinted with permission from Harmon LD. The recognition of faces. *Sci Am.* 1973;229(5):70–82.)

The borders of the squares consist of a mixture of high to low spacial frequencies. If one squints while looking at this figure or puts a blurring lens in front of the eye, the distracting higher frequencies are eliminated and the figure can be identified more easily.[5]

It is sometimes stated that 30 cycles per degree spatial frequency is equivalent to 20/20 Snellen visual acuity. It is argued that the horizontal bars of a 20/20 Snellen *E* corresponds to a 30 cycles per degree grating. Since the vertical thickness of each horizontal bar in the *E* is 1 min of arc, this would give 30 light-plus-dark bar pairs per degree. While roughly true, the size of the *E* and its number of grid lines are much smaller than for the usual stimulus grating. Therefore, predictions of correspondence between grating and Snellen acuity based on this reasoning may not hold up. Also, since Snellen

letters differ among themselves in their line orientation and the presence of curves, some letters are more difficult to identify than others even when they are the same size. Grid stimuli avoid this problem because they have uniform spacing and orientation, and can be given the same overall frame size regardless of detail.

It is possible to determine the MTF for the optics of the eye by directly examining the retinal image produced by a point or line object. However, the clinical measure of object-to-image contrast reduction is usually through an observer's subjective report of contrast threshold. A series of gratings with different spatial frequencies is shown to the subject. At each frequency the grating contrast is reduced until the subject reports the contrast is too low for the gratings to be seen. Contrast sensitivity (1/contrast threshold) is then graphed as a function of spatial frequency, resulting in a *contrast sensitivity function* (*CSF*), which is similar to the MTF used to describe purely optical systems.

The main difference between the CSF for the whole visual system and the MTF for a purely optical system is that the shape of the CSF is determined by the nervous system as well as by the optics of the eye. One might expect a subject's subjective report to be most sensitive to frequencies with the least contrast reduction and follow the MTF for the eye as an optical system. However, the retina and brain tend to filter out low spatial frequencies so that we are less sensitive to them and the CSF falls off for low frequencies[6] (Figure 4.22).

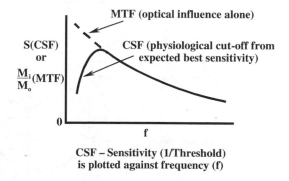

Figure 4.22. Graphs of the modulation transfer function and contrast sensitivity function plotted together. The CSF falls off at lower spatial frequencies as a result of spatial filtering introduced by the visual nervous system.

RETINAL BLUR

When using the Gauss equation for the general case of eyes out of as well as in focus, we have used ℓ for object distance and ℓ' for image distance. However, in order to describe *the* particular object distance that in unaccommodated eyes results in *the* particular image distance in which the image is at the retina we will use k for ℓ and k' for ℓ'. Thus, ℓ and ℓ' are general object and image distances, but k and k' are special object and image distances as shown in Figure 4.23. In this form, K is the dioptric "distance" that an object must be to result in the image being formed at the dioptric "length" of the eye, K'. K, then, is also the dioptric refractive error, and the point at a distance k from the eye is the far point (*pr*, for *punctum remotum*).

We will need to add a pupil to the Emsley reduced eye, which we will assume to be coincident with the cornea and to have a diameter p. Since the cornea is the only refractive surface, the entrance pupil has the same location and size as the "anatomical" pupil.

Then, for an image not on the retina (blurred) of a distant object, by similar triangles we can derive (Figure 4.24):

$$b = p\left(\frac{K}{K'}\right)$$

where b = blur circle diameter at the retina, K' = dioptric power of the eye (approximately +60 D), and K = refractive error of the eye.

Example: For a -5 D *refractive* myopic eye with a 4-mm pupil that views an object at $-\infty$:

$$b = p\left(\frac{K}{K'}\right) = 4\text{ mm }\left(\frac{-5}{+60}\right) = -0.333\text{ mm}$$

Thus, the blur size (b) increases with pupil size (p) and with refractive error (K). This is why placing a pinhole in front of the eye improves VA (up to a point) when there is refractive error. The true pupil diameter (p) of the eye is replaced by the

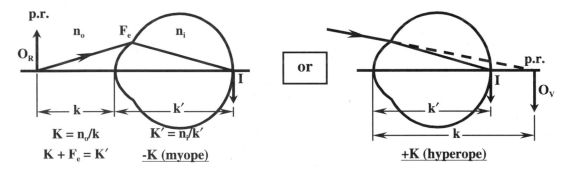

Figure 4.23. For an eye with a given dioptric power (F) and length (k'), there is a unique object distance (k) that will result in the image being in focus on the retina.

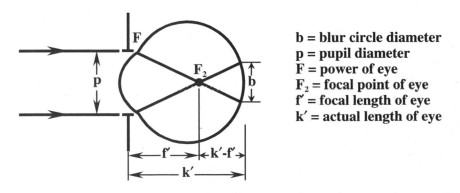

b = blur circle diameter
p = pupil diameter
F = power of eye
F_2 = focal point of eye
f' = focal length of eye
k' = actual length of eye

Figure 4.24. Schematic diagram of the Emsley reduced eye showing the construct used to derive the equation relating retina blur circle size to pupil diameter (p), power (F), and length of the eye (k').

diameter of the pinhole. This also explains why the eye is more sensitive to blur in dim light—the pupil becomes larger. Some optometric tests are used in low illumination so that the patient will perceive blur more readily.

The size of the blur circle on the retina can also be described by its angular size ($\theta_b{}'$) with the apex of the angle at the center of the exit pupil (XP) in the eye. (We can't use the nodal point if the image is out of focus.) This same angular size of blur circle can then be projected into object space for comparison with the overall size of objects that are being viewed, where $\theta_h \approx n\theta_h{}'$ (Figure 4.25).

We can then define the *blur ratio* (*BR*) as the ratio between the angular blur circle diameter ($\theta_b{}'$) and the angular size of the blurred object being viewed ($\theta_h{}'$)[7]:

$$BR = \frac{\theta_b}{\theta_h} \quad \text{or} \quad \frac{b'}{h'} = \frac{b}{h}$$

Obviously, if $\theta_b{}'$ is small relative to $\theta_h{}'$, the object may be identified or resolved. However, if BR is too large, the object will not be resolvable.

There is a strong similarity between the blur ratio and Rayleigh's criterion. If two object points are too close together compared to the size of the projected image blur, they will be seen as one blurred object point rather than as two blurred object points. With Rayleigh's criterion the limiting separation for two just resolvable points is one-half the diameter of the Airy disk diffraction pattern. For resolving power that is limited by blur, the blur circle is analogous to the Airy disk. This suggests that Snellen letters should still be identifiable when the radius of the blur circle ($b'/2$) is less than or equal to the size of the detail being resolved (h') ($b'/2 \le h'$).

Example: How many diopters of misfocus would be expected to blur 20/20 vision, if

$p = 2.5$ mm, and

$h' = 5$ μm (1 min arc or 20/20 detail), and

$b' = 2h' = 10$ μm $= 0.010$ mm.

Since $b' = p(K/K')$, $K = (b'/p)K'$
$K = (0.010/2.5 \text{ mm})(+60 \text{ D}) = 0.24$ D

A practical consequence of the preceding example is that for a given size pupil there is a relationship between VA and diopters of refractive error.

Egger's chart (Table 4.1) shows this for simple myopia and an average size pupil.[8]

Then, on coming down from plus blur during a refraction (an induced myopia) refractionists have an indication of expected dioptric error so that they will be less apt to over minus.

For example, a patient reading 20/25 at some point during the refraction should not require more than –0.25 to –0.50 D of additional minus to read 20/20. The design of the standard Snellen chart makes this possible. In coming down out of plus, each additional –0.25 D of minus should allow the patient to read one additional line on the chart.

Acuity letters agree with Egger's chart if letter size changes geometrically in jumps of $2^{1/3}$ ($= 1.26x$). In other words, it takes three lines to double the letter size. This geometric progression gives a linear relationship between the lowest Snellen line resolved and *low* spherical refractive errors:

$$20/20 \times 1.26^0 = 20/20$$
$$20/20 \times 1.26^1 = 20/25 \quad \text{(3-line change)}$$
$$20/20 \times 1.26^2 = 20/30$$
$$20/20 \times 1.26^3 = 20/40 \quad \text{(i.e., } 1.26^3 = 2 \text{ so } 20/20 \to 20/40)$$
$$20/20 \times 1.26^4 = 20/50$$

When an eye also has astigmatism, the relationship between lens correction and visual acuity is not as clear cut. One might expect that the spherical equivalent of the astigmatism could be used in Egger's chart (e.g., –1.00 D of astigmatism $\approx$ –0.50 D sphere). However, astigmatic blur weights about 0.8 of spherical blur rather than 0.5. (So –1.00 D astigmatic refractive error has about the same effect on acuity as –0.80 D spherical refractive error.)

Table 4.1. Egger's Chart for the Typical Relationship of Unaided Visual Acuity and Amount of Myopia

VA	Diopters of Error
20/20	0.00
20/25	0.25
20/30	0.50
20/40	0.75
20/50	1.00

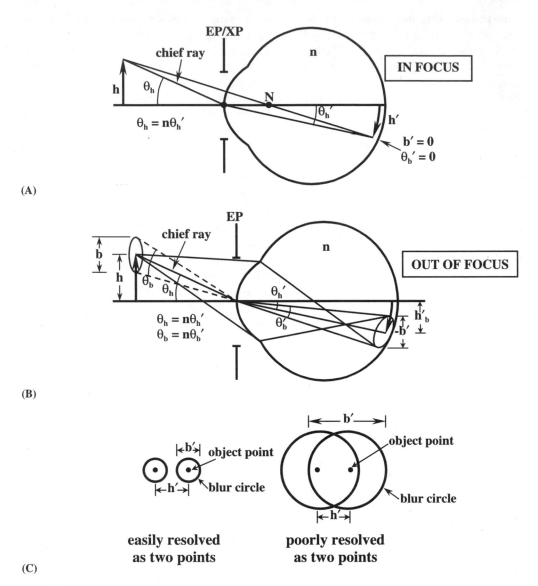

Figure 4.25. (A) For point objects that are in focus on the retina, either the nodal ray or the chief ray will locate the image. However, if the image is not in focus on the retina, only the chief ray goes through the center of the blur circle and accurately defines the location of the blurred image. (B) This diagram illustrates the projection of the angular subtense of the retinal blur circle into object space. Both the angle of the blur circle off the optical axis (θ_b) and its width (h) are increased, approximately, by the factor of the refractive index of the reduced eye. (C) Two retinal image points are perceived as two separate object points if the separation of the images is sufficiently large compared to the blur circle diameters. An arbitrary criterion is that two images will be perceived as two images if the separation between their centers is no smaller than the radius of the blur circles.

DEPTH OF FIELD AND FOCUS

As mentioned in Chapter 1, all optical systems have a critical blur size below which a smaller blur circle either cannot or need not be discriminated from a point image. In the eye, this is due to the physiological limitations of the retina to process detail finer than about one minute of arc—which corresponds to about 20/20 acuity.

The range of distances $(\ell_2 - \ell_1)$ for point objects that gives images less than or equal to the greatest tolerable blur circle diameter is the *depth of field*.

The corresponding range of image distances ($\ell_2{}'$ – $\ell_1{}'$) giving the same blur circle is called the *depth of focus*. The corresponding dioptric depth of field and focus is:

Depth of field in diopters, $L_2 - L_1 = (n_o/\ell_2) - (n_o/\ell_1)$

Depth of focus in diopters, $L_2{}' - L_1{}' = (n_i/\ell_2{}') - (n_i/\ell_1{}')$

where n_o is the index that the object light is in and n_i is the index that the image light is in.

The above concepts can be applied to the Emsley reduced eye. In order for the emmetropic Emsley eye to focus on an object where $|\ell| < |{-}\infty|$ it must increase its power by accommodating so $F = +60 - K$ (where K is the divergence of the object light). For example, if an object is –50 cm in front of the eye $K = -2$ D and $+2$ D of accommodation must be used for a total power of $F = +62$ D (Figure 4.26).

By similar triangles in Figure 4.26:

$$\frac{k' - \ell_1{}'}{b} = \frac{\ell_1{}'}{p}, \ell_1{}' = k' - \left(\frac{b}{p+b}\right)$$

$$k' \approx k' - \left(\frac{b}{p}\right)k'$$

$$\frac{\ell_2{}' - k'}{b} = \frac{\ell_2{}'}{p}, \ell_2{}' = k' + \left(\frac{b}{p+b}\right)$$

$$k' \approx k' + \left(\frac{b}{p}\right)k'$$

The linear depth of focus is then:

$$\ell_2{}' - \ell_1{}' \approx 2\left(\frac{b}{p}\right)k'$$

Example: The human eye can't resolve two image points on the retina that are separated by <5 μm, which is equivalent to a blur circle radius of 0.005 mm (or $b = 0.010$ mm). Suppose $k = -50$ cm (so $K = -2$ D), $k' = +22.22$ mm, and $p = 2.5$ mm. Then $F = +60 - (-2) = +62$ D (Figure 4.27).

$$\ell_2{}' - \ell_1{}' \approx 2\left(\frac{b}{p}\right)k' = 2\left(\frac{0.010\ \text{mm}}{2.5\ \text{mm}}\right)$$

$$(+22.22\ \text{mm}) = 0.178\ \text{mm}$$

Dioptric depth of focus ($L_2{}' - L_1{}'$) and depth of field ($L_2 - L_1$) are about ±0.25 D, which agrees with the observation that patients are usually not sensitive to changes in their prescriptions of less than ±0.25 D, and it is why the minimum power change in phoropters is usually 0.25 D. If an Emsley eye with a 2.5-mm pupil focuses on an object –50 cm in front of it, all objects between 57.0 and 44.8 cm in front of the eye are simultaneously in focus. This is because for images produced by objects in that range of distances, the retinal blur circle *radius* does not exceed 0.005 mm (5 μm).

A patient whose vision is limited to 20/40 by cataracts or retinal pathology has a greater tolerable blur circle diameter and a correspondingly

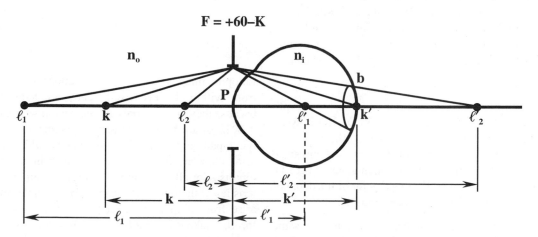

Figure 4.26. Schematic diagram of the Emsley reduced eye showing the construct used to derive the equation relating depth of focus to pupil diameter (p), ocular length (k'), and greatest tolerable blur circle diameter (b).

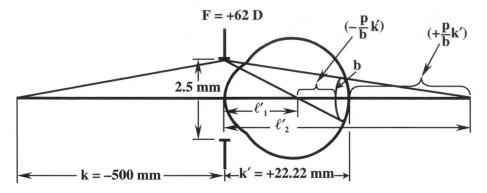

Figure 4.27. Example worked on the Emsley reduced eye to determine depth of focus when the added pupil is 2.5 mm in diameter, the object is 500 mm in front of the eye, and the blur circle diameter is 0.01 mm.

larger depth of field over which blur can't be detected. This is one reason why such patients are difficult to refract. Lens changes in the phoropter simulate different dioptric distances of objects, and the patient can't see differences in blur between lens changes as easily.

Hyperfocal Point

The *hyperfocal point* is that object point that places the most distant point of the depth of field (ℓ_1) at $-\infty$. The distance from the hyperfocal point to the optical system is the hyperfocal distance (k_{hyp}). The concept of the hyperfocal point is of interest to photographers because the greatest depth of field results when a camera is focused on the hyperfocal point. Specifically, if a camera or the eye is focused on the hyperfocal point rather than for infinity, the depth of field will be clear from infinity to half as far from the optical system than if the system were focused exactly on infinity. This is shown in Figure 4.28.

Example: Assume an emmetropic eye has a depth of field of ±0.25 D ($L_1 - L_2 = 0.50$ D). If this eye is focused on $k = -\infty$ ($L = 0$), then ℓ_2, the near point of the depth of field, is $100/-0.25 = -400$ cm since $L_2 = -0.25$ D. If this eye accommodates $+0.25$ D, then $k = -400$ cm and the near point of the depth of field is $100/-0.50 = -200$ cm from the eye.

A corrected ametropic eye can gain the same advantage by focusing on the hyperfocal point. A full Rx makes the ametropic eye effectively emmetropic. Then, if the eye has a depth of field of ±0.25 D, the eye will focus on the hyperfocal point if $+0.25$ D is added to the Rx. For example, a -5.00 D myopic eye would require an Rx of -4.75 D. By taking advantage of the full depth of field, the eye sees object points simultaneously in focus from $-\infty$ to -200 cm with a -4.75 D Rx rather than from $-\infty$ to -400 cm with a -5.00 D Rx.

If a refractionist "pushes plus," he or she automatically makes the retina conjugate with the hyperfocal point rather than with $-\infty$. This then results in the greatest possible linear depth of field. This would not seem to make much difference to a young eye with plenty of accommodative ability. However, a presbyopic eye would especially benefit from this because refracting for the hyperfocal point would reduce the required bifocal add by 0.25 D.

ENTOPTIC IMAGES

Entoptic images are visual sensations that arise from within the eye itself. They are subjective because they are seen only by the person whose eye it is. Most are benign but some are clues to underlying pathology and the clinician should understand their causes and be alert to them in patients' reports. Not all entoptic images arise from characteristics of the optics of the eye; for example, some arise from higher neuronal processing. However, for the sake of completeness, all types will be reviewed here.

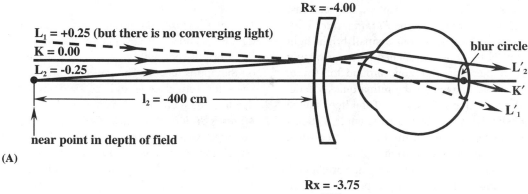

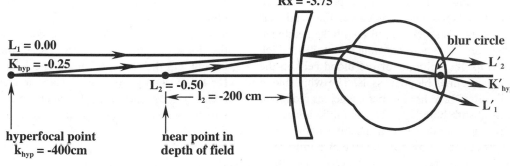

Figure 4.28. (A) This figure shows how half of the dioptric depth of field is lost when the eye is focused precisely on infinity. **(B)** This figure shows how focusing at the hyperfocal point results in the entire range of the depth of field being used and a near point half as far from the eye as for focus at infinity.

Refractive Effects

Small surface changes across the cornea can redirect light outside the retinal image.

1. *Tear film:* When the eye blinks, a horizontal ridge of tears is left momentarily where the lids came together. Some observers report a "shadow" effect seen as a horizontal striation. Mucous strands can do the same thing, but they last longer and move around with the blink.
2. *Corneal corrugations:* Squeezing the lids tightly shut gives transient ridges on the cornea that can give "shadow" streaks, monocular diplopia, and even decreased visual acuity, which in extreme cases can last longer than an hour.

Shadows

A small, bright light source close to the eye produces an out-of-focus patch of light on the retina, which furnishes a good background for projecting shadows of objects and refractive inhomogeneities in the eye. A small light source works best because it produces shadows with mostly umbra and little penumbra so that shadows are more noticeable because of the greater contrast.

1. *Ocular opacities:* Corneal scars, lens opacities, intraocular foreign bodies, vitreal floaters and blood cells would all be expected to cast shadows, but the effect is strongest for opacities nearest to the retina. This is because objects near the retina are more apt to project an umbra rather than just a penumbra onto the retina. Anterior opacities may not be noticed at all by the patient if completely opaque. An example is *asteroid hyalosis,* which is a swarm of calcium soap grains in the vitreous. To the doctor looking in, they look very bright and may make a good view of the fundus difficult due to glare; but because they are opaque, from the retinal side they are dark and the patient may be unaware of them.

2. *Purkinje tree:* Because the retinal blood vessels are in front of the photoreceptors, they can cast a shadow referred to as the *Purkinje tree.* They are normally not seen, but a small bright light can reveal them as a branched pattern stopping short of the avascular zone around the fovea. Since stable images on the retina quickly fade, the Purkinje tree is best seen if the light source is constantly moved over a large angle. Patients sometimes comment on the Purkinje tree when they are examined with bright lights.

3. *White blood cells:* When looking at a bright blue background such as the sky, a person may see bright spots moving along curved lines and their flow may even seem to pulse with the heartbeat. These are thought to be white blood cells, which interrupt the columns of red blood cells in the smaller retinal blood vessels. The white blood cells allow blue light to pass, whereas red blood cells absorb blue light. This entoptic image has been incorporated into a machine known as a blue field entoptoscope to serve as a gross subjective assessment of the function of the retina. Patients look into the blue field generated by the instrument and fixate the center of a cross. They can then report whether they see the objects moving into the four quadrants separated by the cross. If so, the examiner assumes that the patient has functional retina in each of the four quadrants.

Diffraction Effects

1. *Colored haloes:* Corneal edema can be caused by, among other reasons, increased intraocular pressure that forces water into the cornea producing water clefts, which act as diffractive particles. For instance, patients may report colored haloes around small bright lights during episodes of acute glaucoma. Swimming in chlorinated pools and overwear of contact lenses may give a similar effect.

2. *Asterisms:* Small bright objects against a dark background usually have spikes surrounding their geometric images. An example of this is bright stars where the effect is so prominent that artists frequently depict stars with spikes. This effect is assumed to be due to diffraction off the suture lines of the lens.[9]

Pressure Phosphenes

1. *Digital pressure:* If pressure is applied in the dark to the side of the eyeball through the closed lid, a bright spot will be seen in the visual field on the opposite side. The pressure directly activates the retinal cells and the field reversal is due to optical crossed projection.

2. *Moore's lightning streaks:* When the vitreous liquefies with age (*syneresis*), the points of remaining adherence between vitreous and retina may tug on the retina, especially during eye movements. This produces pressure phosphenes, which appear as lightning streaks at points in the visual field that correspond to the locations of adherence. These may be benign, but the clinician should check carefully for the possibility of retinal tears and detachments because they are more likely to occur in patients who experience these events.

Effects Due to Xanthophyll

1. *Maxwell's spot:* If a blue filter is quickly placed in front of your eye as you view a bright, uniform white background, a dark disk appears in the macular area. This is due to a *xanthophyll* pigment (*zeaxanthin*) in the macular retina (*macula lutea*). This acts like a yellow filter, which excludes more of the blue light than the surrounding retina does so that a relatively dark spot appears in the part of the visual field that corresponds to the macula.

2. *Haidinger's brush:* If one looks at a uniform white background through a Polaroid filter, a small yellow, hourglass-shaped figure appears that is centered on the point of fixation. This figure, called *Haidinger's brush,* is due to the birefringence induced by xanthophyll, which is radially polarizing. (A competing theory is that radially oriented receptor cell axons form a birefringent layer in the macula.) This figure fades rapidly due to visual adaptation, but it can be kept in view by rotating the Polaroid filter so that the hourglass also appears to rotate and exposes new retina. A blue background helps to enhance the effect. Haidinger's brush can be used to detect macular edema or to determine whether amblyopic patients fixate with their

foveas since the fovea always corresponds to the center of the hourglass and the center of rotation. Because Haidinger's brush corresponds to the macula, it is sometimes used as a gross subjective test of macular function and sometimes as a training technique in amblyopia to improve fixation. Some observers claim they can see Haidinger's brush in naturally polarized sky light by looking at the zenith during sunrise or sunset while turning their heads. The yellow arms point in the direction of the sun.

Electrical Phosphenes

1. *Blue arcs of the retina:* If a red patch of light is projected against a dim background, blue arcs will be seen following the direction of the optic nerve fibers, but only on the side toward the blind spot. Figure 4.29 shows the appearance of the blue arcs for various locations of the red stimulus. This effect is due to an electrical "short circuit" between the axons from ganglion cells under the red stimulus and ganglion cells encountered along the path of those axons. The effect is subtle, but is a little easier to see if one fixates slightly to the side of the red light. This is sometimes seen when looking at the red LEDs on a digital clock in a darkened room.
2. *Battery stimulation:* If a low-voltage battery (< 10 V) is placed in the mouth between tongue and upper lip in the dark, a faint glow will be seen all over the visual field.

Scotomas

1. *Retinal lesions:* Retinal damage causes visual loss in the corresponding area of the visual field. However, if you observe a retinal lesion with an ophthalmoscope, the expected scotoma will be on the opposite side of the visual field. Patients may be unaware of scotomas since the visual field of the undamaged eye covers for the deficit.
2. *Blind spot:* The blind spot is a 5 × 7-degree scotoma found 15 degrees from the fovea in the temporal field direction. Even though objects disappear if placed in the blind spot (monocularly), observers are entirely unaware that they have a scotoma. If a uniform field is looked at, the visual cortex fills in the vacancy on the basis of the surrounding pattern. This is unlike a scotoma from a retinal lesion where a dark spot is seen against the background. If carefully plotted, the blind spot may have a scalloped appearance as a result of the blood vessels entering and leaving the disc. The blind spot also enlarges with decreasing background illumination.

A common way to plot your own blind spot is to fixate on a spot drawn on a sheet of paper about 30 cm from your eye and observe the tip of a pencil placed about 10 cm *temporal* to the fixated spot. Whenever the pencil tip is moved into the blind spot, it disappears and a mark is made on the paper. A more accurate way to plot your blind spot is to place a spot on a piece of paper and observe the tip of the pen 10 cm *nasal* to the spot with the paper at about 30 cm from your eye (Figure 4.30).

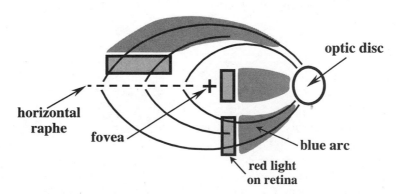

Figure 4.29. The anatomical features corresponding to the perception of blue arcs of the retina.

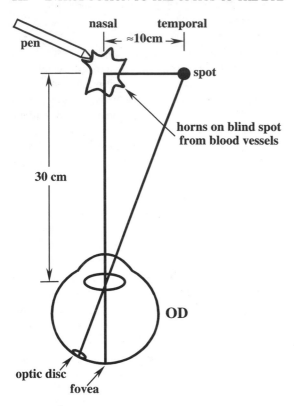

Figure 4.30. A setup for accurately drawing your own blind spot. Note that the pencil tip is centrally viewed while the spot is seen to appear and disappear across the borders of the blind spot.

Your eye follows the pencil tip rather than fixate the spot, and, as the pen is moved around with the eye following, whenever the peripherally located spot disappears, the pen can record the border of the blind spot. This is more precise because the appearance or disappearance of a spot is easier to note than that of the tip of a pencil, and the tip of the pencil, which does the plotting, is observed directly with good acuity.

REFERENCES

1. LeGrand Y. *Light, Colour and Vision.* 2nd ed. London: Chapman and Hall, 1968.
2. Longhurst RS. *Geometrical and Physical Optics.* 2nd ed. London: Longman, 1970.
3. Bennett AG, Rabbetts RB. *Bennett and Rabbett's Clinical Visual Optics.* 3rd ed. Oxford: Butterworth-Heinemann, 1998.
4. Smith WJ. *Modern Optical Engineering: The Design of Optical Systems.* 2nd ed. New York: McGraw-Hill, 1990.
5. Harmon LD. The recognition of faces. *Sci Am.* 1973;229(5):70–82.
6. Van Ness FL, Bouman MA. Spatial modulation transfer in the human eye. *J Opt Soc Am.* 1967;57:401–406.
7. Tunnacliffe AH. *Introduction to Visual Optics.* 3rd ed. London: Association of Dispensing Opticians, 1987.
8. Borish IM. *Clinical Refraction.* 3rd ed. Chicago: Professional Press, 1970;368.
9. Navarro R, Losada MA. Shape of stars and optical quality of the human eye. *J Opt Soc Am.* 1997;14:353–359.

FURTHER READING

Bennett AG, Rabbetts RB. *Bennett and Rabbett's Clinical Visual Optics.* 3rd ed. Oxford: Butterworth-Heinemann, 1998.

Freeman MH. *Optics.* 10th ed. London: Butterworth-Heinemann, 1990.

Hart WM, Jr. Entoptic imagery. In: RA Moses, WM Hart Jr., eds. *Adler's Physiology of the Eye.* 8th ed. St. Louis: Mosby, 1987;373–388.

Pedrotti LS, Pedrotti SJ. *Optics and Vision.* Upper Saddle River, NJ: Prentice-Hall, 1998.

Smith G, Atchison DA. *The Eye and Visual Optical Instruments.* Cambridge: Cambridge University Press, 1997.

Chapter 5
Ocular Biometry

If we place the candlelight about six inches from someone's eye in order that we can see the flame on the cornea when we are sitting to the side of the visual axis of the eye, within the circle of the pupil nearer the periphery, we will see in the back of the pupil a blinking flame, still smaller in its diameter but reversed and of feeble illumination, which we can easily judge, by comparing it with the one on the artificial lens, that it is reflected from the posterior wall of the lens. The front surface of the lens, and partly its inner matter, under the conditions of full transparency we can make accessible for observation if, by looking into the pupil from the side and by placing the light on the opposite side of the eye, the straight lines from the eye to the observer and from the light of the candle shining into the pupil form an obtuse angle. Here one will see elongated image of the flame, which, because it is straight, shows that it is reflected from the convex surface of the lens. —Jan Evangelista Purkinje, 1823 (From Wade NJ. *A Natural History of Vision.* Cambridge, MA: MIT Press, 1998;47.)

In this chapter we discuss some of the common methods for measuring the optical components of the eye. These methods include keratometry to measure the radius of curvature of the anterior surface of the cornea, keratoscopy to assess corneal contour, pachometry to measure corneal thickness, phakometry to determine radii of curvature of the crystalline lens surfaces, ultrasonography and partial coherence interferometry to measure distances between surfaces within the eye, and pupillometry to measure pupil diameter.

KERATOMETRY

Keratometry is a technique for measuring the radius of curvature of the anterior surface of the cornea. The earliest recorded attempt to measure the anterior corneal radius was in 1619 when Christoph Scheiner compared sizes of the images reflected from glass spheres of known radius to the sizes of images reflected from the cornea. Jesse Ramsden, an optical instrument maker, is credited with inventing a keratometer in 1769.[1] In the mid nineteenth century, Helmholtz improved Ramsden's design and developed an instrument similar to the manual keratometers used today.

Keratometry has a variety of clinical uses. It is used in fitting contact lenses. It can serve as an objective method of monitoring corneal changes in anomalies such as keratoconus. Keratometry can be used to measure corneal astigmatism, which can then be used to predict the total astigmatism of the eye. Keratometry has also been used in research to evaluate the contribution of the cornea to refractive development of the eye.

The basic components of a keratometer are (a) an object to be reflected from the cornea, (b) a lens system to give the examiner a magnified view of the reflected image, (c) a system to keep the reflected image in focus, and (d) a system to measure image size.

Optics of the Keratometer

The principle upon which keratometry is based is that the size of a reflected image is a function of the radius of curvature of the surface from which it is reflected. This relationship can be determined by finding the magnification (m), which is the ratio of image size to object size (h'/h). Newton's equation states that the magnification of a reflected image is equal to the focal length of the reflecting surface divided by the distance (x) from the object to the focal point, f/x. Thus,

$$m = h'/h = f/x$$

These distances are illustrated in Figure 5.1.

In keratometry, the distance between the object and the anterior surface of the cornea is quite long relative to the focal length of the anterior corneal surface. The virtual image formed by reflection from the anterior surface of the cornea is very close to the focal point (F) of the corneal surface. As a consequence, d, the distance from the object to the image formed by by reflection from the cornea, is a close approximation to x. Substituting d for x in the preceding formula gives the approximation:

$$h'/h \approx f/d$$

Because the focal length of a mirror is equal to the radius of curvature divided by two, the approximation can be modified to:

$$h'/h \approx (r/2)/d$$

then,

$$r = (2d)(h'/h) = 2dm$$

This equation is known as the approximate keratometer equation. As long as the examiner keeps the image reflected from the patient's cornea in focus, d is held constant. In most keratometers available today, object size (h) is also a constant, so radius of curvature (r) can be determined by mea-suring image size (h'), which is the only unknown in the equation.

Measurement of the Reflected Image

In the B&L style keratometer, a relatively large luminous circular object is placed in front of the eye. Reflection of this light from the anterior corneal surface produces a first Purkinje image, which is a greatly minified virtual image circle located behind the cornea. Because this image is inaccessible to direct measurement, such as with a ruler, keratometers use a telemicroscope to view the image. An objective lens projects a real image of the virtual image between the objective lens and the observer. This image is then observed with an eyepiece and, in theory, could be measured easily. In practice, however, it is difficult to directly mea-sure this image because it is moving.

Even during our best attempts at steady fixation, the eye undergoes constant small involuntary move-ments. For this reason, the keratometer image also moves, and even though the movements are small, they are large relative to the size of the Purkinje image. To overcome the difficulty of measuring a moving target, keratometers employ a doubling principle. Part of the image beam that travels through the keratometer is intercepted by a prism and is deflected. Another part of the beam bypasses the prism and is not deflected (Figure 5.2).

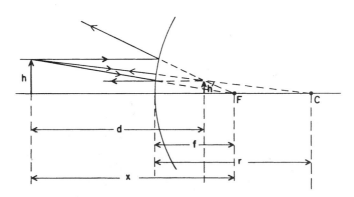

Figure 5.1. Schematic of image formation in keratometry. Image size (h') is proportional to the radius of curvature of the anterior corneal surface (r). The distance from the object to the cornea is relatively longer than depicted here. (h, object size; f, focal length of the anterior surface of the cornea as a mirror). (Reprinted with permission from Goss DA, Eskridge JB. Keratometry. In: JB Eskridge, JF Amos, JD Bartlett, eds. *Clinical Procedures in Optometry.* Philadelphia: Saunders, 1991;136.)

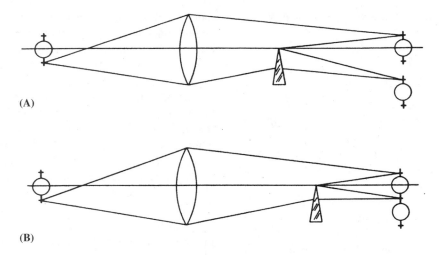

(A)

(B)

Figure 5.2. Variable doubling in the keratometer. (**A**) The prism produces a double image of the object. (**B**) The prism is moved along the axis of the keratometer until the two images are touching. The amount of movement of the prism necessary for this alignment is a function of the image size. (Reprinted with permission from Goss DA, Eskridge JB. Keratometry. In: JB Eskridge, JF Amos, JD Bartlett, eds. *Clinical Procedures in Optometry.* Philadelphia: Saunders, 1991;136.)

This produces a double image as seen through the keratometer eyepiece. As the eye moves, both images still move, but they move together so that their separation remains constant. Then, if the amount of image separation is varied until it equals the image size, the image size could be calculated by noting the prism necessary to do this. Rather than use prisms of different powers to change the image separation, movement of one prism along the optical axis of the keratometer is used to vary the *effective* prism power. The prism is moved until the two images just overlap on one border. The image dimension in the direction of doubling is then equal to the amount of deflection. The keratometer dial that moves the prism could then be calibrated to indicate the amount of prism movement; however, calculations are avoided by calibrating the dial to read the radius of curvature of the cornea directly.

Different keratometers employ either variable or fixed doubling, referring to whether the amount of doubling of the two images can be varied. Most keratometers feature variable doubling, as was described. In instruments that have fixed doubling, object size is varied to obtain a set criterion image size.

Calibration Index

Most keratometers indicate a dioptric power in addition to or instead of a radius. The radius is the more direct measure because it is found by using the keratometer equation. An accurate dioptric power could then be calculated for the anterior cornea by using an assumed corneal refractive index. (For instance, using Gullstrand's value of 1.376 and a radius of +7.7 mm gives an anterior corneal power of +48.83 D.) However, it may be of clinical interest to estimate the *total* corneal power. This calculation requires additional information about the thickness of the cornea and the dioptric power of the posterior corneal surface. Since neither of these quantities is measured by the keratometer, such a calculation must use assumed values for an average eye. Then, as a mathematical shortcut, the total corneal power may be calculated by modeling the cornea as a single refractive surface whose radius is the actual anterior corneal radius as determined by the keratometer, but with a fictitious lower corneal refractive index. The particular fictitious index used for the conversion from radius to dioptric power depends on the assumed values for corneal thickness and power of the posterior corneal surface, as well as on whether the total power is to be the equivalent power or the back vertex power. Most keratometers use a calibration index of 1.3375, although some use calibration index values of 1.336 or 1.332.[2] If the cornea of the Gullstrand schematic eye No. 1 were examined with a keratometer with a calibration index of 1.3375, the dioptric power read from the instrument would be:

$$F = \frac{n' - n}{r} = \frac{1.3375 - 1.00}{+0.0077 \text{ m}} = +43.83 \text{ D}$$

It is unclear why the calibration index of 1.3375 was first established for keratometers, but its use is very long-standing and unlikely to change in the near future. (It may or may not be coincidental that +43.83 D is the back vertex power of the cornea in Gullstrand's schematic eye No. 1.) Although the dioptric power given by a keratometer is only an estimate of the total dioptric power of the cornea, power *differences*, such as changes over time or between meridians, would not be expected to vary greatly from the true difference values.

The Bausch & Lomb Keratometer

We will use the Bausch & Lomb Keratometer as an example of keratometer design. It is perhaps the most widely used keratometer, and its design has been copied by several companies. A schematic cross section of the B&L Keratometer is shown in Figure 5.3, and its optical system is illustrated in Figure 5.4.

The B&L Keratometer varies the amount of doubling but keeps the object size constant. The object, referred to as a mire, consists of a circle flanked by a horizontal pair of plus signs and a vertical pair of minus signs. The mire pattern is made luminous by backlighting a plate, which is opaque except for clear areas in the shape of the mire (see Figure 5.4). The light reflected from the cornea forms a virtual image of the mire behind the patient's cornea. This image is then observed through a hole in the center of the mire plate by a telemicroscope in which an objective lens forms a real image, which is examined through an eyepiece.

The light cone formed by the objective lens passes through two pairs of apertures in an otherwise opaque diaphragm. One pair of holes, oriented horizontally in Figure 5.4 isolates portions of

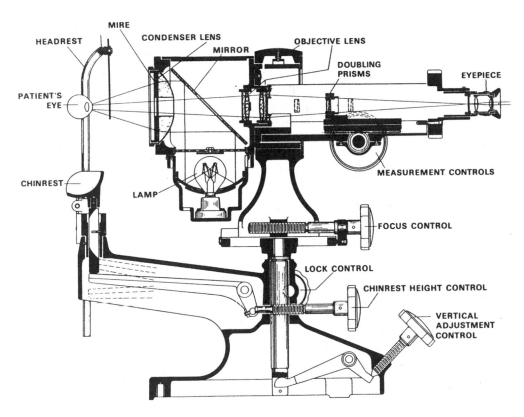

Figure 5.3. Cross section of the Bausch & Lomb Keratometer. (Reprinted with permission from Mohrman R. The keratometer. In: A Safir, ed. *Refraction and Clinical Optics.* Hagerstown, MD: Harper & Row, 1980;455.)

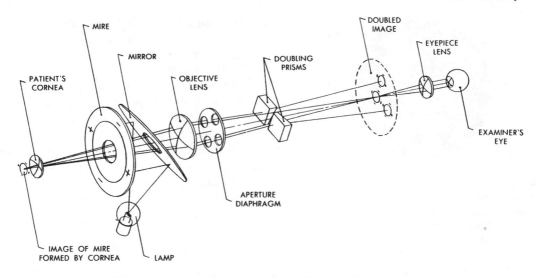

Figure 5.4. Schematic of the optical system of the Bausch & Lomb Keratometer. (Reprinted with permission from Mohrman R. The keratometer. In: A Safir, ed. *Refraction and Clinical Optics.* Hagerstown, MD: Harper & Row, 1980;454.)

the beam so that they go separately through base out and base up doubling prisms. The knobs that move these doubling prisms along the instrument's optical axis are marked to read off the corneal dioptric power in the meridian of doubling for each prism.

The other pair of holes, oriented vertically in Figure 5.4, forms a Scheiner's disc, which is used to assist in focusing the B&L Keratometer. The addition of a Scheiner's disc allows a single image to be seen when the mires are in focus, but two images to be seen when they are out of focus. This gives an additional cue to focus, which can be more sensitive than the blur that results from defocus. The Scheiner's disc principle, described by Christoph Scheiner, is explained in Figure 5.5.

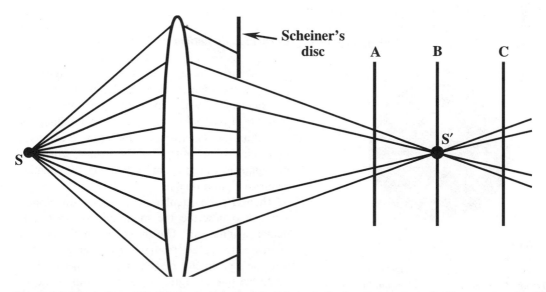

Figure 5.5. Illllustration of the Scheiner's disc principle. Scheiner's disc has two apertures. In this example, *s* is a light source and *s'* is the image of that light source formed by a lens. When a screen is placed at *B* in the plane of *s'*, a single point is seen. When the screen is placed elsewhere, such as at *A* or *C,* two out-of-focus spots of light will be seen.

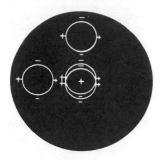

Figure 5.6. Examiner's view through the keratometer after alignment in front of the patient and before focusing. (Reprinted with permission from Mohrman R. The keratometer. In: A Safir, ed. *Refraction and Clinical Optics.* Hagerstown, MD: Harper & Row, 1980;456.)

The examiner's view of the reflected pattern before focusing and aligning the axis is shown in Figure 5.6. The lower right image, whose light went through the Scheiner's disc, appears double because it is out of focus. To obtain focus, the examiner rotates the focus control knob, which changes the distance of the objective lens from the patient's eye, until these images merge. Next the examiner adjusts the instrument for the proper axis of the astigmatism by rotating the entire optical assembly until the axes of the plus and minus signs that flank the prism-doubled mires line up with the central cross.

Then the examiner turns the two knobs that move the doubling prisms in order to superimpose the two plus signs in the lower right and lower left images, and the minus signs in the lower right and the top images (Figure 5.7). When alignment is

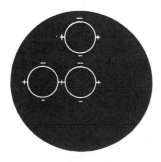

Figure 5.7. Examiner's view through the keratometer when the horizontal doubling prism has been moved to overlap the plus signs on the doubled images. (Reprinted with permission from Mohrman R. The keratometer. In: A Safir, ed. *Refraction and Clinical Optics.* Hagerstown, MD: Harper & Row, 1980;456.)

achieved, the scales on the knobs yield the dioptric keratometer powers in the meridians in which the plus and minus signs are aligned.

The fact that there are two doubling prisms in the B&L Keratometer with axes 90 degrees to one another allows both principal meridians to be measured while the keratometer is rotated to only one position. Keratometers constructed in this way are called one-position keratometers. Keratometers that require rotation from one position to another for measurement of the two principal meridians, are called two-position keratometers.

Area of the Cornea Measured

The area of the cornea that is measured corresponds to the distance on the cornea between the locations where the two plus signs and between where the two minus signs are projected onto the cornea. The separations of these corneal regions vary somewhat with the radius of curvature of the cornea. For the B&L Keratometer the separation of the corneal points is between about 3.0 and 3.2 mm for the most common corneal radii.[2] This area is sometimes referred to as the corneal "cap." Because the mire is a thin circle that is measured at only two points, the validity of the keratometric values for points within the cap are uncertain, and the validity for points outside the cap are unknown.

Corneal Astigmatism

Most corneas have at least some difference in power across their meridians. This results in axial astigmatism in which two separate line images, rather than one point image, are formed along the optical axis. Corneal astigmatism can be corrected by placing a lens in front of the cornea, which has the opposite astigmatism so that the combination achieves a point image.

There is a particular system used in clinical settings to describe the meridian orientations in ocular astigmatism. The meridians of the eye are expressed in degrees from 0 to 180 degrees. We can imagine a protractor placed in a plane perpendicular to the line of sight. Horizontal to the patient's left is 0 degrees (whether the eye in question is the left eye or the right eye) (Figure 5.8).

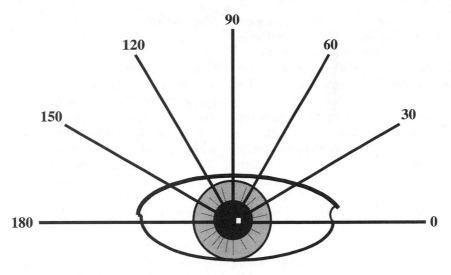

Figure 5.8. The meridians of the eye specified in degrees.

Horizontal to the patient's right is 180 degrees. Vertical is designated as 90 degrees. The meridians of greatest and least power are called the *principal meridians*. These meridians are generally 90 degrees apart, in which case the astigmatism is referred to as regular. Depending on the axis orientation of the principal meridians, astigmatism can be classified as with-the-rule, against-the-rule, or oblique. With-the-rule corneal astigmatism is present when the cornea has its greatest power within 30 degrees of the vertical (90 degrees) meridian (between the 60 and 120 meridians), and the least power somewhere between the 0 and 30 or the 150 and 180 meridians. Against-the-rule corneal astigmatism is present when the cornea has its greatest power within 30 degrees of the horizontal (180 degrees) meridian (between the 0 and 30 or the 150 and 180 meridians) and its least power somewhere between the 60 and 120 meridians. Oblique astigmatism exists when one principal meridian is between 31 and 59 and the other is between 121 and 149.

Astigmatism can be corrected with a cylinder lens—a lens that has power in only one of the principal meridians. And, in fact, the corneal astigmatism is usually recorded as the power of the cylinder lens that would correct it rather than the power of the cornea itself. In a cylinder lens the meridian of maximum power is called the *power meridian* and the meridian of zero power is called the *axis meridian*. For example, if a cylinder lens has zero (plano) power in the 180 meridian and −1.00 D power in the 90 meridian, the axis meridian is at 180 and power meridian is at 90. The clinical notation for astigmatism includes two numbers: the correcting cylinder power and the axis meridian, with an *x* placed between the two numbers to symbolize axis. For the example just given, the notation would be −1.00 × 180. The −1.00 indicates the number of diopters of cylinder power in the correcting lens. The *x* indicates that the number that follows it is the orientation of the axis of the cylinder, in this case 180. Applying the terminology for the orientation of astigmatism, −1.00 × 180 would be with-the-rule. This could also be expressed in terms of plus cylinder power as +1.00 × 90. Examples of against-the-rule astigmatism corrections are −1.00 × 90 or +1.00 × 180.

Keratometry locates the principal meridians of an astigmatic cornea and measures the radius of curvature and dioptric power in those meridians. If a keratometer showed the principal meridians to be oriented at 180 and 90, with 44.00 D in the 180 and 45.00 D in the 90, we would say that the cornea had 1 D of with-the-rule astigmatism. This corneal astigmatism can also be expressed by specifying the cylinder lens that would correct it. For instance, in the preceding example the cornea has 1 D more power in the 90 than in the 180 meridian. This could be compensated for by placing a −1 D cylinder lens in front of the cornea so that the minus cylinder power is aligned in the 90 meridian. This would be written as −1.00 × 180.

The cornea is the main contributor to the astigmatism of the eye, but rarely does the total astigmatism of the eye exactly equal the amount of corneal astigmatism as measured by the keratometer. The reasons that have been given for the fact that corneal astigmatism and total astigmatism are typically not the same include the following: (a) the optical axis of the cornea does not coincide with the line of sight of the eye, effectively making the cornea tilted with respect to keratometer alignment; (b) the posterior surface of the cornea and the crystalline lens may have astigmatism; (c) the crystalline lens may be tilted within the eye with respect to the optical axis of the eye; (d) keratometry is measured at the cornea while correcting lenses are generally placed in the spectacle plane; and (e) the calibration index used in the keratometer differs from the index of refraction of the cornea. The tilt of the cornea and the crystalline lens probably account for most of the difference.[3]

Javal's Rule

Because the cornea is usually the biggest contributor to astigmatism of the eye, and the crystalline lens adds a relatively constant amount, total astigmatism of the eye can be predicted from the corneal astigmatism. Many formulas have been proposed to describe the mathematical relationship between corneal astigmatism and the total astigmatism of the eye. The most common of these is Javal's rule. Javal's rule says that the total astigmatism of the eye can be predicted by multiplying the corneal astigmatism by 1.25 and then adding 0.50 D of against-the-rule astigmatism (assumed to be from the crystalline lens). Again using our example of keratometer powers of 44.00 in the 180 meridian and 45.00 in the 90 meridian, Javal's rule would predict that the eye would have 0.75 D of with-the-rule astigmatism:

total astigmatism = (keratometer astigmatism)
(1.25) + (0.50 D against-the-rule)

total astigmatism = (−1.00 × 180) (1.25)
+ (−0.50 × 90)

total astigmatism = (−1.25 × 180)
+ (+0.50 × 180)

total astigmatism = − 0.75 × 180

Simplification of Javal's Rule

Grosvenor and colleagues[4] note that if one plotted total astigmatism of the eye on the y-axis of a graph as a function of keratometer astigmatism on the x-axis, the relationship could be expressed as an equation for a straight line, $y = mx + b$, where m is the slope and b is the y-intercept. The equation for Javal's rule then could be stated in terms of a slope of 1.25 and a y-intercept of 0.50 D against-the-rule. Grosvenor and colleagues sought to confirm Javal's rule by calculating a regression equation of total astigmatism on keratometer astigmatism using clinical data. They found the slope to be a little less than 1, and the y-intercept to be a little less than 0.50 D against-the-rule.

On that basis, they recommended simplifying Javal's rule by eliminating the step of multiplying by 1.25. For the preceding example their rule would predict 0.50 D of with-the-rule astigmatism:

total astigmatism = (keratometer astigmatism)
+ (0.50 D against-the-rule)

total astigmatism = (−1.00 × 180)
+ (−0.50 × 90)

total astigmatism = (−1.00 × 180)
+ (+0.50 × 180)

total astigmatism = −0.50 × 180

KERATOSCOPY

Keratoscopy is a method used to assess the curvature and topography of the anterior surface of the cornea. Unlike keratometry, which measures only the center of an assumed spherical cornea, keratoscopy can evaluate almost the entire cornea and it can evaluate its asphericity. The clinical uses of keratoscopy include the fitting of contact lenses and the monitoring of corneal changes caused by disease or anterior segment surgery.

A keratoscope consists of a pattern reflected from the anterior surface of the cornea and a viewing system to observe the image from that reflection. The pattern used in most keratoscopes consists of alternating black and white concentric circles, often referred to as a Placido disc named after the nineteenth-century Portuguese oculist.[5] The viewing system may be as simple as a hole in the Placido disc through which the examiner views the reflected image. This system offers only a qualitative assessment of corneal topography. The examiner can observe large amounts of corneal astigmatism or severe corneal distortions. More sophisticated viewing systems allow a more quantitative assessment of corneal topography. Photokeratoscopes use film to capture the image for subsequent measurement but have largely been replaced by digital technology. Videokeratoscopes capture the reflected images on a CCD chip, which inputs them to a computer for instant analysis. Some manufacturers refer to their videokeratoscopes as corneal topographers.

Keratoscopy is based on the principle that the size of a reflected image depends on the radius of curvature of the reflecting surface. If circles are used as objects, the farther that a given point on a given reflected circle is from the center of the entire reflected image, the greater is the radius of curvature at the point on the cornea from which the reflection occurred. In videokeratoscopy the computer uses a polar coordinate system to determine a distance from the corneal apex and an angle for numerous points on each of the circles. The computer system is then programmed to calculate a radius of curvature for each point based on those polar coordinates.

Most videokeratoscopy systems calculate an axial radius of curvature. For axial radius of curvature, the assumption is made that the centers of curvature for all points on the cornea are located on the optical axis of the cornea. This is actually a fiction since it would be true only for a spherical cornea. For aspherical corneas, a more correct radius is the instantaneous radius of curvature, which would be located off the optical axis for all but the central cornea (Figure 5.9). The centers of curvature for a given half meridian of the cornea generally form a caustic curve of points, which lie farther from the optical axis for more peripheral points on the cornea (Figure 5.10). The axial radius of curvature, then, is the location where the instantaneous radius of curvature crosses the optical axis.

The radius of curvature is then converted into a dioptric value based on the keratometer calibration index of 1.3375. Different videokeratoscope manufacturers offer different options for display of the resultant data. The usual presentation mode is dioptric power color-coded maps of the corneal surface based on axial radius of curvature. In these maps, the red end of the spectrum generally depicts greater dioptric powers and the blue end of the spectrum usually indicates lower dioptric powers. Some manufacturers offer the option of maps based on instantaneous radius of curvature. (For some excellent illustrations showing how the color-coded maps of a given cornea can change their appearance depending on the displayed measurement, see Salmon and Horner.[6])

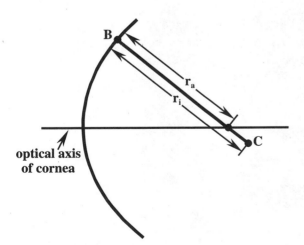

Figure 5.9. Illustration of the axial radius of curvature (r_a) and instantaneous radius of curvature (r_i) at a given point (B) on the cornea. Point C indicates the center of curvature of the cornea at point B.

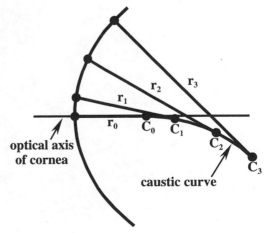

Figure 5.10. Radii of curvature at the corneal apex (r_0) and then at progressively more peripheral points (r_1, r_2, r_3). C_0, C_1, C_2, C_3 are the corresponding centers of curvature.

Figure 5.11 shows the reflected keratoscope rings for a cornea with 3.00 D of astigmatism. Note that the circles are more elongated in the horizontal meridian. That meridian would then be the meridian with greatest radius of curvature. The radius of curvature is 7.48 mm in the 6-degree meridian and 7.01 mm in the 96-degree meridian. Figure 5.12 shows a black-and-white reproduction of the corneal map for that cornea.

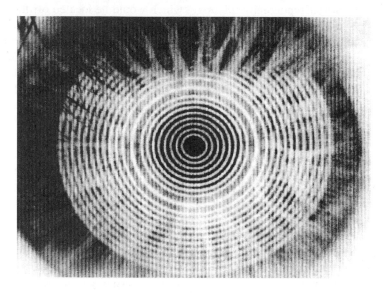

Figure 5.11. Photokeratogram of an astigmatic cornea.

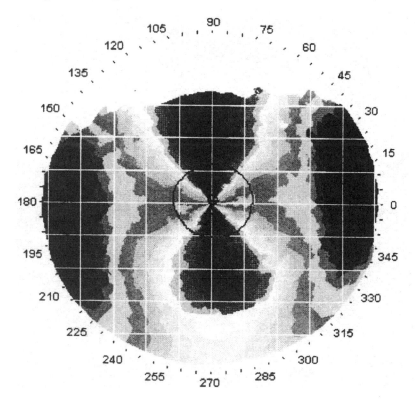

Figure 5.12. Map of the astigmatic cornea shown in the keratograph in Figure 5.11.

Corneal Shape

In most corneas the radius of curvature is shortest in the central portion and progressively lengthens toward the periphery. This is referred to as peripheral flattening. In reality corneas have very complex shapes, but it is useful to fit them to the nearest mathematical conicoid (a surface whose profile is a conic section). Most corneas are fit best by the prolate area of an ellipse (where the optical axis of the cornea is aligned with the major axis of the ellipse). With this orientation the ellipse is most curved in the central portion and less curved in the periphery (Figure 5.13).

Some corneas that have undergone refractive surgery, and a very few normal corneas, are fit best by the oblate region of an ellipse (where the optical axis of the cornea is aligned with the minor axis of the ellipse). An oblate cornea is a cornea with peripheral corneal steepening rather than corneal flattening.

Various index values have been derived from the equations of conic sections in order to assign a one-dimensional number to the surface shapes of corneas. These index values include p-value (p), eccentricity (e), and asphericity (Q).

The p-value (p) is calculated by a formula:

$$p = \frac{2r_0x - y^2}{x^2}$$

where x for a given corneal section is sagittal depth corresponding to the semichord y, as shown in Figure 5.14. The variable r_0 is the radius of curvature

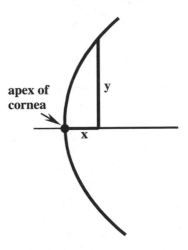

Figure 5.14. In calculation of the p-value to describe corneal shape, x is the sagittal depth for the semi-chord y.

at the apex of the cornea. The other shape indices can be derived from p by:

eccentricity: $e = \sqrt{1-p}$

asphericity: $Q = p - 1$

A p-value less than 1, but greater than 0, indicates a prolate cornea. The more that the p-value is below 1 the greater is the corneal flattening. A p-value of 1 would indicate a circle (in which the radius of curvature is constant), and a p-value greater than 1 would indicate an oblate cornea. (For a brief but very readable account of this confusing topic, see Lindsay et al.[7]) In a study of 220 normal eyes, Guillon and colleagues[8] found an average p-value of 0.85 (standard deviation = 0.15) for the flattest meridian of each eye.

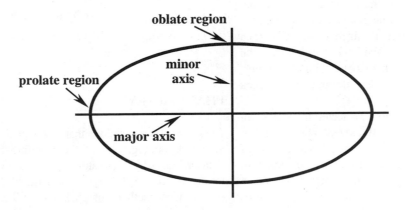

Figure 5.13. The prolate and oblate areas of an ellipse.

PACHOMETRY

Pachometry (or *pachymetry*) is the measurement of corneal thickness. The clinical uses of pachometry include monitoring corneal edema induced by contact lens wear and various corneal conditions, and determining the depth of cuts or ablation in refractive surgery. Corneal thickness can be measured by ultrasound or by optical means.

In ultrasonic pachometry, a probe that produces sound at a frequency high above the range of human hearing is placed on the cornea. Ultrasound directed into the cornea echoes from both the anterior and the posterior surface of the cornea. The difference in echo times is then measured to calculate the time taken for the ultrasound to traverse the cornea. Using a known sound velocity for corneal tissue, corneal thickness is then calculated. Ultrasonic pachometers give more accurate measurements of corneal thickness than optical pachometry, so it has supplanted the use of optical pachometry to a large extent.

The advantage of optical pachometry is that it can be performed with an attachment to a slit lamp biomicroscope,[9] whereas a separate instrument is needed for ultrasonic pachometry. A commercially available optical pachometer is an attachment for the Haag-Streit slit lamp.[10] The instrument masks the illumination beam to form a slit of light so that only a cross section of the cornea is illuminated. This slit beam passes through two glass plates, a bottom plate that is kept perpendicular to the observation axis and an upper plate that can be rotated about a vertical axis. When the upper plate is rotated, the image of the upper corneal section (which passes through the upper plate) is displaced horizontally relative to the lower corneal section. When the doctor turns the plate enough to align the back surface of the upper half image of the cornea with the front surface of the lower half image of the cornea, the amount of displacement equals the projected depth of the beam through the cornea (Figure 5.15).

Figure 5.16 shows how projected thickness can be converted to physical thickness. The amount of rotation of the upper glass plate yields a measure of the lateral projected thickness (*D*) of the cornea. ℓ' is the apparent thickness of the cornea, the distance from the anterior corneal surface to the image of the posterior corneal surface.

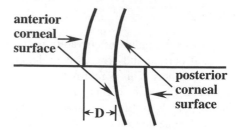

Figure 5.15. Alignment of the split images of the corneal section used for measurement of corneal thickness with optical pachometry. *D* is the lateral projected thickness explained in Figure 5.16.

Apparent thickness ℓ' can be calculated from *D* and θ (θ is 40 degrees in the Haag-Streit pachometer arrangement) as follows:

$$\ell' = D/\sin\theta$$

The actual thickness of the cornea, ℓ, can then be calculated from the apparent thickness, treating the posterior corneal surface as an object imaged through the anterior surface of the cornea. The formula would be:

$$L = L' - F$$

$$n/\ell = n'/\ell' - F$$

where *n* = the index of refraction of the cornea, *n'* = the index of refraction of air, and *F* = the refractive power of the anterior surface of the cornea. For example, if the index of refraction of the cornea is 1.376, and the power of the anterior surface of the cornea is +48.83 D (from Gullstrand's schematic eye No. 1), and we find that ℓ' is 0.37 mm, then the corneal thickness would be 0.50 mm:

$$1.376/\ell = (1.00/{-0.00037}\text{ m}) - 48.83\text{ D}$$

$$\ell = -0.50\text{ mm}$$

PHAKOMETRY

Phakometry is a technique that employs direct observation or photography of the Purkinje images to measure the radii of curvature of the anterior and posterior surfaces of the crystalline lens.[11,12] There are two primary methods of phakometry: Tscherning's method of ophthalmophakometry and comparison

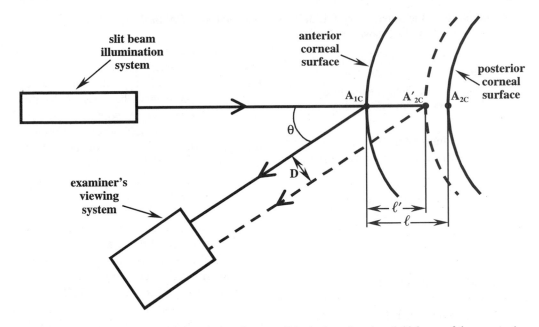

Figure 5.16. Corneal section viewed during optical pachometry. D is the lateral projected thickness of the cornea. Apparent thickness of the cornea is ℓ', the distance from the anterior surface of the cornea (A_{1C}) to the image of the posterior surface of the cornea (A_{2C}').

phakometry. Most research studies today use comparison phakometry. Both methods are based on the principle that the magnification of a reflected image is proportional to the radius of curvature of the reflecting surface. In the case of phakometry, the reflected images are the Purkinje images. In phakometry several assumptions are made: (a) because Purkinje image II is very difficult to see and photograph, the cornea is assumed to be a single refracting surface with its refractive power equal to the keratometer power; (b) index of refraction values for the ocular media are given standard values; (c) the crystalline lens is treated as a homogeneous medium with a single index of refraction; (d) the ocular refracting surfaces are assumed to be spherical rather than aspheric; and (e) the eye is assumed to be a coaxial system with the centers of curvature of the refracting surfaces falling on a single line.[13]

Comparison Phakometry

In comparison phakometry, a photograph is taken of the Purkinje images of a pair of lights. Figure 5.17 is an example of such a photograph.

The separation of the pair of lights is measured for each of the Purkinje images. The apparent radius of a surface is the distance from the surface to the point where an image would be formed of the center of curvature of that surface. The apparent

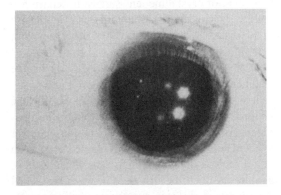

Figure 5.17. Photograph of the Purkinje images used in comparison phakometry. From left to right, Purkinje images IV, III, and I can be seen. (Reprinted with permission from Van Veen HG, Goss DA. A simplified method of Purkinje image photography for phakometry. *Am J Optom Physiol Opt.* 1988;65:906.)

radius of curvature of the anterior crystalline lens surface is determined by the following ratios:

$$\frac{\text{size of Purkinje III}}{\text{size of Purkinje I}} = \frac{\genfrac{}{}{0pt}{}{\text{apparent radius,}}{\text{anterior lens}}}{\genfrac{}{}{0pt}{}{\text{radius of curvature,}}{\text{anterior cornea}}}$$

The apparent radius of curvature of the posterior crystalline lens surface is determined in the same way:

$$\frac{\text{size of Purkinje IV}}{\text{size of Purkinje I}} = \frac{\genfrac{}{}{0pt}{}{\text{apparent radius,}}{\text{posterior lens}}}{\genfrac{}{}{0pt}{}{\text{radius of curvature,}}{\text{anterior cornea}}}$$

Using the solved values for the apparent radii of curvature, the locations of the apparent centers of curvature can be determined. Then the locations of the actual centers of curvature can be determined by where the actual centers of curvature as objects would have to be located in order to be imaged at the locations of the apparent centers of curvature. Finally, the actual radii of curvature are the distances from the actual surfaces to their respective actual centers of curvature.

Usually a three-refracting surface eye with single surface cornea and single index crystalline lens (as in the Gullstrand-Emsley schematic eye) is assumed. The radius of curvature of the anterior corneal surface and the total power of the cornea are obtained from keratometry. The apparent radius of curvature of the anterior crystalline lens surface is determined from the sizes of the first and third Purkinje images; and the apparent radius of curvature of the posterior crystalline lens surface is determined from the sizes of the first and fourth Purkinje images. Then, the actual centers of curvature of the anterior and posterior lens surfaces are located by raytrace using the locations of the apparent centers of curvature as images. For this latter calculation, anterior chamber depth and lens thickness must be obtained from some method such as ultrasonography. The actual radii of curvature are then the distances between the actual crystalline lens surfaces and their actual centers of curvature. As an example, radii of curvature of the crystalline lens of the Gullstrand-Emsley schematic eye are calculated in Appendix 5.1 from its Purkinje image magnifications calculated previously in Chapter 3.

Tscherning's Ophthalmophakometry

Tscherning's ophthalmophakometer is now mainly of historical interest since it has been largely replaced by comparison phakometry. Tscherning's method also compared the sizes of the third and fourth Purkinje images with the first Purkinje image; however, the method of measurement was different.[14] It used two pairs of lamps, a brighter pair for observation of the third and fourth Purkinje images and a dimmer pair for observation of Purkinje image I. For measurement of the radii of curvature of the crystalline lens surfaces, separation of the pair that produced Purkinje image I was varied until the two corneal reflections had the same separation as the two reflections from the anterior and posterior crystalline lens surfaces (Purkinje images III and IV). Tscherning's method of ophthalmophakometry was also used to measure anterior chamber depth and lens thickness. The mathematical calculations were the same as those described for comparison phakometry.

Comments on Phakometry and Purkinje Image Photography

It is easy to identify each image. Purkinje image I is brightest, and both Purkinje images I and III are erect, whereas Purkinje image IV is inverted. Also, Purkinje image III is considerably larger and located farther back than Purkinje images I and IV.

Purkinje image I is easy to photograph due to its brightness and lack of sensitivity to the angles of fixation, camera, and light source. The angles for Purkinje image IV are somewhat more critical since its reflective surface is located behind the pupil so the image can be vignetted. For good results, the subject's fixation is directed toward a point between the light source and the camera so that the reflection will be approximately at the position where the line of sight intersects the crystalline lens surface. Purkinje image III is more difficult to photograph than Purkinje image IV, for at least two reasons. Purkinje image III is less distinct because the anterior lens surface is not as smooth as the posterior lens surface. Also, whereas Purkinje images I and IV are axially close together and can be focused simultaneously, Purkinje image III is located deeper in the eye and is out of focus when photographing Purkinje images I and IV.

The primary use for phakometry is for the study of the contribution of the crystalline lens to refractive errors. Purkinje images have also been used to study crystalline lens changes in accommodation and night myopia. Phakometry systems using commercial photography equipment and video equipment are available.[15,16]

ULTRASONOGRAPHY

Ultrasonography is the most common method for measurement of the distances between ocular surfaces. Ultrasound is an acoustic wave with a frequency higher than the human audible range. (The human ear can detect tones over a range of frequencies from 20 to 20,000 cycles per second.[17]) An ultrasound wave is produced by a transducer through the application of an alternating electrical current to a piezoelectric crystal. The crystal vibrates at a frequency that matches the frequency of the driving current. For ophthalmic ultrasonography, the transducer directs bursts of ultrasound pulses into the eye at about one thousand bursts per second. Each burst contains a train of ultrasound pulses, each pulse lasting about a tenth of a microsecond (10^{-7} second). The intervals between bursts are used to register the echoes coming back into the transducer after being reflected from the surfaces within the eye. The crystal produces electrical energy when it is mechanically vibrated by the returning ultrasound waves. The time between the echoes returning from two axially separated tissue interfaces is measured, and then converted into distance measurements using known velocities of ultrasound in the ocular tissues:

$$d = (V)(t/2)$$

where d = distance, V = velocity, and t = time. Time is divided by 2 in the formula because the time measured is the time for the ultrasound to go into the eye and then return (whereas we require the time for a one-way trip). Velocities of ultrasound in normal ocular tissues are approximately 1640 m/sec for the cornea, 1532 m/sec for the aqueous and vitreous, and 1641 m/sec for the crystalline lens.[18,19]

As long as the medium through which ultrasound travels is homogeneous, no energy is reflected back. However, reflection does occur at the interface of two media with different acoustic impedances. *Acoustic impedance* is defined as the product of the density of the medium and propagation velocity through it. The amplitude of the reflection is proportional to the difference between the acoustic impedances of two media. As a consequence, in the normal eye there are reflections from the major refracting surfaces of the eye and from the retina.

The range of ultrasound frequencies that have been used for various ophthalmic applications is about 5 million to 25 million cycles per second (5 to 25 megahertz, or MHz). As the frequency used is increased, resolution improves but attenuation also increases. *Attenuation* is a progressive loss of ultrasound amplitude as a result of scattering and absorption. Resolution is greater with higher frequencies because the wavelength is shorter. Ultrasonic pachometry requires a higher frequency than is used for measurement of the other intraocular distances, because greater resolution is needed. The frequencies used in ultrasonic pachometry cannot be used to measure axial length because attenuation is too great. Examination of areas of the body other than the eye, such as in obstetrics, generally involve lower frequencies because of the greater attenuation from the longer paths being traversed.

A-Scan Ultrasonography

A-scan, or amplitude modulation, ultrasonography presents a unidimensional display of the amplitude of echoes as a function of time taken for the echo to return to the transducer. Spikes on an oscilloscope trace correspond to echoes from the cornea, the anterior and posterior surfaces of the crystalline lens, and the retina. For A-scan measurements of the entire eye, the anterior and posterior surfaces of the cornea cannot be distinguished. This is because the lower frequencies that must be used to avoid significant attenuation before reaching the retina do not yield sufficient resolution to distinguish both surfaces of the cornea. Figure 5.18 shows an A-scan trace. The main application of A-scan is the measurement of intraocular distances.

Intraocular distances are determined using the formula for distance as a function of time and velocity. Commercially available ultrasound units will give measurements for the distance from the

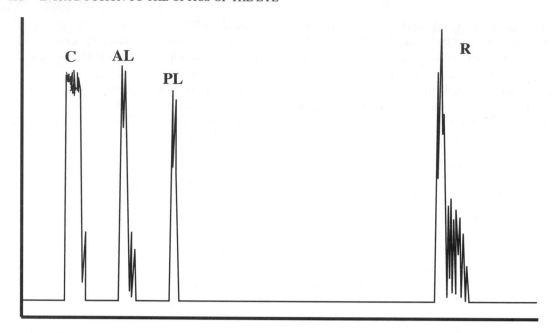

Figure 5.18. Typical pattern of an ophthalmic ultrasound A-scan trace representing the amplitude of the echo as a function of time. The following letters mark the echoes from the surfaces of the eye: *C* = cornea; *AL* = anterior crystalline lens surface; *PL* = posterior crystalline lens surface; *R* = retina.

anterior surface of the cornea to the anterior surface of the crystalline lens (referred to as anterior chamber depth), crystalline lens thickness, and vitreous chamber depth. The sum of these will then be the axial length of the eye. Measurements of axial length and the other intraocular distances are used in studies of the relationship of the ocular optical components to refractive error and in calculations to predict the best lens implant power for replacement of a crystalline lens removed in cataract surgery.

To ensure accuracy of A-scan measurements, it is important to align the ultrasound probe as close as possible with the line of sight of the eye.[20] If the probe is not aligned with the line of sight, the measurement of axial length will usually be too high. Another common source of error in A-scan measurements is to press against the globe with the ultrasound probe rather than to just touch the surface of the cornea, thus depressing the cornea and giving falsely low measures of anterior chamber depth and axial length.

B-Scan Ultrasonography

B-scan is brightness mode, or intensity modulation ultrasonography. It yields a two-dimensional, cross-sectional representation of the eye. In a B-scan probe the beam from the ultrasound transducer sweeps back and forth through a plane, which then is the plane of the cross section of the eye being examined. Different eye cross sections can be observed by changing the orientation of the probe relative to the eye.

The brightness of each spot in the B-scan image is proportional to the ultrasound energy reflected from the corresponding tissue surface. Because ultrasound does not require an optically clear path, B-scan can be used to evaluate portions of the eye that may be obscured from visual inspection by media opacities. The primary uses of B-scan ultrasonography are the detection and localization of conditions such as intraocular tumors, retinal detachment, vitreous hemorrhage, and other intraocular tissue anomalies. B-scan ultrasonography can also be used for the examination of orbital conditions.

PARTIAL COHERENCE INTERFEROMETRY

Partial coherence interferometry (PCI) is a new technique that uses the interference of light to measure axial lengths in the eye.[21,22] It has the potential to achieve measurements ten times as precise as ultrasound. Currently, the Zeiss IOLMaster is the only commercially made pachometer that uses this technology.

Figure 5.19 shows a simplified diagram of PCI. Infrared light from a superluminescent diode is directed through an interferometer. A Fabry Perot interferometer consisting of two parallel, partially transmitting mirrors is used as a simple example. As such, one component of the IR beam goes directly through the two mirrors without reflection. The other component is reflected twice by the two mirrors before it rejoins the direct component. Thus, the reflected component of the beam travels an additional distance that is twice the separation (d) between the two mirrors, and depending on whether the two waves recombine in or out of phase, they have the potential to produce interference fringes. This is similar to the situation in which thin films can produce interference fringes (as described in Chapter 2). However, with a diode light source the difference in distances traveled exceeds the difference in distance over which the light remains coherent (only about 9 μm) so interference fringes *are not* seen.

After leaving the interferometer, the two components of the beam are directed into the eye along its optical axis. Within the eye there is partial reflection off of every refractive surface. Then, if the difference in the *total* number of wavelengths traveled by the two components after going through *both* the interferometer and the eye is less than the number of wavelengths in the coherence length of the light, interference fringes *can be* produced.

The difference in the number of wavelengths between the two beam components that is due to the interferometer equals $2d/\lambda$ (the distance in a round trip between the two mirrors divided by the wavelength of the light in air). However, the difference in the number of wavelengths between the beam components that are reflected off axially separated surfaces within the eye will be greater than the number of wavelengths in the axial thickness (t) of the cornea. The component of the beam that reflects off the posterior cornea will travel $2t$ farther than the component that reflects off the anterior cornea. Since the light that reflects off the posterior cornea encounters the corneal refractive index (n) during its passage, the wavelengths are shortened to $\lambda_n - \lambda/n$, so there are $2nt/\lambda$ wavelengths contained in a round trip through the cornea. The reflected light exiting the cornea rejoins the component reflected from the anterior cornea and is directed by a partially reflecting mirror into a device that can detect the presence of fringes. If the separation of the interferometer

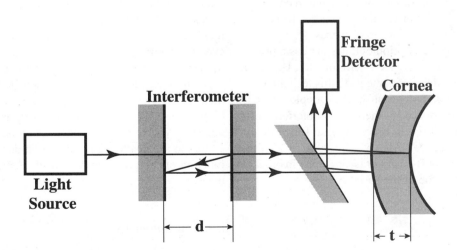

Figure 5.19. A light beam from a diode is directed through an interferometer in order to divide the beam into two coaxial but phase-shifted components. Since the light has a short coherence length no interference fringes result. However, if the beams in being reflected from the anterior and posterior cornea receive an opposite phase shift, the phase shift induced by the interferometer will be nullified and interference fringes will result. When fringes are sensed by the fringe detector the thickness (t) of the cornea equals the separation (d) of the interferometer mirrors divided by the refractive index of the cornea. (The diagram shows the beams as laterally separated only for clarity; they actually coincide.)

mirrors equals the thickness of the cornea times n, then the beam that goes directly through the interferometer and reflects off the back of the cornea will contain the same number of wavelengths as the beam that reflects twice in the interferometer and then reflects off the anterior cornea. Thus, if interference fringes are produced, the corneal thickness can be determined as $t = d/n$ to within an accuracy of plus or minus the coherence length of the light. This is the reason that *partially* coherent light is used. It has a short coherence length, which is necessary for accuracy.

One of the interferometer mirrors is moved to change d between the two mirrors over a continuous range. Then, every time the difference in wavelengths traveled by the two beams in the interferometer matches the difference in the number of wavelengths due to reflection off any two surfaces in the eye (to within the number of wavelengths in the coherence length), interference fringes will be produced as the changing d makes the waves go in and out of phase.

What is really measured is the number of *wavelengths* contained within the axial lengths that separate the different surfaces. Thus, partial coherence interferometry suffers from the same problem as ultrasound. Just as the velocities of the various ocular media in the eye must be assumed in ultrasound in order to convert echo times to distances, the refractive indexes of the various ocular media must be assumed in interferometry in order to convert numbers of wavelengths to distances.

The above description outlines the basic principles of partial coherence interferometry. However, in actual practice, refinements to this technique are usually added. For instance, the Doppler shift in wavelength induced by the moving interferometer mirror can be used in order to make fringe detection more practical. Also, it is feasible to scan the beam much like B-scan ultrasonography in order to generate a profile of the surfaces.

PUPILLOMETRY

Pupillometry is the measurement of the apparent pupil diameter. This is a measure of the image (the entrance pupil) of the anatomical pupil as seen through the cornea, which functions as a magnifying lens, not of the anatomical pupil itself. The apparent pupil is about 12% larger and 0.5 mm closer to the cornea than the anatomical pupil is. Pupil diameter is important in the optical performance of the eye in that increases in pupil size result in greater retinal illumination, allow greater aberration effects, and decrease the depth of field. Very small pupil diameters reduce retinal image quality as a result of diffraction effects. Measurements of pupil diameter are used clinically because differences in pupil size between the two eyes or anomalies in the pupil reaction to light or accommodation can be signs of ocular or neurological disease. There are also various research applications for pupil diameter data, such as the use of pupil diameter as an indicator of mood or alertness. A variety of methods are available for the measurement of pupil diameter.[23]

We can roughly divide these methods into two categories: simple methods and methods using instrumentation.

Simple Methods

Pupil diameter measurements can be as simple as holding a ruler in front of the pupil. A common method for a quick clinical estimate of pupil diameter is to compare the pupil in question to a series of black half-circles on a ruler. The Broca's pupillometer method, which employs two pinholes, is a means by which one can measure one's own pupil diameter. When two pinholes are held close to the eye, they form blur circles on the retina. The edges of the two blur circles appear to just touch when the separation of the two pinholes equals the pupil diameter. Doubling methods, such as with a biprism, use the same principle to measure pupil diameter. When the edges of images doubled with a biprism are just touching, the pupil diameter is a function of the prism power and its distance from the eye.

Instrumentation Methods

Pupil diameter can be measured on photographs. When infrared, rather than visible light, is used, activation of the pupillary light reflex can be avoided. There are some commercial systems that video record the pupil in infrared and feed the image into a computer for analysis. Other methods simply record the amount of light reflected from the iris. Both visible light and infrared are reflected from the iris but transmitted through the pupil. Some systems use this fact in deriving pupil diameter from the amount of a broad beam of infrared being reflected or by monitoring whether a small infrared beam scanned across the pupil and iris is reflected.

APPENDIX 5.1

CALCULATION OF THE CRYSTALLINE LENS RADII OF CURVATURE, USING THE MAGNIFICATIONS OF THE PURKINJE IMAGES IN THE GULLSTRAND-EMSLEY SCHEMATIC EYE AS THE SIZE OF THE PURKINJE IMAGES

These are examples of the calculations done in comparison phakometry.

ANTERIOR CRYSTALLINE LENS RADIUS IN THE GULLSTRAND-EMSLEY SCHEMATIC EYE

The ratio of magnifications of Purkinje images I and III is:

$$\frac{\text{magnification, Purkinje image III}}{\text{magnification, Purkinje image I}}$$

$$= \frac{0.00744}{0.00388} = 1.918$$

Therefore, Purkinje image III is 1.918 times larger than Purkinje image I. The radius of curvature of the cornea is 7.8 mm, so the apparent radius of curvature of the anterior crystalline lens surface is:

$$\text{apparent radius,}_{\text{anterior lens}} = \frac{(\text{size, Purkinje image III})}{(\text{radius, cornea})}{\text{size, Purkinje image I}}$$

$$= (1.918)(7.8 \text{ mm})$$

$$= 14.96 \text{ mm}$$

The apparent radius of curvature of the anterior crystalline lens surface is the distance from the image of the anterior lens surface to the theoretical image of the center of curvature of the anterior lens surface. To find the true radius, it is necessary to follow these steps:

1. Find the location of the image of the anterior lens surface.
2. Find the location of the image of the anterior lens center of curvature.
3. Find the location of the center of curvature.
4. Determine the distance from the center of curvature to the anterior lens surface.

These steps are listed in Table 5.1.

Table 5.1. Steps in Calculation of the Radius of Curvature of the Anterior Surface of the Lens

known from ultrasound: $\overline{A_{1C}A_{1L}}$

known from phakometry photo: $\overline{A_{1L}'C_{1L}'}$ (apparent radius of curvature)

Calculate:

1. $\overline{A_{1L}A_{1L}'}$ (location of the image of the anterior lens surface)
2. $\overline{A_{1C}C_{1L}'}$ (location of the image of the anterior lens center of curvature)
3. $\overline{A_{1C}C_{1L}}$ (location of the anterior lens center of curvature)
4. $\overline{A_{1L}C_{1L}}$ (radius of curvature)

The anterior lens surface is 3.6 mm behind the cornea, so the location of its image is 3.053 mm behind the cornea:

$$L = \frac{n}{\ell} = \frac{1.333}{-0.0036 \text{ m}}$$

$$L = -370.278 \text{ D}$$

$$L' = L_1 + F$$

$$L' = -370.278 \text{ D} + 42.735 \text{ D}$$

$$L' = -327.543 \text{ D}$$

$$\ell' = \frac{1.00}{-327.543} = -0.003053 \text{ m}$$

$$\ell' = -3.053 \text{ mm}$$

The apparent anterior lens radius of curvature is 14.96 mm. The image of the anterior lens surface is 3.053 mm behind the cornea. Therefore, the distance from the cornea to the theoretical image of the anterior lens center of curvature is 18.013 mm:

$$\overline{A_C C_{1L}'} = \overline{A_C A_{1L}'} + \overline{A_{1L}'C_{1L}'}$$

$$= 3.053 \text{ mm} + 14.96 \text{ mm}$$

$$= 18.013 \text{ mm}$$

By the principle of reversibility of light paths, this distance can be used as an object distance for refraction at the cornea in order to find the location of the anterior lens center of curvature. (The principle of reversibility of light paths allows a convenience in calculation. For light being reversed theoretically to go in the opposite direction, image space becomes object space, and object space becomes image space. Image distance is known.

With the direction of light reversed, it becomes the object distance. The calculated image distance is the actual object distance. The alternative way of calculating object distance would be to work through the vergence problem backwards from image distance to object distance.)

$$L = \frac{1.00}{+0.018013 \text{ m}}$$

$$L = +55.515 \text{ D}$$

$$L' = +55.515 \text{ D} + 42.735 \text{ D}$$

$$L' = +98.25 \text{ D}$$

$$\ell' = \frac{1.333}{+98.25}$$

$$\ell' = +0.0136 \text{ m}$$

$$\ell' = 13.6 \text{ mm}$$

The anterior lens center of curvature is 13.6 mm from the cornea, and the anterior lens surface is 3.6 mm from the cornea, so the anterior lens radius of curvature is:

$$\text{radius of curvature} = \overline{A_{1L}C_{1L}}$$
$$= \overline{A_{C}C_{1L}} - \overline{A_{C}A_{1L}}$$
$$= 13.6 \text{ mm} - 3.6 \text{ mm}$$
$$= 10.0 \text{ mm}$$

POSTERIOR CRYSTALLINE LENS RADIUS IN THE GULLSTRAND-EMSLEY SCHEMATIC EYE

The ratio of magnifications of Purkinje images I and IV in the Gullstrand-Emsley schematic eye is:

$$\frac{\text{magnification, Purkinje image IV}}{\text{magnification, Purkinje image I}}$$
$$= \frac{-0.00287}{0.00388} = -0.7397$$

Therefore, if phakometry photographs were taken of this schematic eye, the size of Purkinje image IV would be 74% of that of Purkinje image I. The radius of curvature of the cornea is 7.8 mm, so the apparent radius of curvature of the posterior lens surface is:

$$\begin{array}{l} \text{apparent radius,} \\ \text{posterior lens} \end{array} = \frac{\begin{array}{c} \text{(size, Purkinje image IV)} \\ \text{(radius, cornea)} \end{array}}{\text{size, Purkinje image I}}$$

$$= (-0.7397)(7.8 \text{ mm})$$

$$= -5.77 \text{ mm}$$

The apparent radius is the distance from the image of the posterior lens surface to the theoretical image of the center of curvature of the posterior lens surface. Determining the actual radius of curvature requires:

1. Finding the location of the image of the posterior crystalline lens surface.
2. Finding the location of the image of the posterior lens center of curvature.
3. Finding the location of the center of curvature.
4. Finding the distance from the posterior lens center of curvature to the posterior lens surface.

These steps are summarized in Table 5.2.

Table 5.2. Steps in Calculation of the Radius of Curvature of the Posterior Surface of the Lens

known from ultrasound: $\overline{A_{1C}A_{2L}}$

known from phakometry photo: $\overline{A_{2L}{}'C_{2L}{}'}$ (apparent radius of curvature)

Calculate:
1. $\overline{A_{1C}A_{2L}{}'}$ (location of the image of the posterior lens surface)
2. $\overline{A_{1C}C_{2L}{}'}$ (location of the image of the posterior lens center of curvature)
3. $\overline{A_{1C}C_{2L}}$ (location of the posterior lens center of curvature)
4. $\overline{A_{2L}C_{2L}}$ (radius of curvature)

The posterior surface of the crystalline lens is 3.6 mm behind its anterior surface, which in turn is 3.6 mm behind the cornea. The image of the posterior lens surface is found as follows:

$$L_1 = \frac{n_{lens}}{\ell_1} = \frac{1.416}{-0.0036 \text{ m}} = -393.33 \text{ D}$$

$$L_1' = L_1 + F_{1L}$$

$$L_1' = -393.33 \text{ D} + 8.3 \text{ D}$$

$$L_1' = -385.03 \text{ D}$$

$$\ell_1' = \frac{n_{aqueous}}{L'} = \frac{1.333}{-385.03}$$

$$\ell_1' = -0.0034621 \text{ m}$$

$$\ell_2 = \ell_1' + A_C A_{1L}$$

$$\ell_2 = -0.0034621 \text{ m} + (-0.0036 \text{ m})$$

$$\ell_2 = -0.0070621 \text{ m}$$

$$L_2 = \frac{n_{aqueous}}{\ell_2} = \frac{1.333}{-0.0070621 \text{ m}}$$

$$L_2 = -188.755 \text{ D}$$

$$L_2' = L_2 + F_C$$

$$L_2' = -188.755 + 42.735 \text{ D}$$

$$L_2' = -146.02 \text{ D}$$

$$\ell_2' = \frac{n_{air}}{L_2'} = \frac{1.00}{-146.02 \text{ D}}$$

$$\ell_2' = -0.006848 \text{ m}$$

$$\ell_2' = -6.848 \text{ mm}$$

The image of the posterior crystalline lens surface is 6.848 mm behind the cornea. The apparent radius of curvature of the posterior lens is 5.77 mm. So we can find the location of the image of posterior lens center of curvature as follows:

$$\overline{A_C C_{2L}'} = \overline{A_C A_{2L}'} - \overline{A_{2L}' C_{2L}'}$$
$$= 6.848 \text{ mm} - 5.77 \text{ mm}$$
$$= 1.078 \text{ mm}$$

The theoretical image of the posterior lens center of curvature is 1.078 mm behind the cornea. By the principle of reversibility, the posterior lens center of curvature location can be found by treating its image as an object with refraction at the cornea, and then refraction at the anterior lens surface:

$$L_1 = \frac{n_{air}}{\ell_1} = \frac{1.00}{+0.001078 \text{ m}}$$

$$L_1 = +927.644 \text{ D}$$

$$L_1' = L_1 + F_C$$

$$L_1' = +927.644 \text{ D} + 42.735 \text{ D}$$

$$L_1' = +970.379 \text{ D}$$

$$\ell' = \frac{n_{aqueous}}{L_1'} = \frac{1.333}{+970.379 \text{ D}}$$

$$\ell' = +0.001374 \text{ m}$$

$$\ell_2 = +0.001374 \text{ m} - 0.0036 \text{ m}$$

$$\ell_2 = -0.002226 \text{ m}$$

$$L_2 = \frac{n_{aqueous}}{\ell_2} = \frac{1.333}{-0.002226 \text{ m}}$$

$$L_2 = -598.749 \text{ D}$$

$$L_2' = L_2 + F_{1L}$$

$$L_2' = -598.749 \text{ D} + 8.3 \text{ D}$$

$$L_2' = -590.449 \text{ D}$$

$$\ell_2' = \frac{n_{lens}}{L_2'} = \frac{1.416}{-590.449 \text{ D}}$$

$$\ell_2' = -0.0024 \text{ m}$$

$$\ell_2' = -2.4 \text{ mm}$$

The center of curvature of the posterior lens surface is 2.4 mm in front of the anterior lens surface. The lens thickness is 3.6 mm, so the radius of curvature of the posterior lens surface is:

$$\text{radius, posterior lens} = \overline{A_{2L} C_{2L}}$$
$$= \overline{A_{1L} C_{2L}} - \overline{A_{1L} A_L}$$
$$= -2.4 \text{ mm} - 3.6 \text{ mm}$$
$$= -6.0 \text{ mm}$$

REFERENCES

1. Mandell RB. Jesse Ramsden: inventor of the ophthalmometer. *Am J Optom Arch Am Acad Optom.* 1960;37:633–638.
2. Henson DB. *Optometric Instrumentation.* 2nd ed. Oxford: Butterworth-Heinemann, 1996;107–120.
3. Erickson P. Optical components contributing to refractive anomalies. In: T Grosvenor, MC Flom, eds. *Refractive Anomalies: Research and Clinical Applications.* Boston: Butterworth-Heinemann, 1991;199–218.
4. Grosvenor T, Quintero S, Perrigin DM. Predicting refractive astigmatism: a suggested simplification of Javal's rule. *Am J Optom Physiol Opt.* 1988;65:292–297.
5. Levene JR. The true inventors of the keratoscope and photo-keratoscope. *Brit J Hist Sci.* 1965;2:324–342.
6. Salmon TO, Horner DG. Comparison of elevation, curvature, and power descriptors for corneal topographic mapping. *Optom Vis Sci.* 1995;72:800–808.
7. Lindsay R, Smith G, Atchison D. Descriptors of corneal shape. *Optom Vis Sci.* 1998;75:156–158.
8. Guillon M, Lydon DPM, Wilson C. Corneal topography: a clinical model. *Ophthalm Physiol Opt.* 1986;6:47–56.
9. Douthwaite WA. *Contact Lens Optics and Lens Design.* 2nd ed. Oxford: Butterworth-Heinemann, 1995;119–122.
10. Henson DB. *Optometric Instrumentation.* 2nd ed. Oxford: Butterworth-Heinemann, 1996;150–153.
11. Duke-Elder S, Abrams D. Ophthalmic optics and refraction. In: S Duke-Elder, ed. *System of Ophthalmology, 5.* St. Louis: Mosby, 1970;102–106.
12. Bennett AG, Rabbetts RB. *Clinical Visual Optics.* 2nd ed. London: Butterworth-Heinemann, 1989;477–480.
13. Ludlam WM, Wittenberg S, Rosenthal J. Measurements of the ocular dioptric elements utilizing photographic methods. Part I. Errors analysis of Sorsby's photographic ophthalmophakometry. *Am J Optom Arch Am Acad Optom.* 1965;42:394–416.
14. Tscherning M. *Physiological Optics: Dioptrics of the Eye, Functions of the Retina, Ocular Movements and Binocular Vision.* Philadelphia: Keystone, 1920;50–56, 77–87.
15. Van Veen HG, Goss DA. A simplified method of Purkinje image photography for phakometry. *Am J Optom Physiol Opt.* 1988;65:905–908.
16. Mutti DO, Zadnik K, Adams AJ. A video technique for phakometry of the human crystalline lens. *Invest Ophthalmol Vis Sci.* 1992;33:1771–1782.
17. Yost WA, Nielsen DW. *Fundamentals of Hearing: An Introduction.* New York: Holt, Rinehart, & Winston, 1977;129–141.
18. Lizzi FL, Feleppa EJ. Practical physics and electronics of ultrasound. In: RL Dallow, ed. *Ophthalmic Ultrasonography: Comparative Techniques. International Ophthalmology Clinics.* Boston: Little, Brown, 1979; 19(4):35–63.
19. Thornton SP, Gardner SK, Waring GO III. Surgical instruments used in refractive keratotomy. In: GO Waring III, ed. *Refractive Keratotomy for Myopia and Astigmatism.* St. Louis: Mosby Year Book, 1992; 407–489.
20. Coleman DJ. Ultrasonic measurement of eye dimensions. In: RL Dallow, ed. *Ophthalmic Ultrasonography: Comparative Techniques. International Ophthalmology Clinics.* Boston: Little, Brown, 1979;19(4):225–236.
21. Hitzenberger CK. Optical measurement of the axial length by laser Doppler interferometry. *Invest Ophthalmol Vis Sci.* 1991;32:616–624.
22. Drexler W, Baumgartner A, Findl O, Hitzenberger CK, Sattman H, Fercher AF. Submicrometer precision biometry of the anterior segment of the human eye. *Invest Ophthalmol Vis Sci.* 1997;38:1304–1313.
23. Henson DB. Optical methods for measurement of the ocular parameters. In: WN Charman, ed. *Visual Optics and Instrumentation.* Vol. 1 of J Cronly-Dillon, ed. *Vision and Visual Dysfunction.* Boca Raton, FL: CRC Press, 1991;371–398.

FURTHER READING

Byrne SF, Green RL. *Ultrasound of the Eye and Orbit.* St. Louis: Mosby Year Book, 1992.

Goss DA, Eskridge JB. Keratometry. In: JB Eskridge, JF Amos, JD Bartlett, eds. *Clinical Procedures in Optometry.* Philadelphia: Saunders, 1991;135–154.

Horner DG, Salmon TO, Soni PS. Corneal topography. In: WJ Benjamin, ed. *Borish's Clinical Refraction.* Philadelphia: Saunders, 1998;524–558.

Chapter 6
Optics of Refractive Error Management

. . . when spectacles are used to correct the defects of nature, they do this only by converging the rays which have been spread out or by spreading the rays which are too closely assembled: and experience shows that convex lenses will correct the error of long-sightedness and concave lenses that of short-sightedness. It follows therefore that, in the case of those who are troubled with too long vision, the visual rays ought to be gathered together: while, in the short-sighted, they should be spread apart —Francesco Maurolico, 1554 (From Maurolico F. Photismi de Lumine. transl H Crew. New York: Macmillan, 1940;117–118.)

The glasses needed for this kind of vision [nearsightedness] to enable it to extend out and see from afar have to be more or less concave according to the distance of clear vision. . . . —Benito Daza de Valdes, 1623 (From Daza de Valdes B. *Uso de los Antoios.* libro 1, chapter 6, transl O Pikaza, L Arista, HW Hofstetter. Typescript translation available at the International Library, Archives, and Museum of Optometry, St. Louis.)

In this chapter we examine the basic optics of refractive error and its correction. Clinicians can manage refractive errors in three ways:

1. Lens correction, which uses the placement of spectacle lenses or contact lenses before the eye to provide a clear image on the retina.
2. Developmental control, which uses treatments in an attempt to slow the progression of refractive error (most often myopia).
3. Refractive surgery, which reshapes or adds material to the eye in order to change its power.

To achieve a clear retinal image, there must be a proper match between the dioptric powers of the refractive components of the eye and their axial separations. Eyes that do not have this proper match when distant objects are being viewed are said to have *ametropia*. The amount of ametropia is referred to as *refractive error*, which is the lens power needed to restore focus of parallel rays on the retina when accommodation is relaxed. Eyes that do have the proper match of refractive power and axial length are said to have *emmetropia* and have a refractive error equal to zero, often denoted plano, or pl. Ametropia is divided into three basic categories: myopia (nearsightedness), hyperopia (farsightedness), and astigmatism.

MYOPIA

Myopia is the ametropia in which parallel object rays focus in front of the retina when accommodation is zero diopters; in other words, the second focal point of the eye is in front of the retina. The eye would need either to be shorter or its equivalent power less to have focus on the retina. It is impractical to change the length of the eye, but the effective power of the eye is easily changed by adding lenses. In the example in Figure 6.1, the second focal point is 22.0 mm behind the second principal plane.

Assuming the index of refraction of the vitreous is that for the Gullstrand-Emsley schematic eye, the equivalent power of the eye is:

$$F_e = n'/f' = 1.333/0.022 \text{ m} = +60.59 \text{ D}$$

The distance from the second principal plane to the retina is 22.56 mm. The vergence of light leaving the second principal plane that would result in focus on the retina is:

$$L' = n'/\ell' = 1.333/0.02256 \text{ m} = +59.09 \text{ D}$$

Thus, the eye is too strong to result in focus on the retina and its power would have to be reduced by the amount that F_e is greater than L'. This difference is the refractive error of the eye (RE) at the

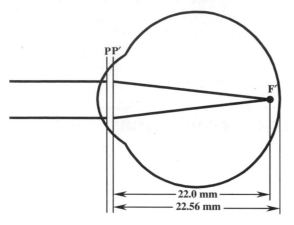

Figure 6.1. An example of an eye with myopia. The second focal point, F', of the eye is in front of the retina. The second focal length is 22.0 mm. The distance from the second principal plane (P') to the retina is 22.56 mm.

were -1.50 D at the first principal plane. This occurs when a real object is -66.7 cm in front of the first principal plane:

$$\ell = n/L = 1.00/-1.50 \text{ D} = -0.667 \text{ m}$$

This example is illustrated in Figure 6.2. The point that is conjugate with the retina when accommodation is relaxed is called the *punctum remotum* (-66.7 cm from the first principal plane in the above example).

The punctum remotum is also known as the far point of accommodation. A person with myopia can readily find his or her punctum remotum by noting the farthest point at which objects can be seen clearly. This is why myopia is commonly known as nearsightedness; near objects can be seen clearly, but distant objects appear blurry.

second principal plane, so RE $= L' - F_e$. In the above example this is:

$$\text{RE} = +59.09 \text{ D} - (+60.59 \text{ D}) = -1.50 \text{ D}$$

In myopia, refractive error is negative in sign. In order for light to be focused on the retina, a minus power lens would need to be used or light with a negative vergence (divergent light) would need to strike the eye. In the preceding case, where the refractive error is -1.50 D, light would be focused on the retina if the vergence of light striking the eye

HYPEROPIA

Hyperopia is the ametropia in which parallel rays from a distant object focus behind the retina when accommodation is zero diopters; that is, the second focal point of the eye is behind the retina. The eye would need to be longer or its equivalent power greater for focus on the retina. Figure 6.3 shows an example of an eye with hyperopia.

With a second focal length of 22.4 mm, the equivalent power of the eye is:

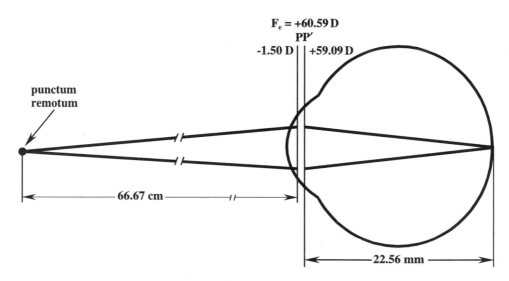

Figure 6.2. The punctum remotum for the eye illustrated in Figure 6.1 is 66.6 cm from the eye. Light from the punctum remotum will have a vergence of -1.50 D. After refraction by the eye (equivalent power $= +60.59$ D), the vergence of light will be $+59.09$ D. This will result in focus on the retina.

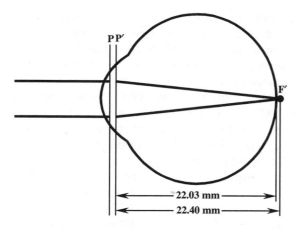

Figure 6.3. An example of an eye with hyperopia. The second focal point (F') of the eye is behind the retina. The second focal length is 22.40 mm. The distance from the second principal plane (P') to the retina is 22.03 mm.

In hyperopia refractive error is positive in sign. That means that for light to be focused on the retina, either a plus power lens would need to be placed in front of the eye or the eye must change its effective power by accommodating. In this example where the refractive error is +1.00 D, the location of the punctum remotum is:

$$\ell = n/L = 1.00/+1.00 = +1.00 \text{ m}$$

The distance of the punctum remotum is +1.00 m from the first principal plane of the eye. The positive sign means that the punctum remotum is located to the right in the diagram in Figure 6.4.

Because this is a virtual object behind the eye, a person with hyperopia cannot use any real object in front of the eye to locate the punctum remotum, as a person with myopia can do.

$$F_e = n'/f' = 1.333/0.0224 \text{ m} = +59.51 \text{ D}$$

The distance from the second principal plane to the retina is 22.03 mm. The vergence of light after refraction by the eye that would yield focus on the retina would be:

$$L' = n'/\ell' = 1.333/0.2203 \text{ m} = +60.51 \text{ D}$$

The refractive error of this eye at the second principal plane is:

$$RE = +60.51 \text{ D} - (+59.51 \text{ D}) = +1.00 \text{ D}$$

ASTIGMATISM

Astigmatism is an ametropia in which there is no point focus anywhere along the optical axis. This refractive error is referred to as axial astigmatism (or simply astigmatism) since, unlike the oblique astigmatism discussed in Chapter 1, it occurs for axial objects. Image formation due to axial astigmatism is similar in appearance to the image formation due to oblique astigmatism. In both types of astigmatism there is an interval of Sturm, which separates two

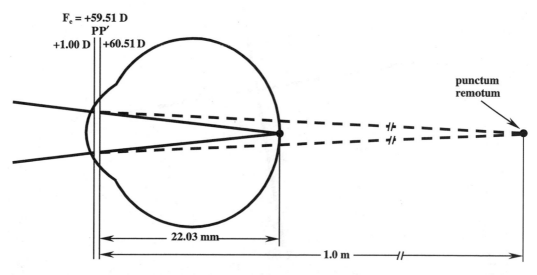

Figure 6.4. The punctum remotum for the hyperopic eye illustrated in Figure 6.3 is 1 m behind the eye. Light striking the eye has a vergence of +1.00 D. After refraction by the eye (equivalent power = +59.51 D), the vergence of light of +60.51 D yields focus on the retina.

line foci that correspond to the principal meridians, and a circle of least confusion within the interval of Sturm. If only spherical lenses were used to correct the astigmatic eye, the best image would be obtained by placing the circle of least confusion on the retina, but even then it would appear blurred in proportion to the amount of astigmatism.

Axial astigmatism occurs when the eye has different refractive powers in different meridians. The two meridians that have the most and least power are referred to as principal meridians, and when 90 degrees apart the astigmatism is said to be regular. In eyes with regular astigmatism, the difference in refractive error between a principal meridian and any other meridian varies as $A \sin^2 \theta$, where A is the total astigmatism and θ is the angle between the two meridians.

One form of graphical notation for refractive error in astigmatism is the optical cross. The optical cross is a simple diagrammatic representation of the two principal meridians drawn with their orientations corresponding to that of the eye as seen from the front. Figure 6.5 shows an optical cross.

The usual notation for refractive error in astigmatism is generally known as the spherocylindrical lens formula. It is not actually a formula, but rather a notation for astigmatic refractive errors which consists of three numbers that correspond respectively to sphere power, cylinder power, and axis (e.g., –2.00 –3.00 x 80). The sphere in the spherocylindrical lens formula is the refractive error in the principal meridian that is specified to be the axis. This can be the refractive error in either of the principal meridians; however, the sign of the cylinder depends on which meridian is chosen. The cylinder is the difference between the powers in the axis meridian and the meridian 90° away from the axis meridian. The angle of the axis is set apart from the cylinder by an x. When the cylinder is a negative number, the notation is said to be in minus cylinder form. When the cylinder is a positive number, the notation is in plus cylinder form. For example, taking the data from the optical cross in Figure 6.5, the refractive error in minus cylinder form is –2.00 –3.00 x 80, and in plus cylinder form it is –5.00 +3.00 x 170.

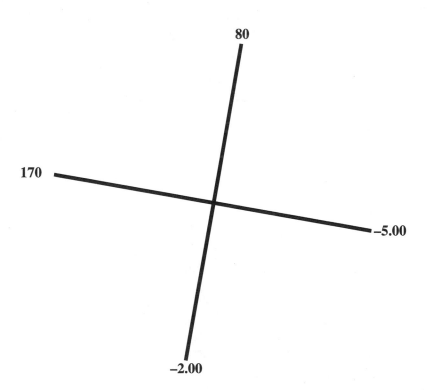

Figure 6.5. The optical cross is a diagram of refractive error in astigmatism that shows the locations of the principal meridians oriented in the same way as the examiner facing the patient as well as the refractive errors in those meridians. In this example, the refractive error in the 80 meridian is –2.00 D and the refractive error in the 170 meridian is –5.00 D.

Another term used in relation to astigmatism is *spherical equivalent*. The spherical equivalent is the average of the refractive errors in the two principal meridians of a spherocylindrical lens. This spherical lens power would place the circle of least confusion on the retina and produce the clearest retinal image possible without correction of the astigmatism. The spherocylindrical lens formula can be used to determine the spherical equivalent by adding the sphere and half the cylinder. For example, the spherical equivalent of the refractive error in Figure 6.5 is –3.50 D.

Classifications of Astigmatism

Astigmatism can be classified by the location of the meridians of maximum and minimum power. The categories in this classification are with-the-rule, against-the-rule, and oblique.

With-the-rule astigmatism is astigmatism in which the most hyperopic or least myopic meridian is within 30 degrees of the horizontal. If the spherocylindrical lens formula is written in minus cylinder form, the axis meridian is the 180 or within 30 degrees of 180 (that is, between 0 and 30 or between 150 and 180).

Against-the-rule astigmatism is astigmatism in which the most hyperopic or least myopic meridian is within 30 degrees of vertical. Using minus cylinder form, the axis meridian is between 60 and 120.

Oblique astigmatism is astigmatism in which one principal meridian is greater than 30 but less than 60 and the other principal meridian is greater than 120 but less than 150.

Astigmatism can also be classified according to where the focal lines at the two ends of the interval of Sturm are located relative to the retina. The categories in this classification are compound myopic, simple myopic, mixed, simple hyperopic, and compound hyperopic astigmatism.

Compound myopic astigmatism is astigmatism in which all meridians are myopic. The entire interval of Sturm is in front of the retina.

Simple myopic astigmatism is astigmatism in which one principal meridian is emmetropic and the other is myopic. In other words, one end of the interval of Sturm is on the retina and the rest of it extends in front of the retina.

Mixed astigmatism is astigmatism in which one principal meridian is myopic and the other principal meridian is hyperopic. The interval of Sturm extends from in front of the retina to behind the retina.

Simple hyperopic astigmatism is astigmatism in which one principal meridian is emmetropic and the other is hyperopic. One end of the interval of Sturm is on the retina and the rest of it is behind the retina.

Compound hyperopic astigmatism is astigmatism in which all meridians are hyperopic. The entire interval of Sturm is behind the retina.

Examples

1. A refractive error of pl –1.00 x 180 would be classified as simple myopic astigmatism and with-the-rule astigmatism. The spherical equivalent is –0.50 D.
2. A refractive error of –1.50 D in the 50 and +2.00 D in the 140 can be written in minus cylinder form as +2.00 –3.50 x 140, or in plus cylinder form as –1.50 +3.50 x 50. It would be classified as mixed astigmatism and oblique astigmatism. The spherical equivalent is +0.25 D.
3. A refractive error of +1.00 –0.50 x 75 can be classified as compound hyperopic astigmatism and against-the-rule astigmatism. The spherical equivalent is +0.75 D.

LENS EFFECTIVITY

Contact Lenses

One way to focus light on the retina of a myopic eye, which has relaxed accommodation, is to place the object at the punctum remotum. Another way is to leave the object in the distance, but place a thin lens (a contact lens) on the cornea, which has the proper power to change the zero vergence of the light from the distant object to the vergence of an object at the punctum remotum. For example, in a myopic eye with a punctum remotum –25 cm from the anterior surface of the cornea, light from the punctum remotum will have a vergence of –4.00 D in the plane of the cornea:

$$L = n/\ell = 1.00/{-0.25} \text{ m}$$

$$L = -4.00 \text{ D}$$

For a hyperopic eye, a physically real object cannot be placed at the punctum remotum because this point is located behind the cornea. However, a plus contact lens on the eye which has the proper power can change the zero vergence of light from a distant object so that rays enter the eye in the direction of the punctum remotum. For example, with a punctum remotum +25 cm behind the anterior surface of the cornea, the corneal plane refractive error will be +4.00 D:

$$L = n/\ell = 1.00/+0.25 \text{ m}$$

$$L = +4.00 \text{ D}$$

This is known as the corneal plane refractive error because it is the power that a thin lens must have to correct the eye if it is placed on the cornea. For thin contact lenses, we can conceive this as adding power to the cornea for the hyperopic eye or subtracting power from cornea for the myopic eye in order to make the eyes the equivalent of emmetropic. However, when the lenses are thick or are displaced from the cornea the powers must be calculated differently.

Spectacle Lenses

Let's return for a moment to the myopic eye with the punctum remotum –25 cm from the anterior surface of the cornea. Focus on the retina is achieved when light has a vergence of –4.00 D at the anterior corneal surface. The necessary power for a contact lens to change the zero vergence of light from a distant object to –4.00 *is* –4.00 D. Therefore, the second focal point of the contact lens was coincident with the punctum remotum. For this contact lens, the second focal length is –25 cm:

$$f_c' = n'/F = 1.00/-4.00 \text{ D}$$

$$f_c' = -0.25 \text{ m}$$

We can also correct this eye with a spectacle lens whose second focal point is coincident with the punctum remotum. However, since a spectacle lens will have a different distance from the punctum remotum than a contact lens will, its necessary focal length, and therefore power, will be different. If a spectacle lens is placed 15 mm in front of the eye, its distance from the punctum remotum and, thus, the second focal length (f_s') will need to be –23.5 cm:

$$f_s' = f_c' - d = -25 \text{ cm} - (-1.5 \text{ cm})$$

$$f_s' = -23.5 \text{ cm}$$

The power of that spectacle lens therefore would be:

$$F = n/f_s' = 1.00/-0.235 \text{ m}$$

$$F = -4.26 \text{ D}$$

This is the spectacle plane refractive error of that eye for a spectacle plane placement 15 mm from the anterior corneal surface. If we instead placed the correcting spectacle lens 12 mm from the cornea, its power (and the 12-mm spectacle plane refractive error) would be –4.20 D:

$$f_s' = f_c' - d = -25 \text{ cm} - (-1.2 \text{ cm}) = -23.8 \text{ cm}$$

$$F = n/f_s' = 1.00/-0.238 \text{ m} = -4.20 \text{ D}$$

This eye could be corrected by many different lenses as long as the lens in question had its second focal point coincident with the punctum remotum (Figure 6.6).

A clear retinal image could even be produced in this eye by a +10 D lens 35 cm from the eye. Readers who have myopia can easily confirm this by holding a +10 D lens 10 cm farther out than the location of their punctum remotum. This is suggested as a demonstration—it is not a practical method of refractive error correction because, for instance, objects will appear upside down!

Now we'll look again at the hyperopic eye with a corneal plane refractive error of +4.00 D. Its punctum remotum was +25 cm behind the anterior corneal surface. If this eye were corrected with a spectacle lens 15 mm from the anterior corneal surface, the power of that spectacle lens would be +3.77 D:

$$f_s' = f_c' - d = +25 \text{ cm} - (-1.5 \text{ cm})$$
$$= +26.5 \text{ cm}$$

$$F = n/f_s' = 1.00/+0.265 \text{ m} = +3.77 \text{ D}$$

From these two examples, we can see that in myopia, corneal plane refractive error is less in magnitude than spectacle plane refractive error. Therefore, to correct a myopic eye, less power is required in a contact lens than in a spectacle lens. In hyperopia, corneal plane refractive error is greater than spectacle plane refractive error. So, to correct a hyperopic eye, more power is required in a contact lens than the spectacle lens.

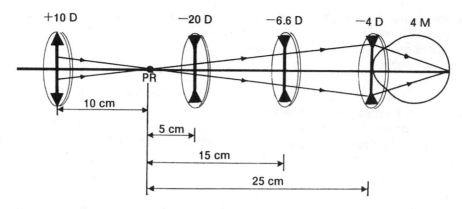

Figure 6.6. Numerous different lenses can correct a refractive error, providing that the second focal point of the lens and the individual's punctum remotum (PR) are coincident. This figure shows some of the possible correcting lenses for an eye with a corneal plane refractive error of –4.00 D. (Reprinted with permission from Michaels DD. *Visual Optics and Refraction: A Clinical Approach.* 2nd ed. St. Louis: Mosby, 1980;221.)

We have so far calculated the power of a correcting lens in a given plane by finding the distance of the plane from the punctum remotum. The following mathematical formula, known as the effective lens formula, avoids the necessity of locating the punctum remotum:

$$F_b = F_a/(1 - dF_a)$$

where F_a is the power of the required lens at the original position, F_b is the power of the lens at the new position, and d is the distance between these two positions as measured in meters. The sign of d will be positive if the lens position is moved toward the eye, and negative if the lens position is moved away from the eye. Because d is multiplied by F_a, the effect of a change in lens position increases as the amount of the refractive error increases. Therefore, an adjustment in lens power in going, say, from a spectacle plane refractive error to a contact lens power is not necessary for low refractive errors of less than about 4.00 D.

The effective power formula can be derived from the relation of the second focal lengths of the lenses at the two positions:

$$f_b' = f_a' - d$$

$$F_b = 1/f_b' = 1/(f_a' - d)$$

$$F_b = \frac{1}{(1/F_a) - d} = \frac{F_a}{1 - dF_a}$$

If we apply the effective power formula to our previous example in which we find the 15-mm

spectacle plane refractive error for an eye with a corneal plane refractive error of –4.00 D, we get –4.26 D, just as before:

$$F_b = F_a/(1 - dF_a)$$

$$F_b = \frac{-4.00 \text{ D}}{1 - (-0.015 \text{ m})(-4.00 \text{ D})}$$

$$F_b = -4.26 \text{ D}$$

Another aspect of lens effectivity is the effect of moving a given lens closer to or farther from the eye. Moving a minus lens farther from the eye will make light less divergent (or more convergent) at the corneal plane. Moving a plus lens farther from the eye will make light more convergent (or less divergent) at the corneal plane. Thus, moving either myopic or hyperopic spectacle lenses farther from the eye will shift their effective power in the plus direction. This is why persons with presbyopia may move their glasses down their nose if their presbyopia is not fully corrected. It is also the reason that myopes who have had increases in their myopia find that they can see distant objects more clearly if they move their lenses closer to their eyes; the effective power shift is in the minus direction.

BACK VERTEX POWER

The position of a spectacle lens is generally expressed as a vertex distance, the distance from the back vertex of the lens to the anterior surface of the cornea. Back vertex focal length is the distance from the back vertex of a lens to its second focal point. Back vertex power is, then, the reciprocal of back vertex focal length:

$$F_v' = 1/f_v'$$

A formula for back vertex power of a lens based on its front surface power (F_1), back surface power (F_2), thickness (d), and index of refraction (n), is as follows:

$$F_v' = \frac{F_1}{1-(d/n)F_1} + F_2$$

The prescription power of both spectacle lenses and contact lenses is specified by back vertex power. The reason that back vertex power is used instead of equivalent power is convenience. The location of the back vertex is directly known, whereas the location of the second principal plane must be calculated. Thus, the use of back vertex focal length (measured from the back vertex) to place the second focal point at the punctum remotum is easier than the use of the second focal length (measured from the second principal plane).

Back vertex power can be modeled by the power of a thin lens that replaces the spectacle lens at its back vertex. If the power of the thin lens is the same as the back vertex power of the replaced spectacle lens, it would have the same second focal point as the spectacle lens and, thus, it would give the same image location for distant objects. Superficially this would seem to be an equivalent lens power, but in reality it would give an accurate image distance only for distant objects. In other words, its power could not be used in the Gauss

equation to find the image locations that correspond to near objects.

SPECTACLE MAGNIFICATION

A spectacle lens in front of an ametropic eye does more than just produce a clear image on the retina. It also changes the size of the clear image compared to the previously blurred image. This is explained by showing that a spectacle lens acts as two Galilean telescopes placed in front of the eye.[1] To understand why this is so, a brief review of Galilean telescopes is given.

Galilean Telescopes

A Galilean telescope in its simplest form consists of two thin lenses, a plus power objective lens and a minus power ocular lens (eyepiece) (Figure 6.7). The objective lens forms an aerial image of a distant object simultaneously at $F_{2(obj)}$ and at $F_{1(oc)}$. Then, the distance (d) between the two lenses equals the focal length of the objective minus the absolute value of the focal length of the ocular. This arrangement is referred to as afocal since parallel light enters and exits the telescope.

$$d = f_{2(obj)} - |f_{2(oc)}|$$

For distant objects the telescopic magnification is:

$$M_{tel} = -\frac{F_{oc}}{F_{obj}} = -\frac{f_{2(obj)}}{f_{2(oc)}}$$

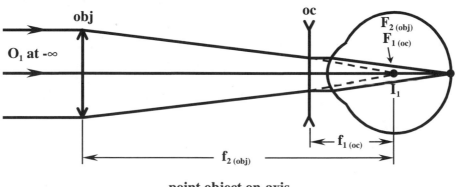

point object on-axis

Figure 6.7. A Galilean telescope set in front of the eye views an object that is on-axis.

Example: A Galilean telescope has a $+0.5$ D objective lens and a -40 D ocular. What is the telescope's length (d) and its magnifying power (M_{tel})?

$$f_{2(obj)} = n/F_{obj} = (1.00/+0.5)(100) = +200 \text{ cm}$$

$$f_{2(oc)} = n/F_{oc} = (1.00/-40)(100) = -2.5 \text{ cm}$$

$$d = f_{2(obj)} - |f_{2(oc)}| = +200 - |-2.5|$$

$$= +197.5 \text{ cm}$$

$$M_{tel} = -(F_{oc}/F_{obj}) = -(-40/+0.5) = +80x \text{ or}$$

$$= -(f_{2(obj)}/f_{2(oc)}) = -(+200/-2.5) = +80x$$

Shape Magnification (M_S)

Since spectacle lenses have a thickness, they form a Galilean telescope in which the front surface is an objective whose power is that of the front surface (F_1) and the back surface power (F_2) is a combination of that of an ocular (F_{oc}) at that location (which produces parallel light) plus a back vertex power (F_V) which is the Rx of the wearer ($F_2 = F_{oc} + F_V$).

For *thin* spectacle lenses, $F_{total} = F_1 + F_2 = F_V$. Also, since spectacle lenses are meniscus, F_1 is plus and F_2 is minus. Then, for a thin spectacle lens, if $F_2 = -F_1$, $F_V = 0$, and this lens would be afocal since, if parallel light enters, parallel light exits, so the Rx would be plano. For thick lenses, however, there is a vergence change over the lens

thickness (t) between the surfaces of power F_1 and F_2 so that for a thick *afocal* lens $F_2 \neq -F_1$.

Example: If $F_1 = +6$ D, $t = 5$ mm ($= 0.005$ m), and $n_2 = 1.50$, what must F_2 be for the thick lens to be afocal? (F_2 will no longer be -6 D since the lens is no longer thin.) (See Figure 6.8.)

$$L_1 + F_1 = L_1'$$

$$0 + (+6) = +6 \text{ D}$$

$$\ell_1' = n_2/L_1' = (1.50/+6)(1000) = +250 \text{ mm}$$

$$\ell_2 = \ell_1' - t = +250 - 5 = +245 \text{ mm}$$

$$L_2 = n_2/\ell_2 = (1.50/+245)(1000) = +6.122 \text{ D}$$
(Vergence has been gained over $F_1 = +6$ D.)

$$L_2 + F_2 = L_2' = 0 \text{ (since an afocal lens is desired)}$$

Therefore, for an afocal lens $F_2 = 0 - (+6.122) = -6.122$ D.

(Note that, unlike for a thin lens, if an afocal thick lens is desired, $F_2 \neq -F_1$.)

This afocal thick lens is a Galilean telescope since F_1 is a plus surface (objective) and F_2 is a more powerful minus surface (ocular). Although the telescope is solid in this case, such a lens can be modeled by two thin lenses of power F_1 and F_2 separated by t/n_2 thickness of air (Figure 6.9).

Then, $M_{tel} = -(F_{oc}/F_{obj})$ applies:

$$M_S = -\frac{F_{oc}}{F_{obj}} = -\frac{-6.122}{+6.00} = +1.02x$$

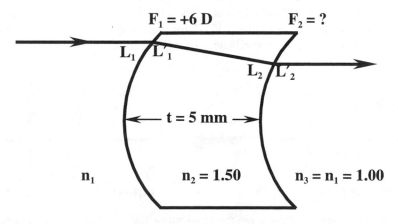

F₁ = +6 D   **F₂ = ?**

L_1 L_1'

L_2 L_2'

$t = 5 \text{ mm}$

n_1 $n_2 = 1.50$ $n_3 = n_1 = 1.00$

Figure 6.8. For a thick spectacle lens to be plano (Rx = 0), the power F_2 of the back surface must differ from the power F_1 of the front surface.

An equivalent equation allows M_{tel} to be found without first finding F_{oc} ($\neq F_2$):

$$M_S = \frac{1}{1 - \left(\dfrac{t}{n}\right)F_1} = \frac{1}{1 - \left(\dfrac{0.005 \text{ m}}{1.50}\right)(+6.00)} = +1.02x$$

There is another equation for spectacle magnification that is even easier to use, but that is only an approximation. It can be shown that $1/(1 - x) \approx 1 + x$ (if $x \ll 1$). Then:

$$M = \frac{1}{1 - dF} \approx 1 + dF$$

Then:

$$M_S \approx 1 + \left(\frac{t}{n}\right)F_1 = 1 + \left(\frac{0.005}{1.50}\right)(+6.00) = 1.02x$$

This thick lens magnification is called *shape magnification* (M_S) because the amount of the magnification depends on the curvature ("shape") of the first surface, which gives F_1 its particular value. An afocal lens can be made from a lens of any F_1 since the last surface F_2 can be made to make L_2' = 0 for $L_1 = 0$.

Spectacle lenses are, of course, usually not afocal. Although $L_1 = 0$ for distance viewing, $L_2' \neq 0$ but has a back vertex power (F_V) equal to the Rx of the wearer. Note, however, that the value of F_2 does not affect M_S since only F_1 is present in the equation.

Power Magnification (MP)

An ametropic eye can be modeled as an emmetropic reduced eye with an additional lens at the cornea that gives the ametropia. For example, if a hyperope is corrected by a +5.00 D spectacle lens placed 12 mm in front of his eye, this could also be corrected by a +5.32 D contact lens at the cornea (due to the difference in effectivity). Then, a +5.00 D spectacle plane refractive error could be simulated by an emmetropic eye fit with a −5.32 D thin contact lens.

This combination of spectacle lens correction and eye can be thought of as a Galilean telescope in which the spectacle lens would be the objective lens (F_{obj} = +5.00 D) and the ametropic component of the eye's power would be the ocular lens (F_{oc} = −5.32 D). Since this forms a telescope, it can be seen that the spectacle lens correction would be expected to change the retinal image size (Figure 6.10).

$$M_{tel} = -\frac{F_{oc}}{F_{obj}} = \frac{-5.32}{+5.00} = +1.064x$$

Thus, the retinal image of the corrected eye would be +6.4% larger than the blurred retinal image in the uncorrected, ametropic eye. This is referred to as *power magnification*.

Since spectacle magnification is based on the comparison of a clear image and a blurred image, the image sizes must be determined by where the *chief ray* strikes the retina. Recall that a chief ray always goes through the center of a blur circle and also goes through the center of the entrance pupil. With the Emsley reduced eye, the EP is at the cornea because this is the only refracting surface, and we are justified in modeling ametropia by a contact lens at the cornea of a reduced eye. However, for real eyes the EP is about 3 mm behind the cornea, so ametropia (F_{am}) would have to be modeled by a lens at the EP plane internally. Then, the distance between the objective (spectacle lens) and ocular (previously a contact lens) is not the vertex distance d, but $d_{EP} \approx d + 3$ mm.

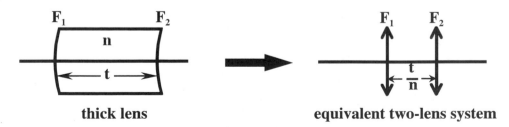

thick lens   **equivalent two-lens system**

Figure 6.9. A single thick lens can be modeled as two thin lenses whose dioptric powers equal the front and back surface powers of the thick lens, but whose separation equals the thickness of the thick lens divided by the refractive index of the thick lens.

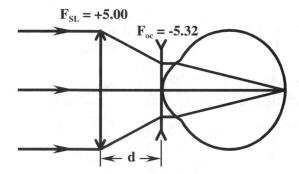

Figure 6.10. An afocal Galilean telescope is placed in front of an emmetropic eye. In this case, it is equivalent to the spectacle lens alone placed in front of a hyperope whose corneal power is 5.32 D too weak.

Example: Given +5 D of hyperopia as measured at the spectacle lens plane 12 mm in front of the cornea, the ametropia could be simulated by a hypothetical minus lens placed at the EP of an emmetropic eye (Figure 6.11).

$$F_{EP} = \frac{n}{f_{EP}} = \frac{1.00}{200 - 15}(1000) = +5.41 \text{ D}$$

This would correct a refractive deficiency of –5.41 D so $F_{oc} = -5.41$ D since F_{oc} is the deficiency. For the resulting telescope magnification:

$$M_P = -\frac{F_{oc}}{F_{obj}} = -\frac{-5.41}{+5.00} = +1.081x$$

For this hyperope, things look +1.081 times as large (8.1% larger) with the spectacles on as with them off. Of course, we are assuming no accommodation, so without the spectacle lens the image would also be blurred.

For myopes, the optics of the eye are too strong and a minus spectacle lens must be used. The model is that of looking through a Galilean telescope in reverse, which gives minification. Looked through in reverse, the minus lens is the objective and the plus lens is the ocular.

Example: Given –5.00 D of myopia as measured at the spectacle lens plane 12 mm in front of the cornea, the ametropia could be simulated by a hypothetical *plus* lens placed at the entrance pupil (EP) of an emmetropic eye (Figure 6.12).

$$F_{SL} = -5.00 \text{ D}, F_{EP} = \frac{1.00}{(-200 - 15)}(1000) = -4.65 \text{ D}$$

The eye is $F_{oc} = +4.65$ D too strong as measured at the EP:

$$M_P = -\frac{F_{oc}}{F_{obj}} = -\frac{+4.65}{-5.00} = +0.93x$$

The spectacle lens minifies the image +0.93x (93% as large or 7% smaller) with the spectacles on compared to with them off.

The equivalent equation to $M_{tel} = -(F_{oc}/F_{obj})$ that eliminates the need for calculating the power

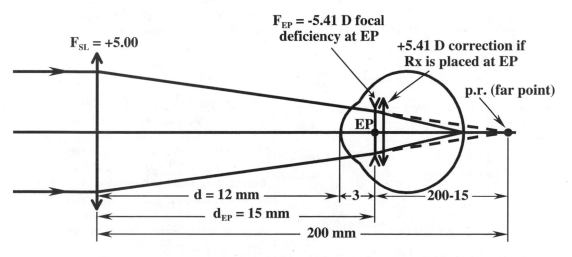

Figure 6.11. A hyperope has a refractive error of +5.00 D as measured at the spectacle lens plane 12 mm in front of the cornea. This ametropia could be simulated by a hypothetical minus lens placed at the EP of an emmetropic eye.

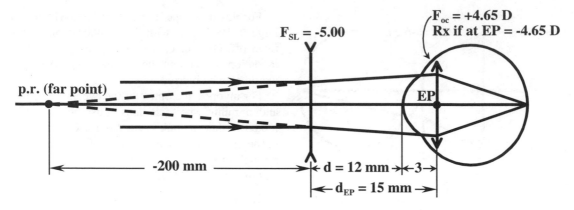

Figure 6.12. A myope has a refractive error of –5.00 D as measured at the spectacle lens plane 12 mm in front of the cornea. This ametropia could be simulated by a hypothetical plus lens placed at the entrance pupil (EP) of an emmetropic eye.

of the lens (F_{oc}) that simulates the ametropia at the EP plane may be used.

d_{EP} is the distance between objective and ocular. Then, $d_{EP} = f_{obj} + f_{oc}$, so $f_{oc} = d_{EP} - f_{obj}$.

$$M_P = -\frac{F_{oc}}{F_{obj}} = \frac{1}{1 - d_{EP}F_{obj}}$$

where d_{EP} is the distance in *meters* from the back vertex of the spectacle lens to the EP plane ($d + 3$ mm).

Example: For a true, full-scale Galilean telescope in which $F_{obj} = +0.5$ D and $F_{oc} = -40$ D:

$$d = f_{obj} - |f_{oc}| = (100/+0.5) - |(100/-40)|$$
$$= +200 - 2.5 = 197.5 \text{ cm, or } 1.975 \text{ meters}$$

$$M_{tel} = -\frac{F_{oc}}{F_{obj}} = -\frac{-40}{+0.5} = +80x$$

$$M_{tel} = \frac{1}{1 - dF_{obj}} = \frac{1}{1 - (1.975)(+0.5)} = +80x$$

Example: For the spectacle lens–corrected hyperope calculated earlier:

$$F_{SL} = +5.00 \text{ D} \text{ and } d_{EP} = 12 + 3 = 15 \text{ mm}$$
$$= 0.015 \text{ meters}$$

$$M_P = \frac{1}{1 - d_{EP}F_{SL}} = \frac{1}{1 - (0.015 \text{ m})(+0.5)}$$
$$= +1.081x$$

This agrees with our previous calculation, but note that F_{oc} (the power of the ametropic lens) need not be known.

Example: For the spectacle lens–corrected myope calculated earlier:

$$F_{SL} = -5.00 \text{ D} \text{ and } d_{EP} = 12 + 3 = 15 \text{ mm}$$
$$= 0.015 \text{ meters}$$

$$M_P = \frac{1}{1 - d_{EP}F_{SL}} = \frac{1}{1 - (0.015 \text{ m})(-5.00)}$$
$$= +0.93x \text{ as found before}$$

Again, note that the main advantage of the new equation over $M = -(F_{oc}/F_{obj})$ is that the spectacle lens effectivity (F_{oc}) at the EP plane doesn't have to be calculated.

The approximate equation based on $1/(1 - x)$ $\approx 1 + x$ (if $x \ll 1$) then gives:

$$M = \frac{1}{1 - dF} \approx 1 + dF$$

For the preceding example with the hyperope, $M_P \approx 1 + d_{EP}F_{SL} = 1 + (0.015 \text{ m})(+5.00) = +1.075x$, which is close to the actual value of $+1.081x$. For the example with the myope, $M_P \approx 1 + d_{EP}F_{SL} = 1 + (0.015 \text{ m})(-5.00) = +0.925x$, which is close to the actual value of $+0.93x$. Note that for an average d_{EP} (≈ 15 mm) this approximate equation implies that there is approximately a 1.5% change in magnification for every diopter change in spectacle lens power.

It must be kept in mind that the approximation is close only if $dF \ll 1$. Try the approximation formula on the example with the full-scale Galilean telescope given earlier where d and consequently dF_{obj} are relatively large.

$$M_{tel} = 1 + dF_{obj} \approx 1 + (1.975 \text{ m})(+0.5)$$
$$= +1.99x$$

This is nowhere near the correct value of $M_{tel} = +80x$ found by the exact equations!

The equation for power magnification depends only on the spectacle lens power and its distance d_{EP} from the EP. In this case, the spectacle lens has been treated as a thin lens (thickness $t = 0$). However, real lenses have a real thickness. Then F_{SL} in the equation is the back vertex power F_V and d_{EP} is the distance in meters between the back surface of the spectacle lens and the EP. As discussed earlier in this chapter, F_V in fact is how a spectacle Rx is specified.

Since this equation depends on the power F_V of the spectacle lens, it is called the power magnification (M_P) formula. So the equation with its proper subscripts is:

$$M_P = \frac{1}{1 - d_{EP}F_V} \approx 1 + d_{EP}F_V, \text{ where } F_V = Rx$$

In summary, a thick spectacle lens can be seen to be a combination of two Galilean telescopes, one that gives M_P, and one that gives M_S. Figure 6.13 models the thick spectacle lens (dashed lines) as two thin lenses of powers F_1, which equals the front surface power, and F_2, which equals the back surface power. F_2 takes part in both telescopes. It has a component F_{afocal}, which is the afocal component where $L_2' = 0$, and F_V, which is the component that corrects the ametropia of the eye.

F_1 = front surface power of the SL.

F_2 = back surface power = $F_{afocal} + F_V$ components.

F_{afocal} = the afocal component, where $L_2' = 0$ and,

F_V = the component which corrects the ametropia of the eye.

F_{am} = the ametropic component of the eye at the EP.

The F_1, t, and n combination forms a Galilean telescope giving M_S (shape magnification) and the F_V and d_{EP} combination forms a Galilean telescope giving F_P (power magnification). Note that F_2 and

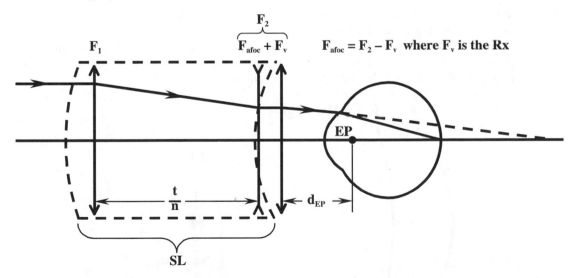

Figure 6.13. A thick spectacle lens is a combination of two Galilean telescopes. This diagram models a thick spectacle lens (dashed lines) as two thin lenses of powers F_1 (which equals the front surface power) and F_2 (which equals the back surface power). F_1 is the power of the objective of the first telescope. F_2 can be broken into two components; one is the power necessary for parallel light to leave the ocular of the first telescope, the other is the power necessary to correct the wearer's refractive error and constitutes the objective power of the second telescope. The refractive state of the eye at the EP constitutes the ocular power of the second telescope.

F_{afocal} are separated only for conceptual reasons and need not be known.

$$M_S = \frac{1}{1 - \left(\dfrac{t}{n}\right)F_1} \approx 1 + \left(\frac{t}{n}\right)F_1$$

$$M_P = \frac{1}{1 - d_{EP}F_V} \approx 1 + d_{EP}F_V$$

The total magnification, $M_{TOT} = (M_S)(M_P)$

$\approx [1 + (t/n)F_1][1 + d_{EP}F_V]$ for example, $(1.05)(1.09) = 1.145$, or 14.5%

$\approx [(t/n)F_1 + d_{EP}F_V](100\%)$ for example, $(0.05 + 0.09)(100\%) = 0.14(100\%)$, or 14.0%

Aniseikonia

Patients can experience a difference in perceived image size between the two eyes, a condition called aniseikonia.[2-4] When this difference (ΔM) exceeds about 3–5%, patients may be bothered by it. Aniseikonia is often caused by a large difference (about 1.5% per diopter) in spectacle Rx between the two eyes. One of the reasons we have discussed spectacle magnification at some length is that aniseikonia can be reduced or eliminated by changing M_S and/or M_P of one or both spectacle lenses.

We cannot predict ΔM just on the basis of a difference in Rx between the two eyes. It is generally determined empirically, the most sensitive technique using a clinical instrument called an eikonometer. Once the percent difference (ΔM) is found between the two eyes, $M_T (= (M_P)(M_S))$ of one or both of the spectacle lenses is changed to give an opposite, corrective ΔM_T.

Recall that:

$$M_P = \frac{1}{1 - d_{EP}F_V} \quad \text{and} \quad M_S = \frac{1}{1 - \left(\dfrac{t}{n}\right)F_1}$$

Our ability to change d_{EP} is limited because there can't be too great a difference in vertex distance between the two lenses if they are mounted in the same frame. F_V is fixed because it is the Rx required for clear vision. This leaves t, n, and F_1 as suitable parameters to change to achieve a ΔM_T. Since all of these apply to M_S, most spectacle correction of aniseikonia involves changes in M_S and not in M_P.

Even if one is not interested in treating aniseikonia, a practical consequence of M_P and M_S is that with an astigmatic lens there will be less difference in magnification between the two power meridia if the cylinder is ground on the back (F_2) rather than the front (F_1) where M_S is affected.

Summary of Equations

Figure 6.14 pictorially reviews the meaning of the parameters used in the spectacle magnification equations.

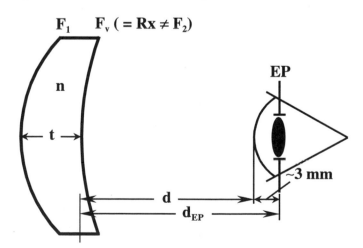

Figure 6.14. Summary diagram pictorially shows the meaning of the various components of the M_P and M_S equations.

$$M_P = \frac{1}{1 - d_{EP}F_V} \approx 1 + d_{EP}F_V \ (d_{EP} \text{ in meters})$$

$$M_S = \frac{1}{1 - \left(\dfrac{t}{n}\right)F_1} \approx 1 + \left(\frac{t}{n}\right)F_1 \ (\tau \text{ in meters})$$

$$M_{TOT} = (M_P)(M_S) \approx \left(d_{EP}F_V + \left(\frac{t}{n}\right)F_1\right)100\%$$

$(d_{EP}$ and t in meters)

REFRACTIVE SURGERY

Refractive surgery is an option for reducing refractive error.[5,6] This can be as simple (in theory) as placing lenses inside the eye, which is a natural extension of the use of spectacle and contact lenses. If a patient has a cataractous crystalline lens removed, a pseudophakic lens may be selected with a power intended to correct any ametropia. The crystalline lens could also be replaced for eyes that are normal except for exceptionally high refractive error. However, these eyes are usually at greater risk for retinal detachment and other side effects of lens removal so the cost-to-benefit ratio is not good. A relatively recent practice is to leave the natural lens in place and to implant a lens in front of the natural lens to correct the refractive error (e.g., the Staar Intraocular Contact Lens).

In the vast majority of cases, refractive surgery has involved changing the radius of curvature of the cornea. The most popular means are by radial keratotomy (RK), photorefractive keratectomy (PRK), and laser-assisted stromal interstitial keratomileusis (LASIK), but less common surgeries are also mentioned here for the sake of completeness.

Corneal Incisions and Sutures

1. *Sutures.* It has been noted in corneal surgery that tightened sutures in the corneal periphery result in a steepening of the central cornea in the meridian that contains the suture. Also, if the suture is loose enough to leave a wound gap, a flattening of the central cornea in that meridian results. This principle has been used to minimize astigmatism induced during corneal trans-

plant surgery or from incisions and preexisting astigmatism during cataract surgery.

2. *Radial keratotomy (RK).* The relaxation effect has been used in radial keratotomy.[7] When a radial cut is made in the periphery of the cornea, the meridian containing the cut becomes less steep centrally and results in less power in that meridian. In RK 4 to 16 radial cuts are placed around the cornea to flatten the cornea equally in all meridians. The deeper they are and the farther they extend toward the central cornea, the more effective the cuts are in changing the corneal power. Therefore, the depth of the cuts is typically 90% of the thickness of the cornea. Since the cuts form radial scars, which scatter light, a 3- to 6-mm central clear zone is left.

3. *Astigmatic keratotomy (AK).* If the cuts are made on one meridian, the effect is a flattening of that meridian. There is also a smaller flattening effect on the corneal meridian perpendicular to the one containing the cuts, but the net effect is to induce a change in the difference in power between the two meridians. For example, cuts in the superior cornea produce against-the-rule astigmatism and can be used to correct with-the-rule astigmatism by equalizing the power in the two meridians.

Circumferential (as opposed to radial) cuts also produce a flattening in the meridian that contains them, but a steepening rather than a flattening in the perpendicular meridian. These "arcuate" or "limbal relaxing" incisions are commonly done following cataract surgery to reduce astigmatism. A combination of radial and circular cuts, which results in power being manipulated in one meridian but left alone in the perpendicular meridian, offers a theoretical way of modifying astigmatism.

There are a number of possible drawbacks to RK and AK. The effect is rather unpredictable and the results can be unstable for a number of years following the surgery. Also, when the pupil dilates in the dark, it may open wide enough to include the scars from the cuts and light will be scattered. This can be a problem especially while driving at night. In addition, the form of the cornea changes so that aberrations (particularly spherical aberration) are induced and contact lenses may be difficult to fit.

Adding Reshaped Material to the Cornea

The following procedures use a button of tissue from a donor cornea or the patient's own cornea to change the power of the cornea. However, with the advent of newer methods these procedures are not performed frequently.

1. *Epikeratophakia.* In epikeratophakia a button of donor cornea is reshaped into a thin lens that can be sutured to the anterior surface of a recipient's cornea. Reshaping is accomplished by freezing the donor cornea, and cryolathing the posterior surface so that the total power is correct. Since freezing kills the donor epithelium, the anterior surface is left with Bowman's layer intact to promote epithelial regrowth. This donor lens is then tucked into an annular pocket around the host cornea and it is sutured into place.

   Epikeratophakia is not an accurate means of gaining emmetropia but it is able to reduce large amounts of ametropia. Therefore, it is usually used only with patients who have high amounts of ametropia whose sight cannot be corrected easily by more common methods. This would include patients who for various reasons can't wear contact lenses.

2. *Keratomileusis.* Keratomileusis is very similar to epikeratophakia but it is a button of the patient's own cornea that is reshaped rather than a donor's cornea. A lamellar section of the patient's anterior cornea is removed, frozen and cryolathed on the back to achieve the desired power change. Then the button is sutured back onto the patient's cornea. It is easier to flatten the cornea than it is to steepen it so greater amounts of myopic than hyperopic ametropia may be eliminated.

3. *Keratophakia.* In keratophakia a lamellar button of a donor's cornea is cryolathed into a lens of a desired power. Then a lamellar section of the patient's cornea is removed and placed over the donor lens and sutured down to form a sandwich. Synthetic lens buttons are also possible. The advantage over keratomileusis is that larger amounts of ametropia can be corrected. This procedure has been largely replaced by epikeratophakia.

Reshaping the Corneal Surface

1. *Photoablation.* The excimer laser produces pulses of UV light in which the individual photons are energetic enough to break molecular bonds in tissues. When argon and fluorine are used as the lasing medium, 193 nm light results. Light not much shorter than this will even be absorbed by air and the excimer beam is immediately absorbed by tissue surfaces, and tissue can be smoothly ablated fractions of a micrometer per pulse with little collateral damage. That makes this laser ideally suited to smoothly sculpting the corneal surface to any desired radius or shape.

   a. *Photorefractive keratectomy (PRK).* PRK refers to the direct sculpting of the anterior corneal surface by excimer laser. The epithelium is first removed either mechanically or with the assistance of a laser. Then the different areas of the corneal surface are exposed to the excimer beam in proportion to the amount of tissue that is to be removed. To correct myopia the beam dwells more on the center of the cornea than the periphery in order to flatten it and reduce its power. Although Bowman's membrane is removed, the epithelium rapidly regrows, probably due to the smoothness of the stromal bed left by the excimer beam. Due to the discomfort experienced by some patients during epithelial regrowth, the possibility of corneal haze, and regression of refractive correction, PRK has largely been replaced by LASIK.

   b. *Laser-assisted stromal interstitial keramileusis (LASIK).* In LASIK a kerotome blade slices off a flap of anterior cornea. The stromal bed underneath is then exposed to the excimer beam to change its radius of curvature and the anterior flap is replaced. Since the epithelium is not disrupted, healing is usually very fast and painless with less variability in visual acuity than PRK immediately following the surgery.

2. *Thermal keratoplasty.* Thermal keratoplasty is used to correct hyperopia. In laser thermal keratoplasty (LTK) a holmium laser produces infrared light, which is focused as a circle of

spots around the corneal periphery. Alternatively, conductive keratoplasty (CK) uses a radio frequency. Both of these methods produce a thermal effect that shrinks the corneal collagen and, similar to the effect of tight sutures, increases the power of the central cornea. Thermal keratoplasty is a useful adjunct to the excimer laser because the excimer laser is not as effective for correcting hyperopia as it is for correcting myopia.

3. *Intrastromal corneal ring segments (ISCRs or Intacs).* Plastic ring segments are threaded through the stroma of the peripheral cornea to produce a tension that can change the radius of curvature and thus the power of the cornea. The advantage of this technique is that it does not disrupt the center of the cornea; it maintains the asphericity of the cornea, and, if necessary, the procedure can be reversed.

Refractive surgery is a very effective and very popular method of reducing refractive error. Patients almost always have improved visual acuity without correction. However, increased spherical aberration and other ocular aberrations have been reported after RK, PRK, and LASIK surgeries.[8-11] Refractive surgery for myopia increases positive spherical aberration because the power of the central cornea is reduced while the power of the peripheral cornea is unchanged or increased. Because of induced aberrations and occasional side effects, such as corneal scarring and haze, visual acuity with lens correction (if necessary) after refractive surgery is sometimes not as good as presurgical visual acuity with lens correction. Some patients have difficulty with night vision after refractive surgery because the pupil enlarges beyond areas of corneal scarring or transition zones between treated and nontreated cornea. Also, a larger pupil does not limit the effect of spherical aberration as much as a smaller light-adapted pupil does.

REFERENCES

1. Keating MP. *Geometrical, Physical, and Visual Optics.* Boston: Butterworth-Heinemann, 1988;279–288.
2. Bannon RE. Aniseikonia. In: A Safir, ed. *Refraction and Clinical Optics.* Hagerstown, MD: Harper & Row, 1980;229–233.
3. Bartlett JD. Anisometropia and aniseikonia. In: JF Amos, ed. *Diagnosis and Management in Vision Care.* Boston: Butterworth-Heinemann, 1987;173–202.
4. Penisten DK. Anisometropia. In: KE Brookman, ed. *Refractive Management of Ametropia.* Boston: Butterworth-Heinemann, 1996;99–121.
5. Waring GO III. Management of myopia: classification of surgical methods. In: T Grosvenor, MC Flom, eds. *Refractive Anomalies: Research and Clinical Applications.* Boston: Butterworth-Heinemann, 1991; 384–396.
6. Bradley A. The changing face of refractive surgery. *Indiana J Optom.* 2000;3:5–12.
7. Waring GO III. *Refractive Keratotomy for Myopia and Astigmatism.* St. Louis: Mosby, 1992.
8. Applegate RA, Hilmantel G, Howland HC. Corneal aberrations increase with the magnitude of radial keratotomy refractive correction. *Optom Vis Sci.* 1996; 73:585–589.
9. Oliver KM, Hemenger RP, Corbett MC, et al. Corneal aberrations induced by photorefractive keratectomy. *J Refract Surg.* 1997;13:246–254.
10. Oshika T, Klyce SD, Applegate RA, et al. Comparison of corneal wavefront aberrations after photorefractive keratectomy and laser in situ keratomileusis. *Am J Ophthalmol.* 1999;127:1–7.
11. Thibos LN, Hong X. Clinical applications of the Shack-Hartmann aberrometer. *Optom Vis Sci.* 1999;76:817–825.

FURTHER READING

Benjamin WJ. Contact lenses: clinical function and practical optics. In: WJ Benjamin, ed. *Borish's Clinical Refraction.* Philadelphia: Saunders, 1998;956–1021.
Douthwaite WA. *Contact Lens Optics and Lens Design.* 2nd ed. Oxford: Butterworth-Heinemann, 1995.
Fannin TE, Grosvenor T. *Clinical Optics.* 2nd ed. Boston: Butterworth-Heinemann, 1996.
Stephens GL. Correction with single vision spectacle lenses. In: WJ Benjamin, ed. *Borish's Clinical Refraction.* Philadelphia: Saunders, 1998;823–882.

Chapter 7

Methods of Measuring Refractive Errors

Two methods have been employed. The first consists in testing the power of vision with glasses of known focal distance. The second in the determination of the refractive condition by means of the ophthalmoscope. For the employment of the first method we require, in the first place, the necessary glasses from 1/80 to 1/2 and from −1/80 to −1/2; in the second place, the necessary objects for testing. The pairs of glasses are kept loose in a box, with a spectacle frame in which they can be placed. It is also convenient to have a black plate of metal of the same size as the glasses, which, placed in the frame, closes one of the eyes. . . . The most suitable objects are letters and numbers. —Frans Cornelis Donders, 1864 (From Donders FC. *On the Anomalies of Accommodation and Refraction of the Eye,* transl. Moore WD. London: New Sydenham Society, 1864;97.)

There are many possible procedures that a clinician may use to measure refractive errors. These may be broadly divided into subjective and objective methods. Subjective methods require a response (typically a verbal response) from the patient. Objective methods do not require a response from the patient, although typically some level of cooperation, such as steady fixation, is necessary.

The most common subjective method is the subjective refraction to best visual acuity. In this method the clinician asks the patient an established series of questions concerning the appearance and clarity of letters and other targets when viewed through lenses of different powers. This technique is time consuming but it is generally agreed that it is more accurate than the objective techniques presently available. It is the preferred method of measuring refractive error for the purpose of prescribing lenses.

The most common objective method is retinoscopy. This technique is commonly used to precede a subjective refraction to gain a preliminary refractive measurement, which is then refined by the subjective refraction to best visual acuity. Under special circumstances retinoscopy and other objective methods of measuring refractive errors are sometimes used alone. For instance, some patients may be unable to respond to standard subjective refraction procedures, as for example in infants, very small children and nonverbal patients. Also, objective refractive procedures may offer advantages when used as research tools.

RETINOSCOPY

Retinoscopy is an objective method of measuring refractive error. Typically, it immediately precedes the subjective refraction to best visual acuity. Clinicians may also use it to prescribe lenses if a subjective refraction is not possible for a given patient. Retinoscopy has also been used in laboratory studies to measure refractive errors in animals. Bowman, Cuignet, Landolt, and Parent were prominent among the early developers of retinoscopy in the second half of the nineteenth century, with additional contributions by Jackson and Wolff at about the turn of the century and Copeland in the first half of the twentieth century.[1,2]

Retinoscopy involves imaging a patch of light onto the patient's retina. This retinal image then becomes an object that diffusely reflects light back through the optics of the eye to form an external image. If accommodation is relaxed, this external image will be formed at the punctum remotum for the eye, and its location can be used to determine the patient's refractive error.

Modern retinoscopes use the filament of a light bulb, powered by a battery in its handle, to form a bright object. In most retinoscopes the bulb uses a long straight filament in order to form a streak-shaped object rather than a spot. This aids in the measurement of astigmatism. A small lens in the handle forms an image of the light bulb's filament. A mirror oriented at 45 degrees to the beam redirects the beam so that it is projected toward the patient at 90 degrees to the handle. This mirror either has a hole in its center or is partly transmissive. This allows the examiner to view the patient's eye through a peephole behind the mirror along the same axis as the image light returning from the patient's eye (Figure 7.1).

We discuss the optics of retinoscopy in terms of an illumination phase (light from the retinoscope incident on the patient's retina) and an observation phase (light emergent from the patient's eye).

Illumination of the Patient's Retina

The distance between the light source and the lens in a retinoscope can be varied so that either convergent or divergent light leaves the retinoscope. This is illustrated in Figure 7.2.

The situation in which divergent light leaves the retinoscope is usually called plane mirror mode. The situation in which convergent light leaves the retinoscope is referred to as concave mirror mode.

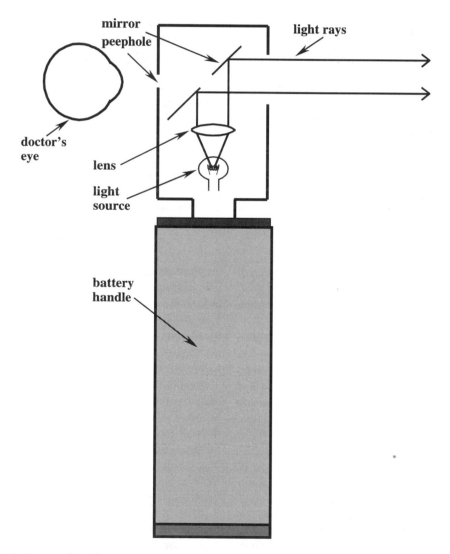

Figure 7.1. Basic features of a retinoscope.

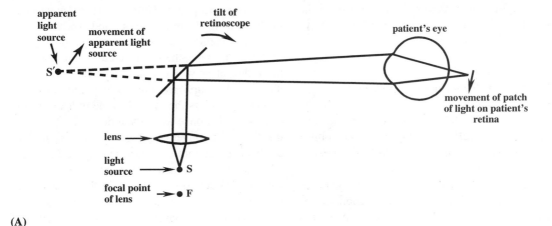

(A)

(B)

Figure 7.2. Illumination of the patient's retina in retinoscopy. (**A**) Plane mirror mode and (**B**) concave mirror mode.

These terms originate historically from the fact that early retinoscopists obtained divergent or convergent light respectively through the use of plane or concave mirrors. In the modern retinoscope, the examiner can shift between plane and concave mirror modes by changing the distance between a converging lens and the light source by moving the retinoscope "sleeve" up and down. On some retinoscopes the sleeve moves the lens closer to or farther from the light source; on other retinoscopes the sleeve moves the light source closer to or farther from the lens. Decreasing the distance between lens and light source sufficiently establishes divergent light (i.e., plane mirror mode) (see Figure 7.2A). Therefore, on retinoscopes in which the sleeve moves the lens, plane mirror mode is established by pulling the sleeve down, which moves the lens toward the light source. In either convergent or divergent mode, the light from the retinoscope is converged by the optics of the patient's eye to form an out-of-focus patch of light on the patient's retina.

Testing procedure in retinoscopy involves tilting the retinoscope, which, in turn, pivots the beam at the mirror of the retinosocpe and moves the patch of light on the patient's retina. In plane mirror mode, the apparent light source is behind the retinoscope. Thus, when the retinoscope is tilted down, the apparent light source moves up and causes the out-of-focus patch of light on the patient's retina to move down (see Figure 7.2A). In concave mirror mode, the apparent light source is between the retinoscope and the patient's eye. Thus, when the retinoscope is tilted down, the apparent light source moves down and causes the out-of-focus patch on the patient's retina to move up (see Figure 7.2B).

Light Emergent from the Patient's Eye

The out-of-focus patch of light on the patient's retina is diffusely reflected and serves as an object for the optics of the patient's eye to form an external image. The appearance of the external image when the examiner's eye is focused on the plane of the patient's pupil is called the retinoscopic reflex. This appears to be located at the patient's pupil, but in reality it is located anywhere in front of or behind the retinoscope. If the patient's accommodation is at a zero level, that external image is formed at the patient's punctum remotum. Therefore, by locating the image, the examiner also locates the punctum remotum and can calculate the patient's refractive error.

One of the aspects of the reflex judged by the examiner in order to determine the location of the external image is the direction of movement of the reflex as the retinoscope is tilted. Most clinicians prefer to use plane mirror mode retinoscopy, so we will discuss motion of the reflex in that mode. If the retinoscope is located between the patient's eye and the patient's punctum remotum, the reflex appears to move down as the retinoscope is tilted down. This is called "with motion." As illustrated in Figure 7.3A, the blurred image of the retinal patch moves up across the retinoscope peephole. Light from the top of the patient's pupil is seen first, followed by lower parts of the pupil. Thus, the reflex appears to move down as the retinoscope is tilted down.

If the patient's punctum remotum is located between the retinoscope and the patient's eye, the reflex appears to move up within the patient's pupil as the retinoscope is tilted down. This is called "against motion." Figure 7.3B illustrates the reason for against motion. As the retinoscope is tilted down, the patch of light on the patient's retina moves down. The lighted patch of the patient's retina forms an image at the patient's punctum remotum. Light from the bottom of the patient's pupil crosses the peephole first and thus is seen by the examiner first. Then light from progressively higher parts of the patient's pupil comes across the retinoscope peephole. Thus, the reflex appears to move up as the retinoscope is tilted down.

If the patient's punctum remotum is in the plane of the retinoscope, there appears to be no motion of the reflex because the reflex appears to fill all of the patient's pupil as soon as the light from the retinoscope enters the eye. Then the reflex seems to disappear all at once when the retinoscope is tilted so that light is no longer entering the patient's eye. This is known as neutrality. As shown in Figure 7.3C, neutrality is observed when the patient's retina is conjugate with the retinoscope peephole. The appearances of against and with motion are shown in Figure 7.4.

If the examiner observes with motion, neutrality can be achieved by adding plus lenses. Neutrality can also be approached by moving farther from the patient; that is, by approaching the punctum remotum. Neutralization of against motion can be achieved by adding minus lenses. When against motion is observed, neutrality can also be approached by moving closer to the patient's eye, again moving toward the punctum remotum. If a clinician changes to concave mirror mode retinoscopy, the retinoscopic reflex goes in the opposite direction as in plane mirror mode, so that with motion indicates minus lenses are needed for neutrality and against motion indicates that neutrality would be obtained with plus lenses.

The astute clinician uses cues in addition to the direction of the reflex in moving toward neutrality. One may deduce from Figure 7.3, that more and more light gets through the retinoscope peephole as the examiner gets closer and closer to neutrality. Therefore, the speed, width, and brightness of the retinoscopic reflex increase as one approaches neutrality. This makes it possible for the experienced clinician to estimate the lens power necessary for neutrality by observing the speed, width, and brightness of the reflex.

Retinoscopy in Astigmatism

In patients with astigmatism there are separate punctum remotum locations for each of the two principal meridians. Therefore, both principal meridians must be neutralized. However, before neutralizing the principal meridians, the examiner must identify which meridians are the principal meridians. If the streak of the retinoscope is not

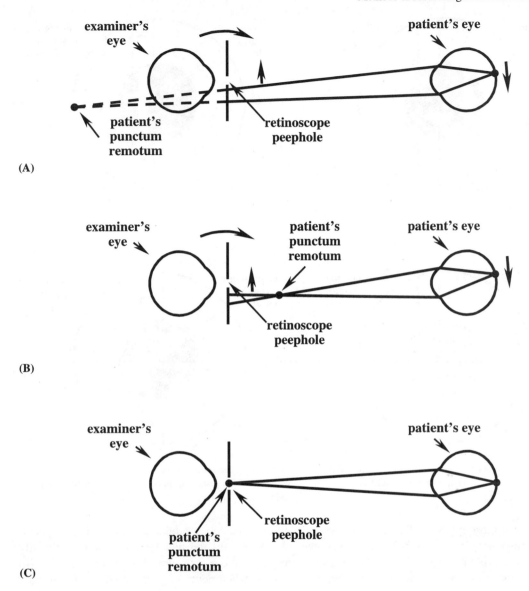

Figure 7.3. Movement of the retinoscopic reflex (**A**) with motion, (**B**) against motion, and (**C**) neutrality.

aligned with one of the principal meridians, the reflex appears to be rotated with respect to the streak on the iris (Figure 7.5).

The examiner then rotates the streak until the reflex is aligned with the streak on the iris. This identifies one of the principal meridians. The other principal meridian, 90 degrees away, can then be neutralized by rotating the streak to a plane perpendicular to the original streak orientation.

Static and Dynamic Retinoscopy

Retinoscopy is referred to as static or dynamic depending on what it is being used to measure. Static retinoscopy is used to measure refractive error. By having the patient look at a distant target and by having plus lenses in place, the assumption is made that accommodation is at zero level. The term *static retinoscopy* comes from that assumption.

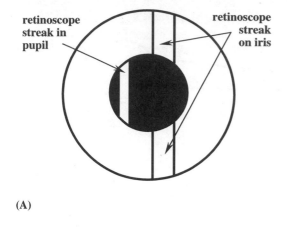

(A)

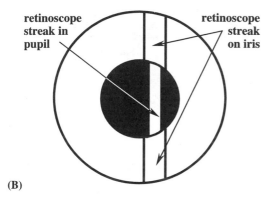

(B)

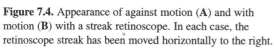

Figure 7.4. Appearance of against motion (**A**) and with motion (**B**) with a streak retinoscope. In each case, the retinoscope streak has been moved horizontally to the right.

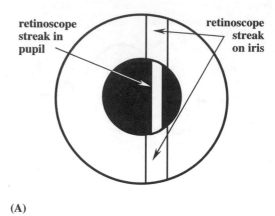

(A)

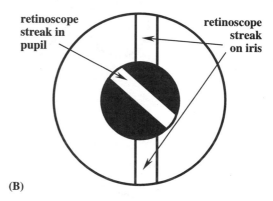

(B)

Figure 7.5. The retinoscopic reflex (**A**) when it is aligned with one of the principal meridians in astigmatism and (**B**) when it is not.

Dynamic retinoscopy is used to measure accommodative response. In this technique, the patient looks at a nearpoint target. There are various dynamic retinoscopy procedures that can then be used to estimate accommodative response.[3]

Calculation of Refractive Error with Retinoscopy

In principle, the punctum remotum could be found by moving the retinoscope closer or farther from the patient until neutrality is reached. Then the refractive error would be the reciprocal of the distance between the retinoscope and the spectacle plane in meters. However, this would be impractical for all but high myopes because the distance would be large, and impossible for hyperopes because the punctum remotum would be a virtual image behind the eye. In actual practice, lenses of

different powers are placed at the patient's spectacle plane until the punctum remotum is optically moved to the retinoscope. This condition is known to exist when neutrality is seen. A simple formula can be written to show the relationship between refractive error, the position of the retinoscope, the power of the lens placed in front of the patient's eye to achieve neutrality, and, if present, the amount of accommodation. The formula is:

$$RE = \frac{1}{-CF} + L + A$$

where

RE = refractive error,

CF = the distance, in meters, of the retinoscope from the patient's spectacle plane when neutrality is observed (i.e., the distance the image of the retinal patch is from the spectacle plane),

L = dioptric power of the lens in the patient's spectacle plane, and

A = accommodation in diopters.

When static retinoscopy is performed, A is assumed to be zero, and $(1/-CF)$ is the power deducted to compensate for the examiner's "working distance," the distance from the retinoscope to the patient's spectacle plane.

Example 1. An examiner does static retinoscopy on a -4 D myope while using a 50-cm working distance. What lens results in neutrality?

$$RE = \frac{1}{-CF} + L + A$$

$$-4\,D = \frac{1}{-0.5\,m} + L + 0$$

$$L = -2\,D$$

Example 2. An examiner does static retinoscopy on a patient while using a 0.67-m working distance, and obtains neutrality with a $+3$ D lens. What is the patient's refractive error?

$$RE = \frac{1}{-CF} + L + A$$

$$RE = \frac{1}{-0.667\,m} + (+3\,D) + 0$$

$$RE = +1.50\,D$$

Example 3. An examiner changes his distance from the patient to obtain neutrality rather than using lenses. Where would neutrality be observed with a -3 D myope looking at a distant target?

$$RE = \frac{1}{-CF} + L + A$$

$$-3\,D = \frac{1}{-CF} + 0 + 0$$

$$CF = 0.333\,m$$

Example 4. An examiner performs dynamic retinoscopy with the retinoscope and the target viewed by the patient 40 cm from the patient's spectacle plane. The patient has -1 D of myopia.

Neutrality is observed with a $+0.50$ D lens. How much accommodation is occurring?

$$RE = \frac{1}{-CF} + L + A$$

$$-1\,D = \frac{1}{-0.4\,m} + (+0.50\,D) + A$$

$$A = 1.00\,D$$

Sources of Error in Retinoscopy

The examiner should align the retinoscope as close as possible to the optical axis of the patient's eye. If this is not done, oblique astigmatism will be introduced, and may be mistaken for axial astigmatism. Due to spherical aberration, the power of the peripheral portions of the patient's pupil is usually different from that of the center of the pupil. Therefore, the examiner should pay attention to the reflex in the center of the patient's pupil and try to ignore the outermost portions of the pupil, particularly when the pupil has been dilated with a pharmaceutical agent. Errors in retinoscopy can also occur if the examiner is not careful about maintaining a constant working distance. Another potential source of inaccuracy in static retinoscopy is failure to maintain the patient's accommodation at a zero level.

BASIC SUBJECTIVE OPTOMETERS

An *optometer* is a device that measures refractive error. Optometers range from very simple devices, which consist of a lens, an object, and a measuring scale, to very sophisticated objective electronic instruments, known as autorefractors. In this section we discuss the most basic subjective optometers. These basic optometers are now seldom used by themselves, but the principles behind them form the basis for the operation of modern autorefractors.

Simple Optometer

The simple optometer places a high plus lens in the subject's spectacle plane. An object on the far side of the lens is moved out until it is blurred, and then moved back toward the lens until it first becomes clear. The vergence of light as it exits the lens is the spectacle plane refractive error. For example, if a +10 D lens is used in the spectacle plane and the object is in focus –25 cm from the lens, the subject's spectacle plane refractive error is +6 D (Figure 7.6).

$$L = 1/\ell$$

$$L = 1/-0.25 \text{ m} = -4 \text{ D}$$

$$L' = L + F = -4 \text{ D} + (+10 \text{ D}) = +6 \text{ D}$$

One disadvantage of the simple optometer is that the subject is aware of the close proximity of the lens and object. This can stimulate some accommodation because one of the cues that induce accommodation is awareness of nearness. Thus the measurements can err in the direction of too little plus or too much minus. Also, the apparent size of the target changes as the object is moved closer to or farther from the lens. One inconvenience of the simple optometer is that the change in vergence of light leaving the lens is not a linear function of the change in object placement; therefore, if a dioptric scale is established to correspond with the object placement, it is not a linear scale.

Young-Porterfield Optometer

The first optometer was described in 1737 by the Scottish surgeon William Porterfield,[4] who also coined the term *optometer.* Improvements in the Porterfield optometer were made by the English physician Thomas Young and described in an 1801 paper. Porterfield's and Young's optometers used the Scheiner double-aperture principle, although they used double slits rather than double pinholes. Young's optometer had a lens with a focal length of four inches (about +10 D) and a thin black line extending from the lens away from the subject. Because of the Scheiner double aperture, the subject sees double lines that form an *x,* which crosses at the object point that will focus on the retina. Young's optometer had a marker that the observer could move along the axis of the instrument to the crossing point of the *x.* Then a scale reading could be made at that point. Figure 7.7 shows a schematic diagram of Thomas Young's optometer.

Badal Optometer

In 1876 Jules Badal described an optometer that now carries his name. In a Badal optometer, the optometer lens is placed such that its second focal point is in the spectacle plane of the subject (or in some other reference plane where the refractive error is to be determined). This arrangement has the advantage that the observer sees no change in angular size of the object as it is moved. Also, unlike the simple optometer, the relation of dioptric power and amount of movement of the object are linear so that each unit of object movement results in an equal change in vergence at the second focal

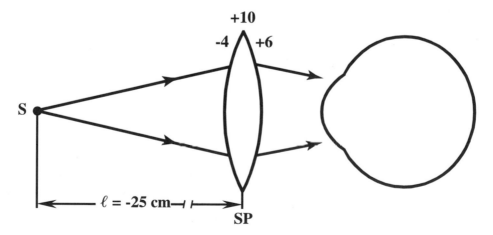

Figure 7.6. An example of spectacle plane refractive error measurement with a simple optometer. The object is in focus with a +10 D lens when the object is –25 cm from the spectacle plane, SP. Therefore, the vergence of light striking the lens is –4 D, and the refractive error (vergence leaving the lens) is +6 D.

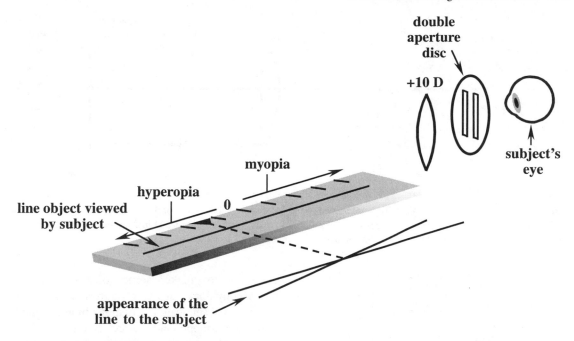

Figure 7.7. Schematic diagram of the Thomas Young's optometer. The line viewed by the subject appeared like an *x* due to the double-aperture disc. The subject moved a marker to the crossing point in the *x*. A scale reading was taken at the marker.

point. For example, if a +10 D lens is placed 10 cm from the spectacle plane, then each 1 cm of object movement will change the vergence of light in the spectacle plane by 1 D (Figure 7.8).

The following three examples show this relationship:

Example 1. The object is in focus 2 cm inside of the first focal point of the +10 D lens. It is therefore 8 cm from the lens.

$$L = 1/-0.08 \text{ m} = -12.5 \text{ D}$$

$$L' = -12.5 \text{ D} + (+10 \text{ D}) = -2.5 \text{ D}$$

$$\ell' = n'/L' = 1/-2.5 \text{ D} = -0.4 \text{ m}$$

The image formed by the lens is 40 cm beyond the lens. Because the spectacle plane is 10 cm closer to the subject than the lens, the image will be 50 cm from the spectacle plane, and thus the vergence of light in the spectacle plane will be –2.00 D:

$$\ell_2 = -0.4 \text{ m} + (-0.1 \text{ m}) = -0.5 \text{ m}$$

$$L_2 = 1/-0.5 \text{ m} = -2.00 \text{ D}$$

Thus a movement of the object of 2 cm toward the optometer lens has changed the vergence of light in spectacle plane by –2.00 D.

Example 2. A 1-cm movement of the object from the first focal point of the lens toward the lens will result in a vergence of –1.00 D in the spectacle plane:

$$L = 1/-0.09 \text{ m} = -11.11 \text{ D}$$

$$L' = -11.11 \text{ D} + (+10.00 \text{ D}) = -1.11 \text{ D}$$

$$\ell' = 1/-1.11 \text{ D} = -0.9 \text{ m}$$

$$\ell_2 = -0.9 \text{ m} + (-0.1 \text{ m}) = -1.0 \text{ m}$$

$$L_2 = 1/-1.0 \text{ m} = -1.00 \text{ D}$$

Example 3. An object 11 cm from the +10 D lens will result in a vergence of +1.00 D in the spectacle plane.

$$L = 1/-0.11 \text{ m} = -9.09 \text{ D}$$

$$L' = -9.09 \text{ D} + (+10.00 \text{ D}) = +0.91 \text{ D}$$

$$\ell' = 1/+0.91 \text{ D} = +1.1 \text{ m}$$

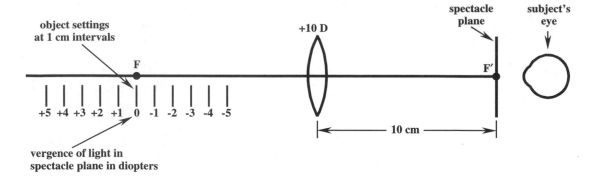

Figure 7.8. Badal optometer with a +10 D optometer lens. F', the second focal point of the lens, is in the spectacle plane. Object placement at the first focal point, F, of the lens results in a vergence of light of 0 D in the spectacle plane. Movement of the object by 1 cm changes the vergence of light in spectacle plane 1 D.

$$\ell_2 = +1.1\ m + (-0.1\ m) = +1.0\ m$$

$$L_2 = 1/+1.0\ m = +1.00\ D$$

OBJECTIVE AUTOREFRACTORS

Objective autorefractors are automated instruments used for the estimation of refractive error. Since they yield essentially the same information as retinoscopy, their readings may be refined by subjective refraction techniques to arrive at a useful lens prescription. Nevertheless, they have certain advantages and disadvantages over retinoscopy. A big advantage of objective autorefraction over retinoscopy is that it can be delegated to a technician, thus saving the busy clinician time. Autorefractors generally do not require a verbal response from patients; they require only that they fixate a target and accommodate accurately. All the operator needs to do is align the instrument and push a button to initiate the measurement. A major disadvantage is that, even though autorefractors give repeatable readings, they may not be as accurate as retinoscopy, especially for high refractive errors.[5] Part of this problem is that, with many autorefractors, the awareness of nearness of the instrument induces proximal accommodation, leading to too much minus or not enough plus in the measurement obtained. Some instruments include fixation objects, which by their appearance or optical path are designed to minimize accommodation. Another disadvantage is that autorefractors do not allow the clinician to make some observations that retinoscopy does, such as variations in pupil diameter that may indicate fluctuations in accommodation. Retinoscopy and autorefraction also share some problems. Neither technique is very effective when performed in cases with very small pupils, unstable fixation, or media opacities.

Although highly sophisticated, most autorefractors rely on the simple principles behind retinoscopy and the Badal optometer. Autorefractors generally incorporate a visible light source for the subject to fixate, some type of electro-optical sensing device, and a microprocessor or computer. Although the fixation target must be seen by visible light, these optometers often use infrared "light" to measure refractive error. This is because infrared radiation is invisible so that it does not distract the patient, nor does it affect the pupil size. However, when infrared radiation is used, a correction factor must be included because chromatic aberration gives the eye different powers for infrared light and visible light.

Basic Principles Used in Autorefractors

Commercial objective autorefractors have been based on various different optical principles including:

1. Scheiner principle
2. Retinoscopic scanning
3. Best focus
4. Knife-edge principle

5. Ray deflection principle
6. Image size principle
7. Wavefront sensing[5–10]

Scheiner Principle

Autorefractors that use the Scheiner principle include the Acuity Systems 6600, Nidek autorefractor, and the Marco AR-800, AR-820, and ARK-900 autorefractors. In these instruments there are two infrared light-emitting diodes rather than the double-aperture Scheiner disc. A Badal optometer system is used for the neutralization of refractive error. An array of photodetectors determines whether the images of the infrared sources are aligned. When they are aligned, the refractive error for that particular meridian is neutralized. The measurement starts with neutralization of refractive error in the 180 meridian. Then the infrared sources and the photodetectors are rotated until the principal meridians are identified, and the refractive errors in the principal meridians are measured.

Retinoscopic Scanning

The operation of the Bausch & Lomb Safir Ophthalmetron, manufactured in the 1970s, was based on the direction of motion of a retinoscope-like streak reflex. The streak is produced by a light source inside a rotating drum, which has slits in it at regular intervals. The reflection of those streaks from the patient's retina is imaged by a Badal optometer lens on two photodetectors. The photodetectors are moved closer to or farther from the lens until the streak hits both photodetectors at the same time, like the neutral movement in retinoscopy. The drum and optometer systems rotate through 180 degrees taking measurements at each 1 degree to produce a plot of refractive error as a $\sin^2$ function of meridian. The examiner can then identify the refractive error at the peak and trough of that $\sin^2$ function to get the refractive errors in the principal meridians, and convert them into the spherocylinder lens formula.

Best Focus

Autorefractors that use the best focus principle include the Dioptron and some of the early Canon and Hoya autorefractors. The Dioptron, for exam-

ple, uses a rotating drum with rectangular gaps at regular intervals through which infrared radiation is directed toward the patient's retina. The light reflected from the patient's retina passes through a mask of alternating opaque and clear stripes before striking a photocell. If the grating projected into the patient's eye is in focus on the retina, it has a high contrast, so that there are alternating bright and dim areas. If it is out of focus, the lower contrast results in the same overall luminance but the bright areas are not as bright. As the reflected bright and dim areas pass across the mask in the instrument's return path, the output of the photocell increases and decreases. The maximum variation in photocell output thus occurs when the contrast of the retinal image is greatest. The lens that focuses light on the retina moves back and forth until the variation in the photocell output is greatest, thus deriving the refractive error for that meridian. The Dioptron measures refractive error in six meridians. Assuming a $\sin^2$ function of refractive error with meridian, the sphere, cylinder, and axis of the patient's refractive error are calculated.

Knife-Edge Principle

An example of an autorefractor based on the knife-edge principle is the Humphrey HARK 599 autorefractor. Before talking about the Humphrey autorefractor, however, we need to discuss the knife-edge principle in general. In this setup, the image of a point source is focused at the edge of a straight opaque surface, or knife-edge. This produces an out-of-focus patch on the retina. If the object point that would focus on the subject's retina (that is, the punctum remotum) is behind the knife-edge, rays passing through the lower part of the pupil will be blocked and thus the upper part of the pupil will appear to be illuminated (Figure 7.9).

If the object point that would focus on the patient's retina is between the eye and the knife-edge, as it would be in higher myopia, the rays passing through the upper part of the pupil are blocked. In this case, the lower part of the pupil appears illuminated (see Figure 7.9).

The Humphrey autorefractor uses the knife-edge principle by using four infrared bar light sources, which act like knife-edges, arranged in a cross pattern. The light from those sources reflected from the patient's retina is analyzed by

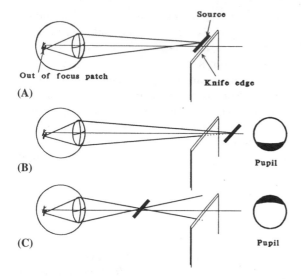

Figure 7.9. An illustration of the knife-edge principle. (A) A light source produces an out-of-focus patch on the subject's retina. (B) If the retina is conjugate with a point beyond the knife-edge, light passing through the lower part of the pupil is blocked. (C) If the retina is conjugate with a point between the knife-edge and the eye, light passing through the upper part of the pupil is blocked. (Reprinted with permission from Henson DB. *Optometric Instrumentation.* 2nd ed. Oxford: Butterworth-Heinemann, 1996;185.)

four photodetectors arranged to produce a four-quadrant photodetection system. The knife-edge principle is used to determine if there is a spherical refractive error. Also, the four-quadrant photodetection system can determine whether the cross is tilted, as it would be if astigmatism were present. The patient's refractive error is neutralized using a combination of three variable power lenses: a sphere; a cross cylinder with principal meridians at 90 and 180; and a cross cylinder with principal meridians at 45 and 135. A cross-cylinder lens is a lens with powers that are equal in magnitude but opposite in sign in the two principal meridians. These cross-cylinder lenses are designed with variable powers such that the principal meridians maintain equal magnitude powers and opposite sign. The powers of the 90 – 180 cross cylinder and the 45 – 135 cross cylinder are varied so that in combination they yield a correction of the patient's astigmatism. The powers of the variable power sphere and the variable power cross-cylinder lenses

are summed to give the sphere, cylinder, and axis of the patient's refractive error.

Ray Deflection Principle

Assuming relaxed accommodation, light from an illuminated patch on the retina of an emmetropic eye exits that eye with rays that are parallel. In a myopic eye, the rays exit the eye convergently because the punctum remotum is in front of the eye. In a hyperopic eye, the rays exit the eye divergently because the punctum remotum is behind the eye. The amount of refractive error determines the vergence of light leaving the eye. Another way to state this is that the amount of refractive error determines how much the rays are deflected from parallelism. In the Canon R-50 autorefractor, photodetectors sense the linear separation of images reflected from the patient's retina. The ray-deflection angle is determined from the linear separation of the images. Refractive errors in three set meridians are determined from the respective ray-deflection angles. The sphere, cylinder, and axis of the patient's refractive error are calculated from the refractive errors in these three meridians.

Image Size Principle

Retinal image size is a function of the amount of uncorrected refractive error. The Topcon RM-A7000 autorefractor measures the size of the retinal image of an annular object produced by passing infrared light through an annular aperture. For analysis of astigmatism, the instrument measures the lengths and orientations of the major and minor axes of an elliptical image on the retina.

Wavefront Sensing

Determining refractive error traditionally means finding the sphere, cylinder, and axis for a lens that when added to the eye would focus the ocular image on the retina. However, these parameters exclude aberrations, and aberrations can also degrade the retinal image if not corrected. It is estimated that if aberrations were also corrected, best visual acuity could theoretically reach 20/8, and there would also be major improvements in contrast sensitivity not reflected by a Snellen visual acuity number. Wavefront sensors measure wavefront error, which includes information not only about sphere, cylinder, and axis, but about all of the imperfections in an optical system that degrade the image. (The concept of wavefront aberration is discussed in Chapter 2.)

As of this writing, several commercial ophthalmic wavefront sensors are available or soon to be marketed. The Dresden Wavefront Analyzer is based on the Tscherning aberroscope in which an evenly spaced grid of object points is projected onto the retina. Aberration is detected as displacements of the image points from their unaberrated positions on the retina as viewed from outside the eye. This is very similar to the Scheiner principle, except that many "pinholes" are used simultaneously and the observations are objective. The Ray Tracing Visual Function Analyzer by Tracey Technologies uses a similar technology, but projects

rays into the eye sequentially. The OPD Scan by Nidek uses a retinoscopy principle.

Most wavefront sensors use the Shack-Hartmann principle, which is described below as an example of wavefront sensing. Examples of instruments that use the Shack-Hartmann principle are The Complete Ophthalmic Analysis System (COAS) by WaveFront Sciences, the Quantum-Light Wavefront Refractor by Zeiss Humphrey, the CustomCornea Wavefront System by Alcon Summit Autonomous, the WaveScan Wavefront System by Visx, Zywave by Bausch & Lomb, and the SureSight Autorefractor that is a hand-held autorefractor by Welch Allyn. The basics of Shack-Hartmann wavefront sensing are shown in Figure 7.10.

A narrow laser beam is directed into the eye along the line of sight so that it illuminates a spot on the fovea. This serves as a luminous point object on the retina, which projects rays through the entire

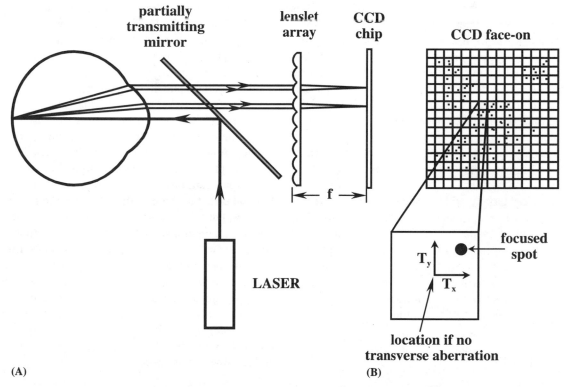

(A)

(B)

Figure 7.10. (**A**) A basic Shack-Hartmann wavefront sensor. Some liberty has been taken in eliminating detail in order to emphasize the basic concepts. In reality, other lenses are included in order to make the entrance pupil of the eye conjugate with the lenslet array, form a fixation target, and so on. (**B**) The pattern of spots imaged onto the CCD chip is shown. The grid shows the boundaries of the individual lenslets. The center of each square is the location of each optical axis. Each spot is the image focused by its corresponding lenslet. The direction and distance that each spot deviates from its lenslet axis is transferred to a computer. The computer interprets this as transverse aberrations, which it transforms into a map of wavefront errors.

pupil of the eye. If the eye is emmetropic and without aberrations, all of the rays will exit the eye in a parallel bundle, that is, with plane wavefronts. This bundle is intercepted by an array of microlenslets where each individual lenslet focuses the part of the beam incident on it onto a CCD chip placed at the focal plane of the lenslets. If the entering beam is truly parallel, then the focused spots will all be located at the image plane *on the optical axis* of each lenslet in the array. To the extent that the spots are displaced from the optical axes, transverse aberrations have been introduced by the optics of the eye, that is, the exiting wavefront was not plane. The CCD detector sends this information to a computer, which calculates the direction and the amount of displacement of each spot from its unaberrated location, and then reconstructs the wavefront shape across the pupil that would have produced this pattern of spots. (The concept of constructing the wavefront on the basis of the transverse aberrations induced by different parts of the total pupil is described in Chapter 2.) Deviations of the true wavefront from the ideal spherical wavefront whose focus is at the retina can be displayed on a computer monitor as a false color map indicating zones of identical wavelength differences. This three-dimensional surface plot is usually fit to an expansion known as a Zernike polynomial whose separate terms can be interpreted as defocus, tilt, cylinder, and numerous other aberrations. The use of the lower-order terms is sufficient to specify a spectacle Rx so a wavefront sensor can be used as an autorefractor. Theoretically, additional terms could be used during refractive surgery to reduce most aberrations and obtain what has been called "superacuity." Also, ophthalmoscopes and fundus cameras are now being developed that incorporate a wavefront sensor to determine the wavefront aberrations of the eye being examined and then correct the aberrations to give unprecedented detailed views of the fundus.[8–10]

PHOTOREFRACTION

Photorefraction is the use of photographic methods for the measurement of refractive errors.[11,12] There are three methods of photorefraction: *orthogonal, isotropic,* and *eccentric.* Orthogonal and isotropic photorefraction are sometimes classified as *point-spread methods of photorefraction*, because they both use a point source of light and measure the spread of the light reflected from the subject's retina. Eccentric photorefraction is also known as *photoretinoscopy* because it is similar in principle to retinoscopy.

Orthogonal Photorefraction

In orthogonal photorefraction a photograph is taken of the point spread of light reflected from the subject's retina. Before passing into the camera lens, light passes through four cylinder lens segments with power axes arranged radially 90 degrees apart. These cylinders produce a cross pattern, which is photographed. The thickness of the cross arms is a function of pupil diameter. The length of opposing cross arms is a function of refractive error, pupil diameter, the distance from the camera to the subject, the power of the photorefractor cylinder lens segments, and the focal length of the camera. Refractive error can be calculated because the other factors are known. One photograph is taken with the cylinder lens segments oriented in the 90 and 180 meridians, and another photograph with the cylinder segments oriented at 45 and 135. The two photographs with the different cylinder lens orientations are used to assess the presence of astigmatism. A third photograph can be taken without the cylinder lens segments in place to get a measure of pupil diameter.

A significant problem with orthogonal photorefraction is that the sign of the refractive error is not obvious, but this can be derived from color photographs of the point spread functions. If the retina is conjugate with a point behind the camera's film plane (or behind the subject's eye as in hyperopia), red rays are at the edge and blue rays are central in the point-spread image. If the retina is conjugate with a point between the camera's film plane and the subject's eye, as in higher amounts of myopia, blue rays are at the edge of the point-spread image and red rays are at the center.

Isotropic Photorefraction

Isotropic photorefraction does not use the cylinder lens segments that are used in orthogonal photorefraction. In isotropic photorefraction three photographs are taken, one with the camera focused on the subject's pupil, one with the camera focused about 0.50 D in front of the pupil, and the third with the camera focused about 0.50 D behind the pupil. The first photograph is used to get a measure of pupil diameter. The second and third photographs are used to measure refractive error from the size of the blurred patch reflected from the subject's retina.

Focusing the camera in front of and behind the pupil provides information on the amount and the sign of the refractive error. In myopia the retina is conjugate with a point in front of the eye. Therefore, the light patch from the retina in the photograph, taken with the camera focused in front of the pupil, is in better focus and is smaller than the light patch in the other photograph. In hyperopia, with accommodation relaxed, the retina is conjugate with a point behind the eye, so the photograph of the light patch taken with the camera focused behind the pupil has better focus and has the smaller diameter. In astigmatism, the photographed patch of light is elliptical; the long and short axes of the ellipse indicate the principal meridians. Neither orthogonal nor isotropic photorefraction can be used to determine high refractive errors.

Eccentric Photorefraction

Eccentric photorefraction is also known as photoretinoscopy because it is similar in principle to retinoscopy. The light source is eccentric to the optical axis of the camera lens. This is similar to tilting the retinoscope and observing the direction of motion of the reflex. In eccentric photorefraction, a photograph is taken of the light reflected from the subject's retina. If the retina is conjugate with the camera, the light fills the pupil just like a neutral reflex in retinoscopy. If the retina is conjugate with a point between the eye and the camera, then an illuminated crescent appears in the pupil on the same side as the light source. This is like the against motion in retinoscopy, because when the light source is directed up across the optical axis of the camera the light crescent appears in the lower part of the pupil. If the retina is conjugate with a point behind the camera, then the illuminated crescent appears in the pupil on the opposite side as the light source. This is like the with motion in retinoscopy.

The portion of the pupil that is not illuminated is a function of the refractive error relative to the camera, the eccentricity of the light source, the distance from the camera to the subject's entrance pupil, and pupil diameter. The commercial eccentric photorefraction instruments are not highly accurate for determination of the amount of refractive error, but are useful for screening for refractive errors.

Uses of Photorefraction

Photorefraction is well suited for assessing refractive error in noncooperative individuals such as infants and children who cannot maintain steady fixation. Because both eyes are photographed at the same time, photorefraction is particularly useful for screening for anisometropia (a difference in refractive errors between the two eyes).

A major disadvantage of photorefraction is that its accuracy is limited. Retinoscopy and autorefraction give better estimates of refractive error. Also the range of refractive errors that can be measured is limited. Since there is no system for controlling accommodation, accommodation can result in an underestimation of hyperopia and an overestimation of myopia.

STANDARD SUBJECTIVE REFRACTION

A routine part of a clinical eye and vision examination is the determination of the lens prescription that would correct the patient's refractive error. The examination sequence generally involves some objective estimate of refractive error such as retinoscopy. This is followed by refinement of the lens correction by a series of lens substitutions and adjustments, along with corresponding questions to the patient concerning the clarity and appearance of objects viewed at a distance of 4 to 6 meters. This procedure is known as the *subjective refraction to best visual acuity*, or sometimes as simply the *subjective refraction*. The subjective refraction results in the sphere, cylinder, and axis values that correct the patient's refractive error. With these lenses in place and accommodation relaxed, the patient can see distant objects clearly because the retina is conjugate with optical infinity.

Subjective refractions are usually performed with the aid of a *phoropter*. A phoropter is an instrument that contains banks of sphere and cylinder lenses and accessory lenses, prisms, occluders, and other devices for refraction and testing binocular vision. The lenses generally progress in steps of 0.25 D; this dioptric change is near the limit that the typical patient can detect. The phoropter is generally mounted on the moveable arm of a stand next to the examination chair. The lens wheels of a standard phoropter are usually rotated manually, but some remote-controlled models have lens wheels that are rotated by motors.

Although the specific procedures and the exact questions asked of the patient may vary somewhat from clinician to clinician, there are three essential components of a subjective refraction, performed in the following order:

1. Monocular subjective refraction and neutralization of astigmatism.
2. Binocular balance.
3. Binocular subjective refraction.

In the first of these steps, monocular subjective refraction and neutralization of astigmatism, each eye is tested separately. Spherical error is neutralized with spherical lenses, and astigmatism is neutralized with cylinder lenses. In order to get correct measures of astigmatism, the spherical component of the refractive error must be approximated first.

The next step of the refractive procedure is the binocular balance. The purpose of this test is to eliminate differences in refractive error between the two eyes that are due to differences in accommodation that occurred during the monocular test. Accommodation is linked in the two eyes such that the stimulation of accommodation in one eye will result in an equal amount of accommodation in the other eye. (This is referred to as consensual accommodation.) Therefore, if the binocular balance procedure is not done correctly, when one eye sees the target clearly, the other eye, which must accommodate the same amount, is accommodated differently from when its refractive error was determined, and it receives a blurred image.

The last step in the subjective refraction is the binocular subjective. The binocular subjective starts with more plus or less minus than the patient's refractive error. This overplussing is sometimes referred to as *fogging*, and it is designed to relax accommodation. Then plus is reduced or minus is increased binocularly until the patient achieves his or her best visual acuity. The endpoint in the binocular subjective is reached when there are no further improvements in visual acuity (and the letters may appear to be getting smaller and darker).

Optical principles of some of the tests that are used as components of or confirmation of the subjective refraction will now be described.

Clock Dial Test

The clock dial test is occasionally used as a preliminary measurement of astigmatism. The name of the test derives from the pattern of the object used for the test, 12 radial lines organized in a clock face pattern.

The test is started with no cylinder lens in front of the patient's eye and with the patient overplussed or fogged. As a result, if astigmatism is present, the interval of Sturm is anterior to the retina. The examiner asks the patient in terms of the hour positions on a clock which lines appear most distinct. Let's consider an example of a patient who requires a refractive correction with the minus cylinder axis in the 180 meridian (and thus its minus power is in the 90 meridian). This means that the eye's vertical (90) meridian has more converging power than its horizontal (180) meridian. The interval of Sturm of a point object formed by this eye would have a horizontal line focus formed by the vertical meridian at its anterior end and a vertical line focus formed by the horizontal meridian at its posterior end. At the start of the clock dial test, then, the vertical line focus would be closer to the retina and thus the vertical line would appear less blurred than the horizontal line (Figure 7.11A). So the patient reports that the lines from 12 o'clock to 6 o'clock are most distinct.

The axis of a minus cylinder lens used to correct this astigmatism would have to be oriented perpendicular to the axis of the clearest line since this places its minus power in the vertical meridian. The examiner can easily determine this axis by multiplying the lower of the two clock face numbers the patient reports by 30. So in our example the clock would read 6:00 or 12:00. Six o'clock (6:00) is the lesser number so the examiner starts increasing minus cylinder power with its axis oriented at

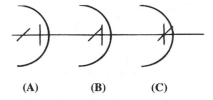

(A)   **(B)**   **(C)**

Figure 7.11. For a patient who has with-the-rule astigmatism, the vertical line focus formed by the horizontal meridian of the eye is closer to the retina than the horizontal line focus formed by the vertical meridian of the eye at the beginning of the clock dial test. (**A**) Addition of minus cylinder axis 180 moves the horizontal line focus posteriorly to narrow (**B**) and then collapse (**C**) the interval of Sturm. (Reprinted with permission from Grosvenor T. *Primary Care Optometry: Anomalies of Refraction and Binocular Vision.* 3rd ed. Boston: Butterworth-Heinemann, 1997;287.)

$6 \times 30 = 180$. This causes the interval of Sturm to narrow as its anterior end, corresponding to the vertical meridian of the eye, moves back (Figure 7.11B). This occurs because the addition of minus cylinder at axis 180 is the addition of minus power in the 90 meridian. When sufficient cylinder power has been added to make all of the radial lines equally distinct, the interval of Sturm has been collapsed and the astigmatism has been corrected (Figure 7.11C). This test is not very precise because it does not provide fine gradations of cylinder axis. However, it gives an initial rough estimate of the cylindrical component of refractive error, which can then be refined by other methods.

Jackson Cross Cylinder Test

The Jackson Cross Cylinder, or JCC, test, proposed by the American ophthalmologist Edward Jackson in 1887, is the most common procedure for the refinement of astigmatism correction. A cross-cylinder lens is a lens with powers that are equal in magnitude but opposite in sign in the principal meridians, usually ± 0.25 D or ± 0.50 D. The JCC test starts with the patient's viewing through the best monocular subjective refraction known at that point, usually obtained by retinoscopy and some brief subjective testing. The JCC lens is placed before the patient's eye, and the patient then compares the clarity of vision with the JCC axis aligned in different meridians. Because the JCC lens creates or exaggerates the interval of Sturm, the patient is told that the views observed on this test may be somewhat blurry.

The JCC test is performed in two stages. First, the axis of the correcting cylinder is determined. Then, the power of the correcting cylinder is determined.

To determine the axis, the JCC lens is oriented so that its principal meridians are placed 45° away from the axis of the cylinder in the phoropter. The Jackson cross-cylinder lens is then "flipped" about the axis of the phoropter cylinder so that the minus power principal meridian of the JCC becomes the plus power principal meridian, and vice versa. If the cylinder axis in the phoropter is not correct, one flip position will give a clearer image than the other. To arrive at the correct axis, the axis of the phoropter cylinder is changed (with the flip axis of the JCC changed in tandem) until the view is equally clear for both flip positions.

To determine the correct cylinder power, one of the principal meridians of the JCC lens is set to coincide with one of the principal meridians of the cylinder in the phoropter. The JCC lens is then flipped about this axis so that the minus power principal meridian of the JCC becomes the plus power principal meridian, and vice versa. The correct cylinder power in the phoropter is obtained when the view is equally clear for both flip positions. For each 0.50 D that the cylinder power in the phoropter is increased or decreased, the spherical power must be changed by 0.25 D of the opposite sign in order to maintain the initial spherical equivalent power. Let's consider, as an example, a situation in which the examiner measures a cylinder of -0.75×80 on retinoscopy, but the patient's actual astigmatism is -1.00×90. Let's also say that the examiner uses a ± 0.25 D JCC lens. For the axis measurement, the principal meridians of the JCC lens are set 45° from the 80 and 170 meridians, so the two flip positions of the JCC lens flip have powers of $+0.25 -0.50$ x 35 and $+0.25 -0.50$ x 125. The side with the minus cylinder axis at 125 is closer to 90, so the patient chooses that one as providing the clearer vision. The examiner then moves the minus cylinder axis on both the JCC lens and the phoropter cylinder lens in that direction. The axis determination is continued until the patient says that the views with the two flip positions of the JCC have equal clarity. At that point, the correct cylinder axis of 90 has been reached.

Next the examiner determines the cylinder power. The JCC lens is rotated so that its principal meridians coincide with the principal meridians of the cylinder in the phoropter. To continue our example, the cylinder in the phoropter is –0.75 × 90, and the powers on the two flips of the JCC lens are +0.25 –0.50 x 90 and +0.25 –0.50 x 180. The –0.50 × 90 JCC cylinder in combination with the –0.75 × 90 phoropter cylinder is –1.25 × 90. We'll call this one choice 1. Choice 2 is –0.50 × 180 in combination with –0.75 × 90, or –0.25 × 90. The combination on choice number 1 (–1.25 × 90) is closer to the patient's actual cylinder correction than the combination on choice number 2 (–0.25 × 90), so the patient picks number 1 as the view with better clarity. Since the JCC lens cylinder on choice 1 was minus cylinder axis 90, the examiner increases the power of the minus cylinder in the phoropter by –0.25 in the horizontal meridian (axis 90). The power is determined by repeating this process until the patient reports the two views to be equal in clarity, or when a reversal occurs on the next cylinder power change.

Red-Green Test

The most common use of the red-green test (also known as the *bichrome test* or the *duochrome test*) is to double-check the spherical endpoint on monocular or binocular subjective refraction. In a standard white light subjective refraction, lens powers are determined to correct the eye for a wavelength near the middle of the visible spectrum. The red-green test makes use of the longitudinal chromatic aberration of the eye to help set the refractive correction at this mid-wavelength. Red and green filters are placed in the projector to bisect the target viewed by the patient, red on one side and green on the other. The target is typically a Snellen chart, in which case the patient sees black letters against a green background on one side of the chart and against a red background on the other side of the chart. The wavelengths transmitted by these filters are selected so that they bracket the wavelength that is desired to be in focus on the retina and are separated from that wavelength by dioptrically equal amounts.

The red-green test starts with the patient over-plussed, thus shifting the longitudinal chromatic interval anterior to the retina. Green light is refracted more by the eye than red, so red light is focused closer to the retina (Figure 7.12A).

The patient looks at the black figures on the red and green backgrounds. Because there is less defocus of the red light than there is of the green light, the edges of the figures on the red side of the chart are more distinct than those on the green side. Plus is then reduced in 0.25 D steps, shifting the chromatic interval posteriorly. The endpoint of the test is reached when the figures on the red and green sides of the chart are equally black and distinct. At this point the red and green foci are dioptrically equidistant from the retina, the green anterior to the retina and the red posterior to the retina (see Figure 7.12B). Some patients go from red being more distinct to green being more distinct in a 0.25 D step, so for them the first green response is the endpoint. This test is very useful but not infallible. For instance, some patients tend to accommodate during the red-green test, so their endpoints are too much minus or not enough plus. It also works poorly if there is uncorrected astigmatism present, because the chromatic interval is then confounded with the interval of Sturm.

The dioptric interval of the wavelength transmissions of the red and green filters should be such that the wavelength used for focus on the retina in

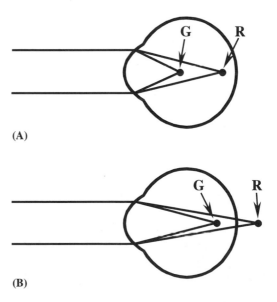

(A)

(B)

Figure 7.12. (A) The chromatic interval between the green focus (*G*) and the red focus (*R*) is anterior to the retina at the beginning of the red-green test. (B) The endpoint of the red-green test is reached when the red and green foci are dioptrically equidistant on either side of the retina.

ordinary white light conditions is at its midpoint. It is often assumed that the wavelength used in ordinary subjective refraction is about 555 nm, because that is the wavelength of maximum photopic sensitivity of the eye.[13] However, during a subjective refraction the distance focus point may be closer to 570 nm,[14] since this is near the peak of the luminosity curve of the incandescent lamps used in examination room projectors. Either way, this difference would be inconsequential because the chromatic aberration between 555 nm and 570 nm is generally less than a tenth of a diopter.

SUBJECTIVE AUTOREFRACTORS

Various automated instruments have been developed to replace the traditional phoropter. The three subjective autorefractors discussed in this section allow the practitioner to perform most or all of the components of a standard subjective refraction.

American Optical SR-III and SR-IV

The American Optical SR-III autorefractor and the later SR-IV autorefractor are self-contained table-mounted instruments based on a design by Guyton.[6,15] A monocular subjective refraction can be performed with this instrument, but a binocular balance cannot. The examiner can make adjustments on the control panel to change the target viewed by the patient, and make other adjustments to change the vergence of light in the patient's spectacle plane and thus neutralize the refractive error. The instrument changes the exiting vergence by moving cylinder lenses and mirrors within the optical system. The cylinder correction refinement procedure uses a Jackson cross cylinder. One interesting feature of this cylinder testing system is that a Maltese cross was used as a target because it was thought that the blur induced by the cross cylinder would be more uniform with that target than with letters. With letters as the target, the patient may choose the position of the cross cylinder that yields less blur in the vertical strokes of letters because letters are more likely to be recognized when the vertical strokes are clear.[12] Also incorporated in the cylinder testing mechanism was simultaneous presentation of both Jackson cross cylinder choices, rather than comparison of clarity before and after a

"flip." Studies of SR-IV testing with adults have found comparable results to standard subjective refraction, but in children the SR-IV sometimes gave too much minus, presumably due to proximal accommodation.[16,17]

Bausch & Lomb IVEX

The Bausch & Lomb Integrated Vision Examination System (IVEX) is a table-mounted computerized instrument that was designed to allow all of the testing that could be performed with a phoropter. The fixation objects, lenses, occluders, prisms, and so on, used for retinoscopy, subjective refraction, accommodation testing, and binocular vision testing procedures such as phorias and fusional ranges, are controlled by a push-button panel operated by the examiner. Retinoscopy can be performed with the examiner on the opposite side of the instrument from the patient. Measures of astigmatism obtained with the IVEX have been reported to agree well with standard subjective refraction; however, a significant number of patients show more minus or less plus with the IVEX than with conventional refraction.[17] Presumably, this is because the IVEX is a large instrument with significant proximity cues that would induce accommodation.

Humphrey Vision Analyzer

The Humphrey Vision Analyzer is an instrument that incorporated a number of new design features.[18–20] It is no longer manufactured but its unique design is interesting and could be incorporated in the development of future instrumentation. The patient and examiner are seated on opposite sides of a table that contains a projection system. The light from the projector is reflected by a concave mirror into the patient's eyes. The distance from the projector to the mirror and the distance from the mirror to the patient's spectacle plane are both equal to the radius of curvature of the mirror (about 3 m).

One of the unique features of the Humphrey Vision Analyzer is the fact that there is no phoropter or other instrumentation directly in front of the patient's eyes. Doing a subjective refraction with a phoropter, a clinician changes the vergence of light in the spectacle plane to match the patient's refractive error by changing the power of the lenses in the phoropter. With the Humphrey Vision Analyzer, the vergence of light in the spectacle plane is changed by changing the vergence of light leaving the projector. One way to illustrate this is to "unfold" the optical system so that the diagram won't show rays reflected from the mirror crisscrossing with the rays that strike the mirror. To unfold this optical system, we replace the concave mirror (which converges light) with a plus lens (which also converges light) that has the same focal length. So in this case the concave mirror with a focal length of 1.5 m (the focal length of a mirror is half its radius of curvature) is replaced with a +0.67 D lens, as shown in Figure 7.13.

For a zero refractive error setting, or in other words, parallel light at the spectacle plane, light would effectively be leaving the first focal point of the lens. As shown in Figure 7.13A, this would be achieved by having a vergence of light equal to +0.67 D leaving the projector.

Light is focused on the retina of an eye with a spectacle plane refractive error of –2.00 D if the vergence of light in the spectacle plane is –2.00 D. So for refraction of a 2.00 D myopia, the vergence of light leaving the projector is changed by –2.00 D to –1.33 D (see Figure 7.13B). As a result, the vergence of light striking the mirror is –0.27 D. The vergence of light leaving the mirror is +0.40 D, forming an image 2.5 m from the mirror or 0.5 m from the spectacle plane. The vergence of light in the spectacle plane is thus –2.00 D.

Another innovative aspect of the Humphrey Vision Analyzer is the lens system in the projector and the subjective refraction procedure. Sphere and cylinder powers are varied using three variable power lenses: a sphere, a cross cylinder with principal meridians at 90 and 180, and a cross cylinder with principal meridians at 45 and 135. The first step in the monocular subjective refraction is the adjustment of the variable power sphere so that the patient sees an acuity chart most clearly. Then the cross cylinders are varied in power to equalize clar-

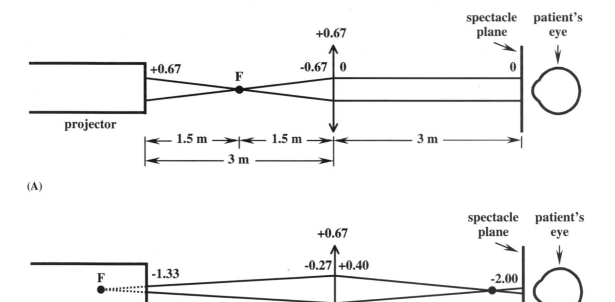

Figure 7.13. Examples of image formation with the Humphrey Vision analyzer projector system. (**A**) For parallel light in the spectacle plane, the vergence of light leaving the projector is +0.67 D. (**B**) For correction of a 2.00 D myopia, the vergence of light leaving the projector is changed by –2.00 D to become –1.33 D.

ity of radial line targets, thus neutralizing astigmatism. The last step in the monocular subjective refraction is to adjust the sphere power to yield the maximum plus or minimum minus to best visual acuity on an acuity chart.

There are separate light paths for the two eyes, making monocular testing possible without the use of occlusion or septums, and also making binocular testing possible. Standard binocular balance and binocular subjective refraction procedures can be followed to complete a full subjective refraction. Because the Humphrey Vision Analyzer does not block the examiner's view of the patient's face like a phoropter does, the examiner can assess whether the patient is squinting or is tilting his or her head. Despite its many innovative and desirable features, the Humphrey Vision Analyzer has not enjoyed wide popularity among practitioners. Perhaps the cost of the unit or the space required for it limited its acceptance.

Comments on Use of Subjective Autorefractors

Although the subjective autorefractors discussed here have incorporated some interesting designs and features, to date they haven't been incorporated in many offices. Perhaps this is because they aren't as convenient or as inexpensive as a simple phoropter. An important limitation of the American Optical SR-III and SR-IV is that they do not give the examiner the capability of performing a binocular balance. A significant drawback of the IVEX is that proximal accommodation occurs in some patients, resulting in too little plus or too much minus in the final refraction.

VALIDITY AND RELIABILITY OF METHODS OF REFRACTION

In this section we discuss the validity and the reliability of various refraction procedures. The *validity* of a measurement is an assessment of how well it measures what it purports to measure; that is, how close the measurement is to the true value of the variable being measured. A synonym often used for validity is *accuracy*. The *reliability* of a measurement is an assessment of its repeatability. A given technique may be highly reliable, but not

highly valid. That is, it could yield the same value almost every time, but it could be consistently too high or too low compared to the actual value. Another technique could be highly valid if enough measurements are taken, but not very reliable. In other words, the measurement would change notably from one reading to another, but when several readings are averaged, a result very close to the true value is obtained.

To assess the validity of various methods used to refract the human eye, we have to assume that there is one method that is known to be valid. Then other methods can be compared to it. Because subjective refraction has been shown through the years to be a very successful method of determining lens prescriptions, it is assumed to be valid and the validity of other refractive methods is based on how well they compare to subjective refraction.

Reliability can be studied by determining how repeatable refractive findings are when repeat measurements are made by the same examiner (intraexaminer reliability) or when different examiners do measurements on the same individuals (interexaminer reliability). Many papers have been written on the validity and reliability of different refractive techniques. We will summarize the results of a survey of those studies.[21]

Reliability data have usually been reported in one of two ways. One method used for testing reliability was to find the percentage of times two examiners (interexaminer) or one examiner on repeat occasions (intraexaminer) agreed within ±0.25 D or ±0.50 D. Another was to determine the 95% limits of agreement. This method uses the principle that 95% of a normal distribution is included in the range of ±1.96 standard deviations either side of the mean. The 95% limits of agreement are found by calculating the standard deviation of repeat measurements and then multiplying it by 1.96. The interexaminer and intraexaminer reliabilities for conventional subjective refraction are very similar. The percentage of times spherical equivalent measurements agreed within ±0.25 D was 63 to 86%. Measurements within ±0.50 D were observed 95 to 98% of the time. In other studies, the 95% limit of agreement for standard subjective refraction ranged from ±0.29 to ±0.63 D.

For retinoscopy, interexaminer comparisons on spherical equivalent or sphere within ±0.25 D were found 58 to 71% of the time. Measurements were within ±0.50 D of each other 81 to 89% of the time. Reliability of sphere or spherical equivalent measurements on various objective autorefractors at the ±0.25 D level were found to be 71 to 94%, and at the ±0.50 D level it has been reported at percentages ranging from 84 to 100%. The 95% limit of agreement reported for different objective autorefractors have ranged from ±0.27 to ±0.72 D.

Agreement of the spherical equivalent or sphere found with various objective autorefractors within ±0.25 D of standard subjective refraction has been reported at 30 to 73%. Agreement within ±0.50 D was 59 to 95%. Agreement of the SR-III, SR-IV, and Humphrey Vision Analyzer subjective autorefractors with conventional subjective refraction are similar. Various studies have reported that 57 to 75% of the time they were within ±0.25 D of the conventional refraction, and 82 to 91% of the time they were within ±0.50 D. It appears that the comparison of the IVEX subjective autorefractor with standard subjective refraction was not as close due to the tendency of the IVEX to overestimate minus. One study found an intraexaminer reliability of 68% (±0.25 D) and 89% (±0.50 D) for the Humphrey Vision Analyzer.

The studies summarized here were performed without cycloplegia (the pharmaceutically induced relaxation of the ciliary muscle to reduce or eliminate accommodation). It may be that the reliability of objective autorefractors would be better with cycloplegia because it should reduce their tendency to overminus. However, reliability of retinoscopy is likely to be reduced with cycloplegia because cycloplegic agents also dilate the pupil. As mentioned, the increased aberration effects with the dilated pupil make the retinoscopic reflex more difficult to assess.

Based on a review of the literature on reliability and validity of refraction, the following conclusions can be reached:[21]

1. A good estimate for both interexaminer and intraexaminer reliability of standard subjective refraction is 95% agreement within about ±0.50 D, and 80% agreement within about ±0.25 D. These levels of agreement are similar for spherical equivalent, sphere, and cylinder values.
2. Because of the limits on reliability of refraction, clinicians should not necessarily change patients' prescriptions by less than 0.50 D on a routine basis. However, there is a significant number of patients who respond very accurately to subjective refraction and can dependably benefit from a 0.25 D change in their prescription.
3. The reliabilities of objective and subjective autorefractors are similar to the reliability of conventional subjective refraction.
4. Some objective autorefractors show a bias in the minus direction compared to standard subjective refraction. Some show a bias in the plus direction. The agreement of objective autorefractors with standard subjective refraction is generally not as good as the reliability of standard subjective refraction. Objective autorefractors can be used as a substitute for retinoscopy (although they do not provide the examiner with clues to the accuracy of the results as in retinoscopy such as observations of the nature of the retinoscopic reflex or fluctuations in pupil diameter). Like retinoscopy, objective autorefractors do not provide for binocular balance testing. Due to these factors, objective autorefractors are not recommended as a substitute for conventional subjective refraction in deriving a lens prescription.

REFERENCES

1. Duke-Elder S, Abrams D. Ophthalmic optics and refraction. In: S Duke-Elder, ed. *System of Ophthalmology, 1.* St. Louis: Mosby, 1970;390–391.
2. Corboy JM. The *Retinoscopy Book: An Introductory Manual for Eyecare Professionals.* 3rd ed. Thorofare, NJ: SLACK:1989;2–6.
3. Daum KM. Accommodative response. In: JB Eskridge, JF Amos, JD Bartlett, eds. *Clinical Procedures in Optometry.* Philadelphia: Lippincott, 1991;677–686.
4. Levene JR. *Clinical Refraction and Visual Science.* London: Butterworth-Heinemann, 1977;10–17.
5. Campbell CE, Benjamin WJ, Howland HC. Objective refraction: retinoscopy, autorefraction, and photorefraction. In: WJ Benjamin, ed. *Borish's Clinical Refraction.* Philadelphia: Saunders, 1998;559–628.
6. Henson DB. *Optometric Instrumentation.* 2nd ed. Oxford: Butterworth-Heinemann, 1996;177–186.
7. Rabbetts RB. *Bennett and Rabbetts' Clinical Visual Optics.* 3rd ed. Oxford: Butterworth-Heinemann, 1998;351–362.
8. Salmon TO, Thibos LN, Bradley A. Comparison of the eye's wave-front aberration measured psychophysically and with the Shack-Hartmann wave-front sensor. *Opt Soc Am.* 1998;15:2457–2465.

9. Thibos LN, Hong X. Clinical applications of the Shack-Hartmann aberrometer. *Optom Vis Sci.* 1999; 76:817–825.

10. Miller DT. Retinal imaging and vision at the frontiers of adaptive optics. *Physics Today.* 2000;53:31–36.

11. Howland HC. Determination of ocular refraction. In: WN Charman, ed. *Visual Optics and Instrumentation.* Vol. 1 of J Cronly-Dillon, ed. *Vision and Visual Dysfunction.* Boca Raton: CRC Press, 1991;399–414.

12. Henson DB. *Optometric Instrumentation.* 2nd ed. Oxford: Butterworth-Heinemann, 1996;187–190.

13. Erickson P. Optical components contributing to refractive anomalies. In: T Grosvenor, MC Flom, eds. *Refractive Anomalies: Research and Clinical Applications.* Boston: Butterworth-Heinemann, 1991;199–218.

14. Rabbetts RB. *Bennett and Rabbetts' Clinical Visual Optics.* 3rd ed. Oxford: Butterworth-Heinemann, 1998;96–97,289–290.

15. Guyton DL. Automated clinical refraction. In: A Safir, ed. *Refraction and Clinical Optics.* Hagerstown: Harper & Row, 1980;505–533.

16. Grosvenor T, Perrigin DM, Perrigin J. Comparison of American Optical SR-IV refractive data with clinical refractive data on a group of myopic children. *Am J Optom Physiol Opt.* 1983;60:224–235.

17. Grosvenor TP. *Primary Care Optometry: Anomalies of Refraction and Binocular Vision.* 3rd ed. Boston: Butterworth-Heinemann, 1996;304–306.

18. Alvarez LW. Development of variable-focus lenses and a new refractor. *J Am Optom Assoc.* 1978;49:24–29.

19. Humphrey WE. Over-refraction and the Vision Analyzer. *Optom Monthly.* 1980;71:563–575.

20. Borish IM, Benjamin WJ. Monocular and binocular subjective refraction. In: WJ Benjamin, ed. *Borish's Clinical Refraction.* Philadelphia: Saunders, 1998; 629–723.

21. Goss DA, Grosvenor T. Reliability of refraction: a literature review. *J Am Optom Assoc.* 1996;67:619–630.

FURTHER READING

Borish IM, Benjamin WJ. Monocular and binocular subjective refraction. In: WJ Benjamin, ed. *Borish's Clinical Refraction.* Philadelphia: Saunders, 1998;629–723.

Campbell CE, Benjamin WJ, Howland HC. Objective refraction: retinoscopy, autorefraction, and photorefraction. In: WJ Benjamin, ed. *Borish's Clinical Refraction.* Philadelphia: Saunders, 1998;559–628.

Grosvenor T. *Primary Care Optometry: Anomalies of Refraction and Binocular.* 3rd ed. Boston: Butterworth-Heinemann, 1996;261–306.

Polasky M. Monocular subjective refraction. In: JB Eskridge, JF Amos, JD Bartlett, eds. *Clinical Procedures in Optometry.* Philadelphia: Lippincott, 1991;174–188.

Chapter 8
Development of Refractive Error

A life spent sitting indoors, bent over a book or a fine manual task, leads to nearsightedness; whereas the person who drinks and sleeps too much, who is given to idleness and daydreams, who ignores what lies before his feet or under his hand, whose gaze is usually directed into the distance, will find that he can no longer see clearly what is close to his face. —Johannes Kepler, 1611 (From Park D. *The Fire within the Eye: A Historical Essay on the Nature and Meaning of Light.* Princeton, NJ: Princeton University Press, 1997;167–168.)

Changes in refractive error occur throughout our lives. This chapter addresses the typical changes and their possible causes. We begin with a general discussion of how the various optical components of the eye contribute to ametropia. Then we discuss the prevalence of refractive errors, typical changes in refractive error during the life span, theories of the cause of development of refractive error, and the possible prevention of refractive error. For the reader who is unfamiliar with the basic statistical concepts in this chapter, Appendix 8.1 offers a brief review.

RELATION OF THE OPTICAL COMPONENTS OF THE EYE TO REFRACTIVE ERROR

Chapter 6 talks about the fact that in myopia the eye is too long for its optical power or it has an optical power that is too great for its length. In hyperopia the eye is too short for its optical power or its optical power is not great enough for its length. When we talk about optical power in this regard we are referring to the combined powers of the cornea and crystalline lens. When we mention length in relation to optical power, we mean the distance from the last of the refracting surfaces to

the retina, that is, the axial depth of the vitreous chamber. Most studies of optical components of the eye report the total axial length of the eye instead of vitreous depth. However, variability in vitreous depth accounts for most of the variability in the total axial length of the eye, so we will consider the studies on axial length to correspond to trends in vitreous depth. To show how ametropia relates to the optical components of the eye, we summarize the results of four lines of investigation: (1) coefficients of correlation of the optical components of the eye with refractive error; (2) comparison of the mean ocular component values in myopia and in emmetropia; (3) a mathematical model to show the amount of refractive error change expected as a result of a given amount of change in the ocular optical components; and (4) measured amount of change in the ocular optical components in myopia progression.

Correlation of Components with Refractive Error

The correlation coefficient of axial length and refractive error has been reported to be around –0.77 in most studies.[1] The negative sign of the correlation coefficient indicates that greater axial length is associated with more minus (myopic) refractive error. (Henceforth, *correlation* here will mean "correlation coefficient.") The relatively high correlation indicates that much of the variability in refractive error is associated with variability in axial length. The square of the correlation is an estimate of the variability of the one factor that is associated with variability of the other. In the case of axial length and refractive error it would be $(-0.77)^2 = 0.59$ or about 59%.

The correlation of the power of the anterior surface of the cornea with refractive error has varied from –0.11 to –0.30 in different studies.[1] The negative sign indicates that greater corneal power is associated with more minus refractive error. These studies were conducted with large numbers of subjects, so the correlations were statistically significant even though they were quite low. In one study the correlation of corneal power and refractive error increased from –0.18 to –0.67 when the effect of axial length was factored out.[2] These findings suggest that corneal power contributes to refractive error but that the contribution of corneal power to refractive errors is much less than that of axial length.

The correlation of crystalline lens power and refractive error has been found to be 0.0 to +0.39 in various studies. The positive correlation means that increasing crystalline lens power is associated with more plus refractive error. This is a paradoxical result because increases in refractive power of the eye would be expected to be associated with myopia.

Mean Ocular Component Values in Myopia and Emmetropia

Another way to look at the contributions of the optical components of the eye to refractive error is to compare mean values for the components in different refractive error groups. In many such studies, not all of the ocular components were measured. We will look at a study that measured radius of curvature of the anterior corneal surface by keratometry, radii of curvature of the crystalline lens by phakometry, and intraocular distances (anterior chamber depth, crystalline lens thickness, and vitreous depth) by ultrasonography.[3] The study was done on 176 young optometry students. The results of the study are summarized in Tables 8.1, 8.2, and 8.3. Tables 8.1 and 8.2 give the means for each of the components, and Table 8.3 gives the statistical significance of the difference between myopes and emmetropes by analysis of variance. Some of the optical components differ by sex, so Table 8.3 also gives the statistical significance of the difference by sex.

Some studies found a slightly greater anterior chamber depth in myopes than in emmetropes, and there appears to be a trend in that direction in this study but the difference was not statistically significant. Anterior chamber depth was about 0.1 mm greater in males than in females. Crystalline lens thickness did not differ significantly by refractive error group or by gender. Tables 8.1 and 8.2 show a notably greater vitreous chamber depth in myopes than in emmetropes. This is consistent with numerous other studies. Vitreous chamber depth was also greater in males than in females.

Several studies found greater anterior corneal surface power in myopes than in emmetropes.[4] Similarly, this study found the radius of curvature of the anterior surface of the cornea to be less in myopes than in emmetropes. The corneal radius was also less in females than in males.

The radius of curvature of the anterior surface of the crystalline lens did not differ by refractive error group or by sex. The posterior lens radius came

Table 8.1. Ocular Optical Components in Emmetropic and Myopic Females

Component	Emmetropes			Myopes		
	N	Mean	SD	N	Mean	SD
Anterior chamber depth (mm)	19	3.72	0.32	44	3.80	0.28
Crystalline lens thickness (mm)	19	3.69	0.31	44	3.66	0.23
Vitreous depth (mm)	19	15.83	0.64	44	16.85	0.77
Corneal radius (mm)	19	7.60	0.22	44	7.57	0.20
Anterior lens radius (mm)	18	9.57	0.94	37	9.78	1.11
Posterior lens radius (mm)	18	–5.68	0.50	37	–5.83	0.57
Crystalline lens power (D)	18	21.48	1.50	37	20.56	2.45
Retinoscopy (D)	19	+0.17	0.36	44	–3.42	2.20

The principal meridian nearest vertical was used for corneal radius and retinoscopy.
Reprinted with permission from Goss DA, Van Veen HG, Rainey BB, Feng B. Ocular components measured by keratometry, phakometry, and ultrasonography in emmetropic and myopic optometry students. *Optom Vis Sci.* 1997;74:489–495.

Table 8.2. Ocular Optical Components in Emmetropic and Myopic Males

Component	Emmetropes			Myopes		
	N	Mean	SD	N	Mean	SD
Anterior chamber depth (mm)	34	3.86	0.28	71	3.92	0.31
Crystalline lens thickness (mm)	34	3.63	0.25	71	3.62	0.24
Vitreous depth (mm)	34	16.33	0.62	71	17.13	0.94
Corneal radius (mm)	34	7.77	0.26	71	7.63	0.22
Anterior lens radius (mm)	32	10.05	0.86	66	9.88	1.16
Posterior lens radius (mm)	32	−5.93	0.43	66	−6.10	0.59
Crystalline lens power (D)	32	20.35	1.07	66	20.39	1.69
Retinoscopy (D)	34	+0.25	0.36	71	−2.87	2.14

The principal meridian nearest vertical was used for corneal radius and retinoscopy.
Reprinted with permission from Goss DA, Van Veen HG, Rainey BB, Feng B. Ocular components measured by keratometry, phakometry, and ultrasonography in emmetropic and myopic optometry students. *Optom Vis Sci.* 1997;74:489–495.

Table 8.3. Statistical Significance (*p* values) of the Difference in Ocular Optical Components between Emmetropes and Myopes and between Females and Males (data in Tables 8.1 and 8.2) (Tested by analysis of variance.)

Component	Refractive Group	Gender
Anterior chamber depth	0.197	0.010
Crystalline lens thickness	0.695	0.213
Vitreous depth	<0.001	0.008
Corneal radius	0.008	0.009
Anterior lens radius	0.854	0.212
Posterior lens radius	0.086	0.005
Crystalline lens power	0.315	0.111

Reprinted with permission from Goss DA, Van Veen HG, Rainey BB, Feng B. Ocular components measured by keratometry, phakometry, and ultrasonography in emmetropic and myopic optometry students. *Optom Vis Sci.* 1997;74:489–495.

close to being significantly greater in magnitude in myopes than in emmetropes. This would be a lower surface power in myopes than in emmetropes, which would be consistent with the paradoxical correlation of crystalline lens power and refractive error discussed earlier. The posterior lens radius was less in females than in males. Some studies found crystalline power to be less in myopes than in emmetropes,[5] but this study did not.

Mathematical Model to Predict Effects of Changes in the Ocular Components on Refractive Error

Another approach that can be taken to evaluate the effects of changes in the ocular optical components on refractive error is to trace rays through a schematic eye to determine the refractive error change when a given ocular component is changed. Erickson[6] traced the vergence of light backward through the eye starting from the retina and exiting from the cornea, in effect treating the retina as an object imaged by the paraxial optics of the eye. The vergence of light emergent from the cornea is then equal in magnitude, but opposite in sign, to the corneal plane refractive error. Appendix 8.2 uses the Gullstrand-Emsley schematic eye to demonstrate use of this method to calculate the refractive error.

Erickson[6,7] used this method on the Gullstrand schematic eye No. 1 to calculate the changes in refractive error that resulted from systematic changes in a given component. Table 8.4 shows the effects of 0.1-mm changes in the axial positions of the various ocular surfaces. Note that the largest change in refractive error would occur as a result of an increase in vitreous depth by moving the retina posteriorly. Moving the retina back 0.1 mm would induce a refractive error shift of –0.28 D.

Table 8.4 also indicates that the amount and direction of refractive error change depends on how a given intraocular distance is changed. For example, if anterior chamber depth is increased by 0.1 mm by shifting the cornea anteriorly, refractive error changes toward *myopia* by 0.14 D. In contrast, if anterior chamber depth is increased 0.1 mm by shifting the crystalline lens posteriorly, refractive error changes toward *hyperopia* by 0.13 D. Changes in crystalline lens thickness can also induce myopic or hyperopic shifts depending on what other intraocular distance is changing.

Table 8.5 shows the changes in the refractive error of the Gullstrand schematic eye No. 1 when the refractive index is increased by 1%. The largest change in refractive error would occur with an index change in the lens core. The next largest refractive error change would result from a change in index of refraction of the vitreous.

Erickson also studied how refractive error would change when radii of curvature of the refracting surfaces are varied. Table 8.6 gives the refractive error changes that result from increasing the corneal radii of a schematic eye with corneal parameters the same as in the Gullstrand schematic eye No. 1,[7] and from increasing crystalline lens radii in the Gullstrand-Emsley schematic eye. Flattening of the anterior corneal surface, or the ante-

Table 8.5. Changes in Refractive Error in the Gullstrand Schematic Eye No. 1 Resulting from 1% Increases in Index of Refraction of the Various Ocular Media

Medium	Refractive Error Change (D)
Cornea	+0.17
Aqueous	–0.82
Anterior lens cortex	+0.23
Crystalline lens core	–2.81
Posterior lens cortex	+0.19
Vitreous	+1.67

Data taken from Erickson P. Optical components contributing to refractive anomalies. In: T Grosvenor, MC Flom, eds. *Refractive Anomalies: Research and Clinical Applications.* Boston: Butterworth-Heinemann, 1991:199–218.

rior or posterior crystalline lens surfaces, causes changes in the hyperopic direction, but the largest refractive error change for a given change in radius comes from changing the curvature of the anterior corneal surface.

Measured Changes in the Ocular Components

The fourth approach to looking at the contribution of the ocular optical components in ametropia is to measure changes in the ocular optical components with age. This approach has been used most often in investigations of the increases of myopia in

Table 8.4. Effects of Changes in Intraocular Distances on the Refractive Error of the Gullstrand Schematic Eye No. 1 (Each change increases by 0.1 mm.)

Variable Increased	Method of Increase	Accompanying Increase in Axial Length (mm)	Change in Refractive Error (D)
Corneal thickness	Into anterior chamber	0	–0.03
	Anterior surface displacement	0.1	–0.17
Anterior chamber depth	Change in corneal position	0.1	–0.14
	Change in lens position	0	+0.13
Crystalline lens thickness	Into anterior chamber	0	–0.04
	Into vitreous chamber	0	+0.09
	No change in chamber depth	0.1	–0.18
Vitreous chamber depth	Change in retina position	0.1	–0.28
	Change in lens position	0	–0.13

Reprinted with permission from Erickson P. Optical components contributing to refractive anomalies. In: T Grosvenor, MC Flom, eds. *Refractive Anomalies: Research and Clinical Applications.* Boston: Butterworth-Heinemann, 1991;199–218.

Table 8.6. Changes in Refractive Error Resulting from 0.2-mm Increases in the Magnitude of the Radius of Curvature (i.e., flattening of the surface whether convex or concave)

Refracting Surface	Refractive Error Change (D)
Anterior cornea	+1.24
Posterior cornea	–0.16
Anterior crystalline lens	+0.13
Posterior crystalline lens	+0.26

Data from Erickson P. Mathematical model for predicting dioptric effects of optical parameter changes in the eye. *Am J Optom Physiol Opt.* 1977;54:226–233.

childhood and young adulthood commonly known as myopia progression. In a study in Denmark,[8] the correlation of refractive error change with vitreous depth change between 10 and 18 years of age in children who had been born with normal birth weight was –0.76. In that study there were 23 eyes that had refractive error changes greater than 2.5 D (all toward myopia) between the ages of 10 and 18 years.[9] In those 23 eyes anterior chamber depth increased an average of +0.13 mm, crystalline lens thickness increased an average of +0.04 mm, and vitreous depth increased an average of +1.44 mm. These mean changes in anterior chamber depth and crystalline lens thickness were similar to those for children who had lesser amounts of refractive error change, but vitreous depth increases were less in children who had lesser refractive error changes.

Another study that gives longitudinal data on changes in some of the ocular components is a study from Japan reporting changes in 1 year in a group of myopes.[10] For 18 eyes of 7- to 10-year-olds, the mean increase in myopia was 0.60 D (SD = 0.27). Corneal power decreased negligibly by an average of –0.06 D (SD = 0.08). Crystalline lens power decreased by –0.36 D (SD = 0.31). This decrease would not contribute to the increase in myopia; instead it would cause a tendency away from myopia. The increase in myopia can be accounted for by the average increase in axial length of 0.32 mm (SD = 0.11), which presumably would be due mostly to increases in vitreous depth.

Some studies of myopia progression in young adulthood found significant correlations between corneal power increase and myopia increase.[4] However, the corneal changes were small so that corneal steepening would contribute only slightly to increasing myopia. In one study of 16 persons who had onset of myopia in young adulthood, the correlation coefficient of refractive error change with change in vitreous depth was –0.77, with the amount of the vitreous depth increase appearing to account for most of the increase in myopia.[11]

Overview of Ocular Optical Component Contribution to Refractive Error

Each of the four approaches to understanding the contribution of the ocular optical components to refractive error point to vitreous depth as the major contributor to refractive error.

A secondary contributor to refractive error is the power of the anterior surface of the cornea. Differences in the radii of curvature and index of refraction of the crystalline lens seem to be of minor importance. However, changes in the index of refraction of the crystalline lens, along with swelling, are presumably the cause of the refractive error fluctuations experienced by persons with uncontrolled diabetes.[12]

EPIDEMIOLOGY OF SPHERICAL REFRACTIVE ERRORS

In this section we discuss the epidemiology of refractive errors and the factors that affect the prevalence of refractive errors. The greatest influence on the distribution of refractive errors is age.

Prevalence of Refractive Errors with Age

An instructive graphical summary of the change in the distribution of refractive error with age was presented by Everson[13] (Figure 8.1).

Even though the studies Figure 8.1 summarized are somewhat old now, the basic trends are the same as those identified by more recent summaries of the literature.[14] In this figure there are several histogram frequency distributions with percentage of eyes on the y-axis and refractive error on the x-axis. Histogram A is a frequency distribution of refractive error in newborn infants. Distributions from the eyes of progressively older individuals are displaced up and to the right. The horizontal solid lines represent zero percent for each histogram.

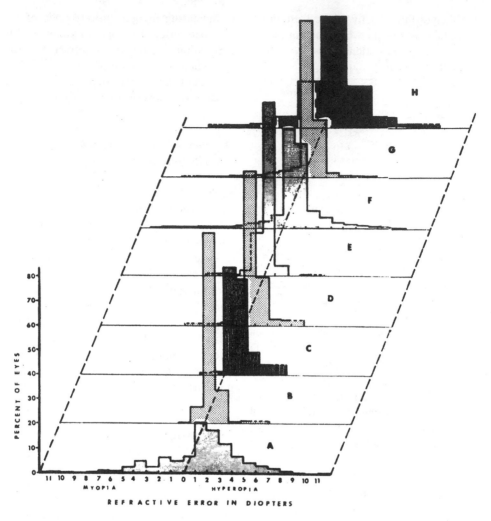

Figure 8.1. Frequency distribution histograms of refractive error at different ages. Histogram A is for newborns. Histogram H is for elderly persons. Histograms B through F are for intermediate ages from 5 to 7 years in Histogram B to the 20s in Histogram F. The solid horizontal line on each histogram is 0%. The dashed line extending up and to the right indicates zero refractive error. (Reprinted with permission from RW Everson. Age variation in refractive error distributions. *Optom Weekly.* 1973;64:200–204.)

The dashed line going up and to the right through the middle of each distribution indicates zero refractive error at the point where it crosses the solid horizontal line for each histogram. The scales are the same on each histogram for both the *x*-axis and the *y*-axis.

Histogram A is a distribution of refractive errors of Arkansas infants 30 hours old measured by retinoscopy under atropine cycloplegia. There is a wide range of refractive errors, extending from –12 to +12 D. Myopia was found in 25% of the eyes.

In the first few months of life, both myopic and hyperopic refractive errors start shifting toward emmetropia. This reduces the variability in refractive error. By about the time children enter school, the variability of refractive error is less than at any other time in the human life span. Histogram B gives the data for 950 boys, ages 5 to 7 years, tested by retinoscopy without cycloplegia on school screenings near Los Angeles. The distribution is more sharply peaked than one would expect from a normal distribution (it is leptokurtic). The vast majority of refractive errors is in the range from 0 to +1.0 D. The total range of refractive errors is much less than in Histogram A. The age group in Histogram C, 6 to 8 years of age, is very similar to that in Histogram B. Histogram C is a distribution of cycloplegic refractions of 154 Caucasian boys and 179 Caucasian girls in Washington, D.C. Most of the refractive errors were in the range from 0 to +2 D. As in Histogram B, the range in Histogram C is narrow.

Histogram D is the refractive error distribution for a sample of 12- to 16-year-olds in Washington, D.C., measured under cycloplegia. The total range of refractive errors is wider than at earlier ages. The most common refractive error is 0 to +1 D. There are noticeably more myopic refractive errors than in Histograms B and C. Histogram E is based on school screening retinoscopy data for 728 Los Angeles area boys with ages of 13 to 14 years. The distribution is leptokurtic with a peak at 0 to +1 D, but there are more myopes than in Histograms B and C. In Histogram F for 1,033 male British military recruits and in Histogram G for more than 2,500 male Swedish military recruits, the distributions are still leptokurtic, but the ranges are wider than in the previous distributions with the exception of the newborns. The peaks are again at 0 to +1 D.

The data in Histograms A through G were collected using samples that should be representative of their populations. For example, children examined on a school screening should be representative of the total population. However, it is difficult to obtain data for an unselected sample of adults. Histogram H was taken from a sample of older adults consisting of more than 700 individuals in a Philadelphia institution for the elderly and indigent. The median age was 74 years. The refractive errors were given in 2 D groupings as opposed to the 1 D groupings in the other histograms. The peak was at 0 to +2 D, but the distribution does not appear to be as leptokurtic as in Histograms B through G. The range of refractive errors is wide.

The trends that can be observed in Figure 8.1, and that are supported by other studies are:

1. A wide range of refractive errors extends from high myopia to high hyperopia among newborns.
2. Variability in refractive errors appears to be at its minimum at about 5 to 6 years of age.
3. With the exception of the newborns, the distributions are leptokurtic.
4. The peak in most distributions is at 0 to +1 D.
5. The variability of refractive errors is greater among older adults than among persons in their 20s.

6. The prevalence of myopia increases from 5 or 6 years of age through young adulthood.

In summarizing numerous studies on the prevalence of myopia at different ages, Grosvenor[15] proposed a classification of myopia based on age-related prevalence and age of onset. Figure 8.2 shows how the prevalence of myopia changes with age in the United States and the four categories in Grosvenor's classification of myopia.

The four categories are defined as follows:

1. *Congenital myopia* is myopia that is present at birth and is high enough in amount that it persists through the emmetropization period of early childhood and throughout the rest of life. Its prevalence is 1 to 2% at all ages.
2. *Youth-onset myopia* has its onset between about 5 years of age and physical maturity. The prevalence of myopia gradually increases through the school-age years until it reaches about 20% in the late teens.
3. *Early adult-onset myopia* is myopia that has its onset after physical maturity and up to about 40 years of age. Myopia prevalence continues to increase during the early adulthood years and reaches about 30 to 35% by about 40 years of age.

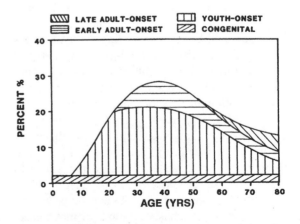

Figure 8.2. Graphical representation of the prevalence of myopia of −0.50 D or greater with age, with myopia classified as congenital, youth-onset, early adult-onset, and late adult-onset. (Reprinted with permission from Grosvenor T. A review and a suggested classification system for myopia on the basis of age-related prevalence and age of onset. *Am J Optom Physiol Opt.* 1987;64:545–554.)

4. *Late adult-onset myopia* has its onset after about 55 years of age due to changes in the nucleus of the crystalline lens. Most people have a shift in refractive error toward hyperopia after about 40 or 45 years of age. As a result some youth-onset myopes and early adult-onset myopes with low amounts of myopia lose their myopia after age 40 or 45. This accounts for the decline in myopia prevalence after 40 years of age in Figure 8.2.

Factors That Affect Prevalence of Refractive Errors

Most studies of the factors that affect the distribution of refractive errors have looked specifically at the association of various factors with the prevalence of myopia.[14,16] Some studies found higher prevalences of myopia among females than among males, but this has not been consistent. Prevalences of myopia are higher among Americans of European ancestry than among African Americans. Some very high prevalences of myopia have been reported among Asians, but these results may have been affected by the association of myopia and educational level.

Numerous studies have observed an association of myopia and near work. Myopia is more common in persons who have occupations involving near work, spend more time doing near work, have higher educational achievement and more years of education, and have better reading ability. Myopes tend to perform better on intelligence tests. Hyperopia has often been found to be associated with poor reading ability.[17] Myopia is more common in persons with higher socioeconomic status.

Myopia is more common among persons with a family history of myopia. Familial resemblance is probably due in part to inheritance and in part to common life style factors. Identical twins tend to be more alike in refractive error than fraternal twins.[14] Pedigree studies of human myopia have failed to identify a consistent mode of inheritance, probably due to at least two factors—the influence of environment and near work and the likely fact that growth and development of the refractive apparatus of the eye is guided by multiple genes.

CHANGES IN SPHERICAL REFRACTIVE ERROR DURING THE LIFE SPAN

Different stages in the human life span have characteristic trends in the change of refractive error.[18–20] Here we discuss the typical refractive changes in the following stages of life: (a) infancy and early childhood, (b) school-age years, (c) early adulthood from the late teens to about 40 years of age, and (d) later adulthood, starting at about 40 years of age.

Infancy and Early Childhood

Both the myopia and to a lesser extent the hyperopia present early in infancy decrease toward emmetropia in the first few years of life, with most of the change occurring in the first year. As a result, the prevalence of emmetropia increases. This is generally referred to as emmetropization.

School-Age Years

Although many children have fairly stable refractive error throughout the school-age years, some trends have been identified. Some children with hyperopia have decreases in hyperopia. For example, in one study in Finland,[21] hyperopic children had a mean rate of refractive error change of –0.12 diopters per year (D/yr), with a standard deviation (SD) of 0.14 D/yr and a range of rates from +0.11 to –0.45 D/yr. In contrast, myopic children had a mean rate of change of –0.55 D/yr (SD = 0.27, range = 0 to –1.63 D/yr). For 30 children who were hyperopic and then became myopic, the mean refractive error change rates were –0.21 D/yr (SD = 0.21) when they were hyperopic and –0.60 D/yr (SD = 0.45) when myopic.

The largest refractive error changes in the school-age years are the increases in myopia known as myopia progression. Once myopia appears in childhood, it increases in amount until it typically slows or stops in the mid to late teens.[22] Figure 8.3 shows typical patterns of myopia progression.

Rates of myopia progression vary considerably from one child to another. In a study in which data were taken from five optometry practices in the

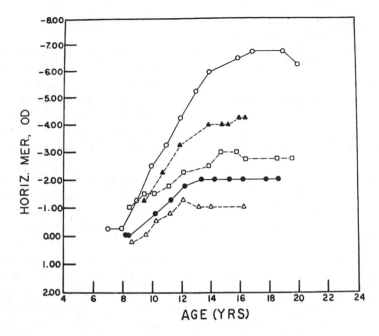

Figure 8.3. Typical patterns of childhood myopia progression. Each set of common symbols represents the data for one person. The y-axis is the refractive error in the principal meridian nearest horizontal in the right eye. (Reprinted with permission from Goss DA, Winkler RL. Progression of myopia in youth: age of cessation. *Am J Optom Physiol Opt.* 1983;60:651–658.)

central United States, the mean rates of childhood myopia progression were –0.40 D/yr (SD = 0.24, range = –0.01 to –1.09) in boys and –0.43 D/yr (SD = 0.25, range = +0.12 to –1.52) in girls.[23] A frequency distribution of the rates is given in Table 8.7.

Factors that have been reported to be associated with higher rates of childhood myopia progression include earlier age of onset, esophoria at near (convergent misalignment of the lines of sight of the two eyes when binocular fusion is prevented, such as by covering one eye), ophthalmoscopically visible myopic changes in the posterior segment of the eye, higher intraocular pressure, greater amount of time spent on reading and near work, and less time spent on outdoor activities.[20]

Young Adulthood

For most people, the time span from the late teens or early 20s to about 40 years of age is the period of most stability in refractive error.[19,20] The most common refractive change in this time period is the

Table 8.7. Frequency Distribution of Childhood Myopia Progression Rates for Patients from Five Optometry Practices in the Central United States

Range of Rates (D/yr)	Number of Males	Number of Females
+0.20 to 0.00	0	4
–0.01 to –0.20	37	20
–0.21 to –0.40	51	48
–0.41 to –0.60	41	44
–0.61 to –0.80	15	23
–0.81 to –1.00	12	7
–1.01 to –1.20	2	1
–1.21 to –1.40	0	0
–1.41 to –1.60	0	1

Reprinted with permission from Goss DA, Cox VD. Trends in the change of clinical refractive error in myopes. *J Am Optom Assoc.* 1985;56:608–613.

onset and progression of myopia. Some hyperopes have small increases in their hyperopia.

Rates of young adulthood myopia progression are generally less in magnitude than the rates of childhood myopia progression. Using patient records from five optometry practices in the central United States, one study[24] classified patterns of change in myopia in young adulthood as adult stabilization, adult continuation, and adult acceleration. Figure 8.4 shows an example of each of these patterns. *Adult stabilization* is characterized by stable refractive error in young adulthood after childhood myopia progression. This pattern was found in 68% of the males and 87% of the females in the records collected from those practices.

Adult continuation is characterized by continuation of myopia progression in young adulthood but at a slower rate than in childhood. The adult continuation pattern was found in 25% of the males and 13% of the females. In *adult acceleration* there is either onset of myopia in young adulthood or the rate of young adulthood myopia progression is greater than the rate of childhood myopia progression. The adult acceleration pattern was found in 6% of the males and none of the females in the records from the five general optometry practices. It is likely that the adult continuation and adult acceleration patterns would be more common in some populations, such as graduate students or military cadets.[16]

Later Adulthood

Most persons have hyperopic shifts after the age of 40 or 45 years. Because of this the prevalence of hyperopia increases and the frequency of emmetropia decreases after 40 or 45 years of age. A study from a California optometry practice reported a median refractive error of +0.18 D for patients aged 45 to 49 years and a median of +1.02 D for those aged 75 and older.[25]

The hyperopic direction of this shift is difficult to reconcile with what is known about the growth of the crystalline lens during adulthood. The adult lens increases its axial thickness approximately linearly with age as new fibers are added to its front and back surfaces, whereas its equatorial diameter remains nearly constant. This results in a steepening of the front and back surfaces so that the aging lens begins to resemble the young accommodated lens. Since this should result in a shift toward myopia with age, rather than hyperopia, this effect is sometimes referred to as the "lens paradox." One possible explanation is that the refractive index of the lens may decrease during this period. For persons who develop age-related nuclear cataracts, there are shifts in refractive error in the myopic direction.

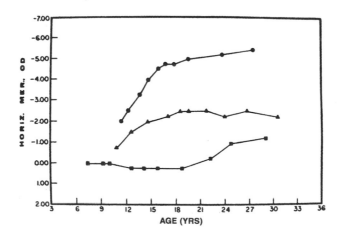

Figure 8.4. Examples of the adult stabilization (triangles), adult continuation (circles), and adult acceleration (squares) patterns of myopia progression. Each set of common symbols represents the data for one person. The *y*-axis is the refractive error in the principal meridian nearest horizontal in the right eye. (Reprinted with permission from Goss DA, Cox VD. Trends in the change of clinical refractive error in myopes. *J Am Optom Assoc.* 1985;56:608–613.)

PREVALENCE AND CHANGES IN ASTIGMATISM

As with spherical refractive errors, the most important factor in the prevalence of astigmatism is age.[14,20,26] In this section we discuss the prevalence of and changes in astigmatism in the same four age groups as for spherical refractive errors. Some other factors related to astigmatism prevalence are also discussed.

Infancy and Early Childhood

There is a high prevalence of astigmatism in neonates in the first weeks of life. In studies of Caucasian neonates, against-the-rule astigmatism is two to four times more common than with-the-rule astigmatism. This astigmatism decreases over the first few months of life, so that most of the infants who had significant astigmatism as neonates have spherical or nearly spherical refractive errors by 2 to 5 years of age.

School-Age Years

Most children entering school do not have astigmatism. Then, the prevalence and amount of astigmatism tend to increase slightly during the school-age years. In a study in California[27] based on retinoscopy during school screening, 81% of children at about 6.5 years of age had zero astigmatism and 72% of children at about 12.5 years of age had zero astigmatism. Astigmatism tends to increase slightly in childhood with reported average rates of change ranging from 0.03 to 0.06 D/yr.

Young Adulthood

With-the-rule astigmatism is more common than against-the-rule astigmatism among young adults. From the limited data on changes in astigmatism in young adults, it appears that the change in astigmatism is minimal—an average change of 0.1 to 0.3 D occurring in the 20 years between 20 and 40 years of age.[20]

Later Adulthood

Starting at about 40 years of age, astigmatism starts changing in the against-the-rule direction due to a steepening of the horizontal meridian of the cornea relative to the vertical meridian. On average, persons who have with-the-rule astigmatism have decreases in their astigmatism, persons who have against-the-rule astigmatism have increases in their astigmatism, and persons without astigmatism develop against-the-rule astigmatism. The change averages about 0.2 to 0.3 D every 10 years.[26] As a result of this change, against-the-rule astigmatism becomes more common than with-the-rule astigmatism by 50 or 60 years of age.[28,29]

Other Factors in Astigmatism Prevalence

Several papers have reported the prevalence of with-the-rule astigmatism to be very high in Western American Indian tribes.[30] Prevalences of 1.00 D or greater with-the-rule astigmatism exceeding 30% have been observed in Navajo, Sioux, Cheyenne, and Zuni sample populations.

The etiology of most cases of astigmatism is uncertain. One theory that has received some attention concerns the effects of lid tension on the cornea. It is clear that some manipulations and conditions of the eyelids can induce changes in corneal curvature and astigmatism.[4,31] However, attempts to relate measured eyelid tension to corneal astigmatism have failed to show a correlation.[32]

EMMETROPIZATION

As discussed earlier, the distribution of refractive errors is more sharply peaked and closer to emmetropia than would be expected by chance. It is theorized that this is due to a growth process, referred to as *emmetropization*, which is under feedback control from the quality of the retinal image. Emmetropization is most active in young eyes and occurs in the human eye mainly in the first years of life. Emmetropization is thought to be accounted for by two factors: (1) a natural tendency for the ocular components of the eye to grow together toward emmetropia without the need of feedback, and (2) an ocular growth mechanism that is highly dependent on visual feedback control and that fine-tunes the refractive state of the eye.[1,33,34]

In the first factor, the natural growth of the components of the eye as the eye enlarges tends to counterbalance the effects that each separate component has on refractive error. The component changes that occur during childhood include (1) an overall lengthening of the eye, including vitreous depth, which can continue through puberty; (2) an increase in corneal radius of curvature, which occurs mostly in the first few months of life; and (3) a decrease in crystalline lens power, which is fastest during early childhood. Of all the components, the increase in vitreous depth has the largest potential to affect the refractive state. By itself, vitreous depth increase would cause a change toward myopia. An increase in the corneal radius would decrease the corneal power and, by itself, would cause a change toward hyperopia. And an increase of the crystalline lens radii of curvature would cause a decrease in lenticular power, which, by itself, would cause a change toward hyperopia. The normal growth of all of these components tends to guide the eye toward approximate emmetropia; but an additional mechanism, the second factor, is necessary to explain the exquisite fine-tuning of the refractive state toward emmetropia.

Evidence that emmetropization involves an active vision-dependent feedback system comes from several types of studies:

1. *Form deprivation.* Studies from a variety of animal species show that depriving an animal of clear form vision interferes with emmetropization and produces myopia via abnormal axial elongation of the eye. One such manipulation is to diffuse the retinal image, such as by placing translucent diffusers (like miniature Ping-Pong balls) over the eye or by suturing an eyelid shut. Although ethical considerations prevent such manipulations on humans, there are natural conditions that block or diffuse normal transmission of light to the retina. Such conditions as congenital cataracts, lid hemangiomas, ptosis, neonatal lid closure, vitreous hemorrhage, and retrolental fibroplasia all result in a high incidence of myopia in infants and children.

2. *Deprivation reversal.* Chicks with induced refractive errors recover toward emmetropia if the inducing factor is removed while the animal is young. Hyperopia can be induced in chicks by dark rearing, and myopia can be induced by form deprivation. When the dark rearing is ceased at an early age (during the "sensitive period"), chicks with induced hyperopia respond by accelerating the normal increase in vitreous depth and thus decreasing hyperopia. When form deprivation is stopped within the sensitive period, the eye slows its rate of vitreous depth increase and, therefore, recovers from the induced myopia.

3. *Lens manipulation.* Studies with chicks, tree shrews, and monkeys show that when the retinal image is moved by placing lenses in front of the eye, there is an adjustment in refractive development that tends to reduce the distance between image and retina. Plus lenses (which move the image forward) tend to slow the axial elongation of the eye and cause refractive error changes in the hyperopic direction. Minus lenses (which move the image backward) are observed to accelerate axial elongation of the eye and cause refractive error changes in the myopic direction. These studies may have some implications for lens prescription strategies for humans. For example, if minus lenses cause myopic shifts in axial length, one might expect that delaying prescription of plus lenses for hyperopia might encourage the emmetropization process to reduce the hyperopia. These observations have led to the "defocus theory" of emmetropization.

The defocus theory maintains that a consistently defocused image on the retina, due to a mismatch of dioptric power and axial length, results in a feedback signal that is used to adjust the rate of growth of the posterior segment of the eye until the focal point and retina more nearly coincide. If the focal point is anterior to the retina, the normal rate of axial growth is slowed while the normal growth of the cornea and lens continue. This results in an increase in the focal length of the eye until the focal point reaches the retina. If the focal point is posterior to the retina, axial growth is accelerated until the retina is moved posteriorly enough to meet the focal point. Blur alone appears to be a potent and adequate stimulus that can lead to elongation of the young eye. For instance, if monkeys are reared in the dark so that there is no retinal image at all, axial changes are not induced by lid suture.[35] This suggests that the feedback for eye growth comes from a defocused image rather than simple light deprivation.

THE ETIOLOGY OF REFRACTIVE ERROR

Any theory of the etiology of refractive error should be consistent with the results of studies on the optics and epidemiology of refractive errors in humans, the recognized patterns of refractive development, and the results of animal studies in which refractive errors have been induced. And a theory of ametropia should be compatible with theories of emmetropization. Thus if we look at myopia etiology, a theory should incorporate axial elongation of the eye as the primary physical change responsible for the myopia, some role of near work in inducing the myopia, and some role of visual input in guiding the axial elongation of the eye. We can identify two main categories of myopia theories: accommodation/mechanical theories and defocus/humoral theories.

Accommodation/Mechanical Theories

One suggested mechanism is that accommodation might change the mechanical forces on the sclera and ciliary body. These forces would, in turn, produce permanent changes in the axial length of the eye. For instance, Young[36] reported increases in vitreous pressure in the eyes of monkeys during near viewing. From this, Young proposed an accommodation theory in which an increased vitreous pressure produced by prolonged periods of near work stretches the sclera and leads to a longer axial length and consequent myopia. However, this theory appears to be counter to studies that have found that accommodation results in decreases in intraocular pressure measured at the cornea.[37] In addition, experiments with chickens suggest that the physical action of accommodation could not be the only factor. When the Edinger-Westphal nucleus in chicks (the motor nucleus that controls accommodation) is lesioned, plus and minus lenses have the same effects on axial growth as in nonlesioned chicks.[38]

Defocus/Humoral Theory

The defocus experiments with animals have led many persons to accept the defocus theory as the most likely mechanism by which near work could influence myopia development. Myopia may be a form of emmetropization for near viewing. Myopes as a group tend to underaccommodate for near objects to a greater extent than emmetropes do.[39–41] If the accommodative response is significantly less than the accommodative stimulus, the near object being viewed would have its best focus somewhere behind the retina. Perhaps myopia develops to move the retina closer to the point of best focus.

The emmetropic mechanism may be controlled by a local chemical signal in the retina. Studies with chicks show that image blur in only part of the visual field results in local axial growth confined to the corresponding part of the retina.[33] Thus, the control of axial growth can be confined to local regions of the retina. This axial growth may be due to changes in the extracellular matrix of the sclera, which make it grow or make it more capable of being stretched by the natural pressure in the eye. One may surmise that when retinal ganglion cells are not stimulated adequately by high-contrast borders (which requires a clear image), a local chemical signal is released that itself, or through a cascade of reactions, diffuses through to the sclera, causing it to weaken and stretch or to grow. This potential for growth is greatest in the young eye, so manipulations of the focal plane generally do not work on adult animals. However, adult humans show continued susceptibility to axial myopia due to intense near work (e.g., studying by college students).

It may be more than coincidental that development of myopia tends to cease or slow at a time when collagen in both sclera and bone stops developing. The proposed humoral control must be due primarily to a local rather than to a circulating hormone since image manipulation in just one eye has little or no effect on emmetropization of the other eye. Also, as mentioned previously, if blur is restricted to a local area of the retina, only that area elongates. These observations suggest that there may be a pharmacological way to arrest the development of myopia in individuals who by genetics and/or environment are disposed to it. The defocus theory of myopia development in humans is still speculative. Because of differences in ocular physiology and anatomy, rates of ocular development, patterns of use of the eyes, and so on, the applicability of the animal results to human myopia still is open to question.[42,43]

Mechanical and humoral theories are not necessarily incompatible. For example, the humoral signal might allow the sclera to be stretched more easily by the natural vitreous pressure, while mechanical effects could increase the vitreous pressure to make this effect more potent.

IMPLICATIONS FOR REFRACTIVE ERROR CONTROL

The environmental factor that appears to have the greatest impact on refractive development is near work. As discussed earlier, greater prevalence of myopia is associated with more near-work activity. Perhaps it is possible to train the eye to respond better to near work or to prescribe lenses for better near-work performance in order to influence refractive development.

If the defocus theory is correct, it does suggest the possibility of preventing myopia or slowing its progression. For example, vision training to improve the accuracy of accommodation might help to prevent myopia or to slow myopia progression. Another way to compensate for a poor accommodative response is to use a bifocal or progressive addition lens. These lenses have more plus power (or less minus power) in the lower, reading, portion of the lens than in the top of the lens used for distance viewing. The additional plus power would move the image formed from a near object, which tends to lag behind the retina, closer to the retina.

Many papers have been written on the use of bifocal lenses to slow childhood myopia progression.[44–46] Some report partial success in controlling myopia while others report a lack of success. It is possible that bifocals slow myopia progression in a particular subset of children but not in others. As Table 8.8 shows, five of six studies found myopia progression rates to be at least 0.1 D/yr lower with bifocals than with single vision lenses in children with esophoria at near. (Esophoria is the inward misalignment of the lines of sight of the two eyes with respect to the object of regard when binocular fusion is prevented. Exophoria is the outward misalignment of the two eyes with respect to the object of regard when binocular fusion is prevented. A small amount of exophoria, about 3 prism diopters, is the normal condition for near viewing.)

There was little or no reduction in myopia progression rates in children with exophoria. One possible explanation for better myopia control with bifocals in esophoria than in exophoria is that the accommodative response tends to be less in

Table 8.8. Mean Rates of Childhood Myopia Progression in Diopters per Year and Number of Subjects (*n*) Wearing Single Vision Lenses (SV) and Bifocal Lenses (BF) in Six Studies

Study	SV		BF	
	n	**Mean**	**n**	**Mean**
Esophoria				
Roberts and Banford	167	−0.48	65	−0.28
Goss	10	−0.54	35	−0.32
Goss and Grosvenor	7	−0.51	18	−0.31
Jensen	8	−0.69	10	−0.62
Fulk and Cyert	14	−0.57	14	−0.39
Fulk et al.	39	−0.50	36	−0.40
Orthophoria and Exophoria				
Roberts and Banford	181	−0.41	17	−0.38
Goss	36	−0.44	21	−0.45
Goss and Grosvenor	25	−0.44	47	−0.42
Jensen	41	−0.55	41	−0.44

Results for subjects with esophoria at near and with orthophoria and exophoria at near are presented separately. (Standard deviations of the rates were generally between 0.2 and 0.3.)

Compiled from Goss DA. Effect of spectacle correction on the progression of myopia in children: a literature review. *J Am Optom Assoc.* 1994;65:117–128; Grosvenor T, Goss DA. *Clinical Management of Myopia.* Boston: Butterworth-Heinemann, 1999;113–128; Fulk GW, Cyert LA, Parker DE. A randomized trial of the effect of single vision vs. bifocals on myopia progression in children with esophoria. *Optom Vis Sci.* 2000;77:395–401.

esophoria than in exophoria, so the images from near objects lag farther behind the retina. Another possible explanation is that patients with esophoria are more compliant with the use of the bifocals for near work because the bifocals reduce or eliminate esophoria and make near vision more comfortable.

If the defocus theory applies to the development of human myopia, some of the old admonishments about not holding the book too close or about not reading in dim illumination may be good advice after all.

APPENDIX 8.1

STATISTICAL CONCEPTS IN THE STUDY OF REFRACTIVE ERROR

This appendix reviews some basic statistics that are used in the discussion of refractive error in Chapter 8. This appendix also discusses a computational method for handling spherocylinder data.

MEASURES OF CENTRAL TENDENCY AND VARIATION

Common measures of central tendency include the mean, median, and mode. The arithmetic mean is usually referred to as the average. The arithmetic *mean* is the sum of the measured values divided by the number of items or individuals. The *median* is the value of the middle item when the items are arranged in numerical order. When there is an even number of items, the median is the mean of the values of the middle two items. The *mode* is the value that occurs most frequently in a set of numerical data.

Standard deviation is an index of the variation within a sample. The formula for standard deviation (SD) takes into account how far each value differs from the mean of the sample and how many subjects or items are in the sample:

$$\sqrt{\frac{\sum(x_i - \bar{x})^2}{(n-1)}}$$

where,

$\bar{x}$ = the value of the mean for the subjects in the sample,

x_i = the value for subject $i = 1,2,3, \ldots$, and

n = the number of subjects.

FREQUENCY DISTRIBUTIONS

A *frequency distribution* is a presentation of the frequency of numerical data arranged according to magnitude. It can be in tabular or graphical form. It indicates the frequency of occurrence of a given magnitude of some variable. In graphical form, the frequency is on the y-axis and the magnitude of the variable being studied is on the x-axis.

Various terms are used to describe the shapes of frequency distributions. A *normal distribution* is the specific shape of frequency distribution that results from random variation. This distribution is often referred to as a bell-shaped curve. The mean, median, and mode are coincident at one point, and the curve is symmetrical about that point. In a normal distribution, the mean ± 1 SD contains 68.3% of the sample, the mean ± 2 SD contains 95.5% of the sample, and the mean ± 3 SD contains 99.7% of the sample. A frequency distribution is *leptokurtic* if it has a sharper peak than a normal distribution. If a variable has a distribution with leptokurtosis, it suggests that the variable does not exhibit random variation.

CORRELATION COEFFICIENTS

A *correlation coefficient* is a statistic that specifies the closeness of two related variables. Correlation coefficients can range from 0 (no correlation at all) to 1.0 (prefect correlation), although in biological systems correlation coefficients are very rarely, if ever, equal to 0 or 1.0. A correlation coefficient with a positive sign indicates that both variables increase together, a direct relation. A correlation coefficient that has a negative sign indicates an inverse relation, that is, one variable increases as the other decreases or the negative value of one variable increases as the positive value of the other increases.

Different correlation coefficient formulas are used for different types of data. For continuous data (noncategorical, nonrank data) such as refractive error, axial length, vitreous depth, corneal power, and so on, the correlation coefficient used is the Pearson product moment coefficient of correlation. If the correlation coefficient is squared, one obtains an estimate of the variability of one parameter that is related to variability of the other parameter. For example, if the correlation coefficient is 0.8 (a very high correlation for biological systems), one can say that 64% of the variability of one parameter is related to variability of the other parameter.

PREVALENCE AND INCIDENCE

The terms *prevalence* and *incidence* are often used in clinical studies. Although these terms have different meanings, they are often confused. The *prevalence* of a given condition is the percentage of a population that has that condition at a certain point in time. *Incidence* is the percentage of a population that develops a given condition within a particular period of time. In other words, prevalence represents the number of existing cases, regardless of the time or age of onset, while incidence represents the number of new cases. For example, let's say that we find that 15 out of 100 11-year-olds have myopia. Prevalence is 15%. Then say we test these same children after 1 year, and we find that those 15 children still have myopia and another 3 have developed myopia. Incidence is 3% and prevalence is now 18%.

COMPUTATIONAL METHOD FOR STATISTICAL ANALYSIS OF SPHEROCYLINDER DATA

The expression of astigmatism correction as cylinder and axis essentially makes use of a polar coordinate system. Polar coordinates are not convenient for performing statistical calculations. One way to convert the sphere, cylinder, and axis of spherocylinder lens data into a form in which statistical computations can be performed is conversion into three components[1,2]:

1. The spherical equivalent, symbolized below as *M*.
2. A 90–180 cross cylinder (J_0).
3. A 45–135 cross cylinder (J_{45}).

J_0 expresses the powers in the principal meridians of the 90–180 cross cylinder. To find J_0, one can divide the difference between the power in the 180 meridian and the power in the 90 meridian by 2. If the cross cylinder, for example, has powers of +0.25 D in the 180 and –0.25 D in the 90, then J_0 is +0.25. If the cross cylinder has powers of –0.50 D in the 180 and +0.50 D in the 90, then J_0 is –0.50. To find J_0 from sphere, cylinder, and axis in minus cylinder form, one can use the following formula:

$J_0 = (-C/2)(\cos 2\alpha)$, where C = cylinder power, and α = cylinder axis.

The J_{45} value is an index of the powers in the principal meridians of the 45–135 cross cylinder. J_{45} can be found by dividing the difference between the power in the 45 meridian and the power in the 135 meridian by 2. For example, if the cross cylinder has a power of +0.25 D in the 45 and a power of –0.25 D in the 135, J_{45} is equal to +0.25. If, for another cross cylinder there are powers of –1.00 D in the 45 and +1.00 D in the 135, J_{45} is –1.00. A formula to find J_{45} from sphere, cylinder, and axis in minus cylinder form is:

$$J_{45} = (-C/2) (\sin 2\alpha)$$

Example: The *M*, J_0, and J_{45} components of –1.50 –0.50 x 30 are:

$$M = S + (C/2) = -1.50 + (-0.50/2)$$

$$M = -1.75$$

$$J_0 = (-C/2)(\cos 2\alpha) = (- (-0.50)/2)(\cos 60)$$

$$J_0 = (+0.25)(0.5)$$

$$J_0 = +0.125$$

$$J_{45} = (-C/2)(\sin 2\alpha) = (- (-0.50)/2)(\sin 60)$$

$$J_{45} = (+0.25)(0.866)$$

$$J_{45} = +0.217$$

Once spherocylinder data are broken down into their *M*, J_0, and J_{45} components, statistical calculations can be performed. Resultant *M*, J_0, and J_{45} values can then be recombined back into sphere, cylinder, and axis in minus cylinder form using the following formulas:

$$S = M \sqrt{\left(J_0^{\,2} + J_{45}^{\,2}\right)}$$

$$C = 2\sqrt{\left(J_0^{\,2} + J_{45}^{\,2}\right)}$$

$$\alpha = (\tfrac{1}{2})\tan^{-1}\left(J_{45}/J_0\right)$$

Example: Conversion of spherical equivalent = –1.75, J_0 = +0.125, and J_{45} = +0.217 back into sphere, cylinder, and axis in minus cylinder form is as follows:

$$S = M + \sqrt{\left(J_0^2 + J_{45}^2\right)}$$

$$S = -1.75 + \sqrt{0.062714} = -1.75 + (+0.25)$$

$$S = -1.50$$

$$C = -2\sqrt{\left(J_0^2 + J_{45}^2\right)}$$

$$C = -2(+0.25)$$

$$C = -0.50$$

$$\alpha = \left(\tfrac{1}{2}\right)\tan^{-1}\left(J_{45}/J_0\right)$$

$$\alpha = \left(\tfrac{1}{2}\right)\tan^{-1}(1.736)$$

$$\alpha = \left(\tfrac{1}{2}\right)(60)$$

$$\alpha = 30$$

Appendix References

1. Salmon TO, Horner DG. A new subjective refraction method: the meridional polarized vernier optometer. *J Am Optom Assoc.* 1996;67:599–605.
2. Thibos LN, Wheeler W, Horner D. Power vectors: an application of Fourier analysis to the description and statistical analysis of refractive error. *Optom Vis Sci.* 1997;74:367–375.

APPENDIX 8.2

CALCULATION OF THE REFRACTIVE ERROR OF THE GULLSTRAND-EMSLEY SCHEMATIC EYE USING THE ERICKSON VERGENCE METHOD

To aid in our understanding of the contribution of the individual ocular optical components to refractive error, a simple computational method for deriving refractive error from component values would be useful. Erickson has developed such a method.[1-4] In this model, the vergence of light is traced backward through the eye starting at the retina. In other words, the retina is treated as an object imaged by the paraxial optics of the eye. The vergence of light emergent from the cornea is equal in magnitude, but opposite in sign, to the corneal plane refractive error.

To demonstrate this method, the refractive error of the Gullstrand-Emsley schematic eye is calculated from its component data. Our convention of light going from left to right is maintained by turning the eye so that the retina is to the left of the ocular optics. The first refraction thus occurs at the posterior surface of the crystalline lens. The object distance is the distance from the retina to the posterior lens surface (-16.69 mm), and the index of refraction in object space is the index of the vitreous (1.333). Therefore, the vergence of light striking the posterior lens surface is:

$$L_1 = \frac{n_1}{l_1} = \frac{1.333}{-0.01669 \text{ m}} = -79.8682 \text{ D}$$

The vergence of light leaving the posterior lens surface (image vergence) is the sum of the object vergence and the dioptric power of the posterior lens surface:

$$L_1' = L_1 + F_{2L}$$

$$L_1' = -79.8682 \text{ D} + (+13.778 \text{ D})$$

$$L_1' = -66.0902 \text{ D}$$

Image space is the crystalline lens ($n = 1.416$), so image distance is:

$$\ell_1' = \frac{n_1'}{L_1'}$$

$$\ell_1' = \frac{1.416}{-66.0902 \text{ D}}$$

$$\ell_1' = -0.021425 \text{ m}$$

The second refraction occurs at the anterior surface of the crystalline lens. The object distance for this refraction is the sum of the first image distance and the thickness of the crystalline lens:

$$\ell_2 = (-0.021425 \text{ m}) + (-0.0036 \text{ m})$$

$$\ell_2 = -0.025025 \text{ m}$$

Object space is now the crystalline lens ($n = 1.416$). The vergence striking the anterior lens surface is:

$$L_2 = \frac{n_2}{\ell_2}$$

$$L_2 = \frac{1.416}{-0.025025 \text{ m}}$$

$$L_2 = -56.5834 \text{ D}$$

Image vergence, the vergence of light leaving the anterior lens surface, is the sum of the object vergence and the dioptric power of the anterior crystalline lens surface:

$$L_2' = L_2 + F_{1L}$$

$$L_2' = (-56.5834 \text{ D}) + (8.27 \text{ D})$$

$$L_2' = -48.3134 \text{ D}$$

Image space is in the aqueous ($n = 1.333$). The image distance is:

$$\ell_2' = \frac{n_2'}{L_2'}$$

$$\ell_2' = \frac{1.333}{-48.3134 \text{ D}}$$

$$\ell_2' = -0.02759 \text{ m}$$

The third refraction occurs at the cornea. The object distance is the sum of the image distance for the second refraction and the anterior chamber depth:

$$\ell_3 = (-0.02759 \text{ m}) + (-0.0036 \text{ m})$$

$$\ell_3 = -0.03119 \text{ m}$$

Object space is in the aqueous ($n = 1.333$), so the vergence of light striking the cornea is:

$$L_3 = \frac{n_3}{\ell_3}$$

$$L_3 = \frac{1.333}{-0.03119 \text{ m}}$$

$$L_3 = -42.74 \text{ D}$$

The vergence of light leaving the cornea is the sum of the object vergence and the dioptric power of the cornea:

$$L_3' = L_3 + F_c$$

$$L_3' = (-42.74 \text{ D}) + (+42.74 \text{ D})$$

$$L_3' = 0 \text{ D}$$

The corneal plane refractive error calculated by this method is the same as that calculated previously using equivalent powers and principal planes:

$$RE_{cp} = -L_3'$$

$$RE_{cp} = 0 \text{ D}$$

Appendix References

1. Erickson P. Mathematical model for predicting dioptric effects of optical parameter changes in the eye. *Am J Optom Physiol Opt.* 1977;54:226–233.
2. Erickson P. Complete ocular component analysis by vergence contribution. *Am J Optom Physiol Opt.* 1984; 61:469–472.
3. Erickson P. Optical components contributing to refractive anomalies. In: T Grosvenor, MC Flom, eds. *Refractive Anomalies: Research and Clinical Applications.* Boston: Butterworth-Heinemann, 1991;199–218.
4. Goss DA, Erickson P. Effects of changes in anterior chamber depth on refractive error of the human eye. *Clin Vision Sci.* 1990;5:197–201.

REFERENCES

1. Goss DA, Wickham MG. Retinal-image mediated ocular growth as a mechanism for juvenile onset myopia and for emmetropization: a literature review. *Doc Ophthalmol.* 1995;90:341–375.
2. van Alphen GWHM. On emmetropia and ametropia. *Ophthalmologica.* 1961;142(suppl):1–92.
3. Goss DA, Van Veen HG, Rainey BB, Feng B. Ocular components measured by keratometry, phakometry, and ultrasonography in emmetropic and myopic optometry students. *Optom Vis Sci.* 1997;74:489–495.
4. Grosvenor T, Goss DA. Role of the cornea in emmetropia and myopia. *Optom Vis Sci.* 1998;75: 132–145.
5. Rosenfield M. Refractive status of the eye. In: WJ Benjamin, ed. *Borish's Clinical Refraction.* Philadelphia: Saunders, 1998;2–29.
6. Erickson P. Optical components contributing to refractive anomalies. In: T Grosvenor, MC Flom, eds. *Refractive Anomalies: Research and Clinical Applications.* Boston: Butterworth-Heinemann, 1991;199–218.
7. Erickson P. Mathematical model for predicting dioptric effects of optical parameter changes in the eye. *Am J Optom Physiol Opt.* 1977;54:226–233.
8. Fledelius HC. Changes in eye refraction and eye size during adolescence, with special reference to the influence of low birth weight. In: HC Fledelius, PH Alsbirk, E Goldschmidt, eds. Third International Conference on Myopia. *Doc Ophthalmol Proc.* 1981;28:63–69.
9. Fledelius HC. The growth of the eye from the age of 10 to 18 years: a longitudinal study including ultrasound oculometry. In: JM Thijssen, AM Verbeek, eds. Ultrasonogrpahy in Ophthalmology. *Doc Ophthalmol Proc.* 1981;29:211–215.
10. Tokoro T, Kabe S. Relation between changes in the ocular refraction and refractive components and development of the myopia. *Acta Soc Ophthalmol Jpn.* 1964;68:1240–1253.
11. Grosvenor T, Scott R. Three year changes in refraction and its components in youth-onset and early adult-onset myopia. *Optom Vis Sci.* 1993;70:677–683.
12. Goss DA. Refractive changes in diabetes. In: DA Goss, LL Edmondson, eds. *Eye and Vision Conditions in the American Indian.* Yukon, OK: Pueblo Publishing, 1990;53–59.
13. Everson RW. Age variation in refractive error distributions. *Optom Weekly.* 1973;64:200–204.
14. Zadnik K, Mutti DO. Incidence and distribution of refractive anomalies. In: WJ Benjamin, ed. *Borish's Clinical Refraction.* Philadelphia: Saunders, 1998; 30–46.
15. Grosvenor T. A review and a suggested classification system for myopia on the basis on age-related prevalence and age of onset. *Am J Optom Physiol Opt.* 1987; 64:545–554.

16. Working Group on Myopia Prevalence and Progression. *Myopia: Prevalence and Progression.* Washington, D.C.: National Academy Press, 1989.

17. Garzia RP, Franzel AS. Refractive status, binocular vision, and reading achievement. In: RP Garzia, ed. *Vision and Reading.* St. Louis, 1996;111–131.

18. Goss DA. Childhood myopia. In: T Grosvenor, MC Flom, eds. *Refractive Anomalies: Research and Clinical Applications.* Boston: Butterworth-Heinemann, 1991;81–103.

19. Grosvenor T. Changes in spherical refraction during the adult years. In: T Grosvenor, MC Flom, eds. *Refractive Anomalies: Research and Clinical Applications.* Boston: Butterworth-Heinemann, 1991;131–145.

20. Goss DA. Development of the ametropias. In: WJ Benjamin, ed. *Borish's Clinical Refraction.* Philadelphia: Saunders, 1998;47–76.

21. Mäntyjärvi MI. Change of refraction in schoolchildren. *Arch Ophthalmol.* 1985;103:790–792.

22. Goss DA, Winkler RL. Progression of myopia in youth: age of cessation. *Am J Optom Physiol Opt.* 1983;60:651–658.

23. Goss DA, Cox VD. Trends in the change of clinical refractive error in myopes. *J Am Optom Assoc.* 1985;56:608–613.

24. Goss DA, Erickson P, Cox VD. Prevalence and pattern of adult myopia progression in a general optometric practice population. *Am J Optom Physiol Opt.* 1985;62:470–477.

25. Hirsch MJ. Changes in refractive state after the age of forty-five. *Am J Optom Arch Am Acad Optom.* 1958; 35:229–237.

26. Lyle WM. Astigmatism. In: T Grosvenor, MC Flom, eds. *Refractive Anomalies: Research and Clinical Applications.* Boston: Butterworth-Heinemann, 1991; 146–173.

27. Hirsch MJ. Changes in astigmatism during the first eight years of school: an interim report from the Ojai longitudinal study. *Am J Optom Arch Am Acad Optom.* 1963;40:127–132.

28. Hirsch MJ. Changes in astigmatism after the age of forty. *Am J Optom Arch Am Acad Optom.* 1959; 36:395–405.

29. Anstice J. Astigmatism: its components and their changes with age. *Am J Optom Arch Am Acad Optom.* 1971;48:1001–1006.

30. Goss DA. Astigmatism in American Indians: prevalence, descriptive analysis, and management issues. In: DA Goss, LL Edmondson, eds. *Eye and Vision Conditions in the American Indian.* Yukon, OK: Pueblo Publishing, 1990;61–76.

31. Goss DA. Corneal curvature and topography alterations due to the effects of the eyelids and lid conditions. *Br J Optom Disp.* 1994;2:471–474.

32. Wilson G, Goss DA, Vaughan WA, Roddy KC. Corneal toricity, lid tension, intraocular pressure, and ocular rigidity in North American Indians. In: DA Goss, LL Edmondson, eds. *Eye and Vision Conditions in the American Indian.* Yukon, OK: Pueblo Publishing, 1990;77–84.

33. Wallman J. Retinal factors in myopia and emmetropization: clues from research on chicks. In: T Grosvenor, MC Flom, eds. *Refractive Anomalies: Research and Clinical Applications.* Boston: Butterworth-Heinemann, 1991;268–286.

34. Wildsoet CF. Active emmetropization: evidence for its existence and ramifications for clinical practice. *Ophthal Physiol Opt.* 1997;17:279–290.

35. Raviola E, Wiesel TN. Effect of dark-rearing on experimental myopia in monkeys. *Invest Ophthalmol Vis Sci.* 1978;17:485–488.

36. Young FA, Leary GA. Accommodation and vitreous chamber pressure: a proposed mechanism for myopia. In: T Grosvenor, MC Flom, eds. *Refractive Anomalies: Research and Clinical Applications.* Boston: Butterworth-Heinemann, 1991;301–309.

37. Mauger RR, Likens CP, Applebaum M. Effects of accommodation and repeated applanation tonometry on intraocular pressure. *Am J Optom Physiol Opt.* 1984;61:28–30.

38. Schaeffel F, Troilo D, Wallman J, Howland HC. Developing eyes that lack accommodation grow to compensate for imposed defocus. *Vis Neurosci.* 1990; 4:177–183.

39. Gwiazda J, Thorn F, Bauer J, Held R. Myopic children show insufficient accommodative response to blur. *Invest Ophthalmol Vis Sci.* 1993;34:690–694.

40. Goss DA, Zhai H. Clinical and laboratory investigations of the relationship of accommodation and convergence function with refractive error: A literature review. *Doc Ophthalmol.* 1994;86:349–380.

41. Gwiazda J, Bauer J, Thorn F, Held R. A dynamic relationship between myopia and blur-driven accommodation in school-aged children. *Vision Res.* 1995; 35:1299–1304.

42. Zadnik K, Mutti DO. How applicable are animal models to human juvenile onset myopia? *Vision Res.* 1995;35:1283–1288.

43. Smith EL III. Environmentally induced refractive errors in animals. In: Rosenfield M, Gilmartin B, eds. *Myopia and Nearwork.* Oxford: Butterworth-Heinemann, 1998;57–90.

44. Goss DA. Effect of spectacle correction on the progression of myopia in children: a literature review. *J Am Optom Assoc.* 1994;65:117–128.

45. Grosvenor T, Goss DA. *Clinical Management of Myopia.* Boston: Butterworth-Heinemann, 1999;113–128.

46. Fulk GW, Cyert LA, Parker DE. A randomized trial of the effect of single vision vs. bifocals on myopia progression in children with esophoria. *Optom Vis Sci.* 2000;77:395–401.

FURTHER READING

Grosvenor T, Goss DA. *Clinical Management of Myopia.* Boston: Butterworth-Heinemann, 1999.

Ong E, Ciuffreda KJ. *Accommodation, Nearwork and Myopia.* Santa Ana, CA: Optometric Extension Program, 1997.

Rosenfield M, Gilmartin B, eds. *Myopia and Nearwork.* Oxford: Butterworth-Heinemann, 1998.

Chapter 9
Ocular Accommodation

Make a number of perforations with a small needle in a piece of pasteboard, not more distant from one another than the diameter of the pupil of the eye . . . if it is held close to one eye, while the other is shut, as many images of a distant object will be seen as there are holes in the pasteboard . . . at a certain distance, objects do not appear multiplied when they are viewed in this manner.
—Christoph Scheiner, 1619 (From Wade NJ. *A Natural History of Vision*. Cambridge, MA: MIT Press, 1998;39.)

Accommodation is the process by which the crystalline lens changes its power. Increased accommodation increases the total dioptric power of the eye and moves the ocular image anteriorly. This ability to increase the ocular power allows the eye to keep a clear image on the retina when closer objects are viewed. It also allows hyperopes, whose image of distant objects is behind the retina when the eye is unaccommodated, to clear what would otherwise be a blurred retinal image. The amount of accommodation available is highly dependent on age and somewhat on training. In this chapter we look at the mechanism of accommodation, how is it measured, how it changes through life, and some of the factors that affect the amount of its response.

MECHANISM OF ACCOMMODATION

The crystalline lens is a viscoelastic bundle of collagen-filled cells contained in a thin elastic shell known as the lens capsule. The lens and its capsule are suspended from an encircling ciliary muscle by strands of tissue called zonules. The ciliary muscle is the inner part of the larger ciliary body, which is a ringed structure that originates just posterior to the edge of the cornea, and ends at the most anterior border of the retina (Figure 9.1). The zonules attach to the lens capsule at the equator of the lens (equatorial zonules), and also just anterior and posterior to the equator of the lens (anterior and posterior zonules).

The crystalline lens increases its power by shortening the radii of curvature of its refractive surfaces. We know that this is accomplished by action of the ciliary muscle through the zonules, but we do not know the precise mechanism by which it does this. Historically there have been many theories about the mechanism of accommodation. Each can be tested by how it explains the known changes that occur in the eye during an increase in accommodation. Any valid theory must be consistent with the following observations:

1. The ciliary muscle contracts.
2. The radius of curvature of the central portion of the anterior surface of the crystalline lens decreases, thus increasing its dioptric power.
3. The radius of curvature of the posterior surface of the crystalline lens also decreases, but it accounts for much less change in power than the anterior surface.
4. The thickness of the crystalline lens increases.
5. The anterior surface of the crystalline lens moves forward toward the cornea.

Presently the most accepted theory of accommodation is that of Helmholtz.[1]

Helmholtz Theory

According to the Helmholtz theory, during accommodation the ciliary muscle contracts, which causes its diameter to decrease and the ciliary muscle as a whole to move forward. This decrease in

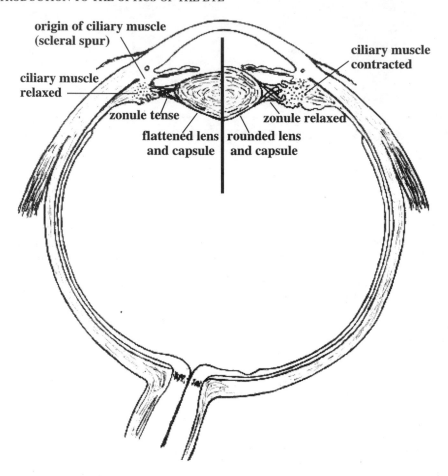

Figure 9.1. Cross-sectional diagrams of the eye showing the basic elements of the changes in the eye during accommodation according to the Helmholtz theory of accommodation. The two cross sections are placed next to each other for comparison. The left diagram shows the unaccommodated eye, and the right diagram shows the accommodated eye. (Modified from Stark L. Presbyopia in light of accommodation. *Am J Optom Physiol Opt.* 1988;65:411.)

diameter reduces the tension on the anterior zonules so that they do not pull so much on the capsule and crystalline lens. This allows the lens to elastically reduce its diameter, which results in steeper surface curvatures, more so on the anterior than the posterior surface. This results in an increase in the net dioptric power of the lens due mainly to the decreased radius of curvature on the anterior surface of the lens.

When a distant object is viewed, the ciliary muscle relaxes. The ring of the ciliary muscle around the eye increases in diameter, thus increasing the tension on the zonules. The zonules pull on the capsule and crystalline lens more, which increases the equatorial diameter of the lens so that it becomes thinner and flatter. Most of the flattening is of the

anterior surface of the lens, which is most responsible for decreasing the lens's dioptric power.

Competing Theories

A theory attributed primarily to Tscherning in the late nineteenth century, but suggested earlier by Cramer, proposed that the crystalline lens alters its shape during accommodation because the vitreous pushes forward against it.[2] According to this theory, the change in shape is mainly on the anterior surface of the lens because the posterior surface of the crystalline lens is constrained from changing in shape by the force on it from the vitreous. Cramer, and also Coleman,[3] suggested that the vitreous is pulled forward by the action of the ciliary muscle on the choroid to which the vitreous is attached. In a new theory proposed by Schachar,[4,5] the ciliary muscle accomplishes accommodation by *pulling* on the zonules, which in turn exert an outward force on the equator of the lens. Although this would result in an *increase* in the equatorial diameter of the lens, the central area of the anterior lens surface is assumed to steepen, which increases its power, while the peripheral area is assumed to flatten, which decreases its power. Most of the outward tension on the lens is assumed to be from the equatorial zonules, while the anterior and posterior zonules would serve to stabilize the lens. An experiment that found decreases in equatorial diameter of the lens during accommodation in monkeys contradicts the Schachar theory and supports the Helmholtz theory.[6]

EFFECTIVE STIMULI

Four types of conditions have been identified as effective stimuli for accommodation: (1) blur, (2) proximity, (3) binocular retinal disparity, and (4) empty field.

Blur

Accommodation occurs to improve the contrast and clarity of the retinal image. This is sometimes called *optical reflex accommodation*. Optical reflex accommodation can be demonstrated by observing the changes in accommodation that occur when spherical lenses are introduced in front of the eye.

Proximity

Accommodation can also occur in response to the awareness of nearness to an object. This is often referred to as *proximal accommodation*. Awareness of proximity is responsible for the increases in accommodation that often occur when looking into instruments held close to the eye. An example of this is the viewfinder on a camera. To compensate for this, minus lenses are sometimes incorporated into camera sights. This *instrument myopia* is also the cause of too much minus in prescriptions determined by some autorefractors.

Binocular Retinal Disparity

Retinal disparity exists when the image of an object being looked at binocularly does not fall on the foveas of both eyes. A vergence eye movement, rotation of the lines of sight of the two eyes either toward each other (convergence) or away from each other (divergence), occurs to eliminate retinal disparity. For any given object distance, the visual nervous system coordinates the level of accommodation with the amount of vergence. Convergence is associated with an increase in accommodation and divergence is associated with a decrease in accommodation.

Empty Field

When there is no visual input to stimulate accommodation, accommodation does not go to a zero level as one might expect, but rather to an intermediate level. This occurs when there is an empty visual field and also in darkness. The accommodation that occurs in darkness is known as the *dark focus of accommodation*. The dark focus of accommodation is responsible for the phenomenon of *night myopia* in which the eye tends to accommodate too much for a given object distance when lighting levels are low. One study found a mean dark focus of 1.52 D (SD = 0.77).[7]

PUNCTUM PROXIMUM AND AMPLITUDE OF ACCOMMODATION

Earlier we defined the punctum remotum, or far point, as the farthest object point that can result in clear vision. The *punctum proximum*, or near point, is the closest object point that can result in clear vision. In other words, the punctum proximum is the object point whose image is in focus on the retina when the eye's full amount of accommodation is being used, a value referred to as the *amplitude of accommodation*. This can be measured as the maximum dioptric amount of accommodation that an eye can exert and is calculated as the difference between the dioptric values corresponding to the punctum remotum and the punctum proximum.

The dioptric values of the punctum remotum and punctum proximum must be referenced to a specific plane such as the spectacle lens or contact lens plane. From a theoretical standpoint, the first principal plane of the eye is a logical reference plane for amplitude of accommodation because it is close to the crystalline lens and would closely match the actual dioptric power changes of the lens. A formula for principal plane amplitude of accommodation (AA_p) is:

$$AA_p = (1/k_1) - (1/k_2)$$

where k_1 = the distance from the first principal plane to the punctum remotum and k_2 = the distance from the first principal plane to the punctum proximum.

Since $1/k_1$ is the refractive error referenced to the principal plane (RE_p), the formula can also be written as:

$$AA_p = RE_p - (1/k_1)$$

The location of the first principal plane of a given eye is usually not known so a more practical reference plane, such as the corneal plane or the spectacle plane, is usually employed. Clinically, the most common reference plane is the spectacle plane. Although its location varies with the actual placement of a spectacle lens, the spectacle plane is on average about 13 mm in front of the cornea. The spectacle plane amplitude of accommodation can be computed in the same way as the principal plane amplitude of accommodation.

Example 1: An eye with the punctum remotum −50 cm in front of the spectacle plane and a punctum proximum −8 cm in front of the spectacle plane would have a spectacle plane amplitude of accommodation (AA_s) of:

$$AA_s = (1/k_1) - (1/k_2) = (1/-0.5 \text{ m}) - (1/-0.08 \text{ m})$$
$$= +10.5 \text{ D}$$

Example 2: The spectacle plane amplitude of accommodation of an eye with a spectacle plane refractive error of +2.50 D and a punctum proximum −50 cm in front of the spectacle plane would be:

$$AA_s = RE_s - (1/k_1) = +2.50 \text{ D} - (1/-0.5 \text{ m})$$
$$= +4.50 \text{ D}$$

Clinically the way that the amplitude of accommodation is often measured is to have patients view through lenses that correct their refractive error and then find their near point of accommodation through the lenses. The reciprocal of the distance in meters from the near point of accommodation to the spectacle plane is then the spectacle plane amplitude of accommodation in diopters.

EFFECT OF AGE ON AMPLITUDE OF ACCOMMODATION

The amplitude of accommodation declines throughout life until at about 50 or 60 years of age the amplitude of accommodation becomes zero. (A nonzero measurement after these ages based on the subject's report of blur is typical because of the depth of field of the eye.) The largest collections of data on amplitude of accommodation as a function of age are the cross-sectional data of Donders (1864) and Duane (1922). Figure 9.2 shows Duane's well-known graph of amplitude versus age.

From Duane's cross-sectional data, it appears that the decline in amplitude occurs at a fairly constant rate until the mid 40s when it seems to

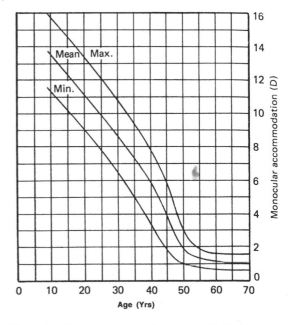

Figure 9.2. Monocular spectacle plane amplitude of accommodation from the data of Duane (1922). (Reprinted with permission from Bennett AAG, Rabbetts RB. *Clinical Visual Optics.* 2nd ed. London: Butterworth-Heinemann, 1989;140.)

decrease at a faster rate. However, the limited longitudinal data available in the literature suggest that decrease in amplitude with age in the 40s is also linear.[8,9] (Perhaps the difference could be explained by the fact that Duane's data was cross-sectional and was taken from a clinical, and thus self-selected, sample.) Assuming a linear decline in amplitude, Hofstetter[10,11] derived the following formulas for expected amplitude as a function of age, using the data of Donders, Duane, and Kaufman:

Maximum amplitude = 25 − 0.4 (age)

Probable amplitude = 18.5 − 0.3 (age)

Minimum amplitude = 15 − 0.25 (age)

Clinicians often use the minimum amplitude formula to assess whether a patient has an abnormally low amplitude of accommodation.

Because the amplitude of accommodation declines with age, nonmyopic people eventually have difficulty seeing clearly during near-point tasks. Although amplitude of accommodation declines gradually, a patient may feel that his loss has been sudden once his amplitude of accommodation no longer comfortably includes his reading distance. The blur during near vision resulting from the normal decrease in amplitude of accommodation with age is known as *presbyopia*. Presbyopia is sometimes quantitatively defined as an amplitude of accommodation less than 5 D, which is the point at which many patients become symptomatic. This usually occurs at about 40 or 45 years of age. Presbyopia that has advanced to the point that the ability to accommodate is completely absent is known as *absolute presbyopia*. As noted earlier, absolute presbyopia is reached between 50 and 60 years of age. The treatment for presbyopia is the addition of plus power to the distance Rx for use when viewing near objects. This is usually in the form of reading glasses, bifocal spectacles, or multifocal spectacle lenses.

Various theories have attempted to explain why amplitude of accommodation decreases with age, but the actual cause is unknown. The crystalline lens adds fibers and continues to enlarge in both its axial and equatorial dimension throughout one's life. A common theory of presbyopia is that continued enlargement makes the lens harder and more difficult to deform due to changes in the lens sub-

stance. Other possible causes or contributors to presbyopia include changes in the geometry of the zonules and their attachments to the lens, and changes in the elastic properties of the lens capsule.[12–16]

ACCOMMODATIVE RESPONSE

The dioptric *accommodative response* (the actual amount of accommodation) increases as the dioptric *accommodative stimulus* (the amount of accommodation required for exact focus of an object on the retina) increases.[17] This is often presented graphically, as in Figure 9.3.

In Figure 9.3, the accommodative response is presented as a function of the accommodative stimulus. If the accommodative response perfectly matched the accommodative stimulus, the function would be a 45-degree straight line starting at the origin (shown by the uninterrupted line on the graph). In reality the function has a more complex shape. A typical accommodative response/accommodative stimulus function is represented by the

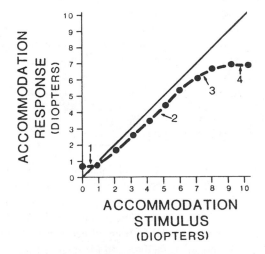

Figure 9.3. A plot of typical accommodative response data as a function of accommodative stimulus (dashed line). The solid diagonal line is a 1-to-1 line where accommodative response would be equal to accommodative stimulus. (Reprinted with permission from Ciuffreda KJ, Kenyon RV. Accommodative vergence and accommodation in normals, amblyopes, and strabismics. In: CM Schor, KJ Ciuffreda, eds. *Vergence Eye Movements:Basic and Clinical Aspects.* Boston: Butterworth-Heinemann, 1983;102.)

dotted/dashed line in Figure 9.3. At low accommodative stimulus levels (labeled 1 in the figure), accommodative response may actually exceed accommodative stimulus. This is referred to as a *lead of accommodation.* At intermediate accommodative stimulus levels (labeled 2 in the figure), the dioptric accommodative response is typically less than the dioptric accommodative stimulus. This is referred to as a *lag of accommodation.* The curve is fairly linear in this section, and the slope here is usually a little less than 1.0, so the lag of accommodation increases somewhat as the stimulus increases. An individual can perceive clear vision even though a lag of accommodation exists because of the depth of focus of the eye. At higher stimulus levels (labeled 3 in the figure), the accommodative response does not increase at the same rate because the maximum amount of accommodation is being approached. When the full amplitude has been reached, the response plateaus (labeled 4 in the figure). The shape of the curve can be changed. For example, decreases in target luminance or target contrast decrease the slope. The use of an artificial pupil to increase the depth of focus also decreases the slope.

Accommodative response/accommodative stimulus functions vary considerably from one individual to another. For instance, there can be differences in slope, lag of accommodation, the point where the curve crosses the 1-to-1 line, and the amplitude.[18]

CLINICAL MEASURES OF ACCOMMODATION

A full clinical examination of a patient's vision usually includes assessment of accommodative function. Clinical tests of accommodative function include four categories of measurement: (1) amplitude of accommodation, (2) lag of accommodation, (3) accommodative facility, and (4) relative accommodation. Poor performance on one of these types of tests does not predict poor performance on another, so a complete clinical workup of accommodation in a nonpresbyopic patient would include tests from each of these categories.[19–21] The following is a brief overview of these four types of tests:
1. Amplitude of accommodation is usually measured clinically using a *push-up test* in which the distance of letters near best visual acuity is decreased until patients report the first blur.
2. Lag of accommodation can be assessed clinically using various retinoscopic procedures. When retinoscopy is used to test accommodation for near objects, it is called *dynamic retinoscopy.* For dynamic retinoscopy the patient views a near-point test card at a typical near-point working distance. This establishes a known accommodative stimulus. This card has a hole in it through which the examiner does retinoscopy to determine the accommodative response.
3. Testing accommodative facility provides an index of how quickly accommodation can change. Plus and minus lenses are successively placed before patients' eyes while they change their accommodation as quickly as they can in order to keep a near object clear. Accommodative facility is usually measured as the number of cycles (from plus to minus and back to plus) that patients can complete in a given period of time.
4. Relative accommodation is a measure of the lens powers that can be introduced over the patient's refractive correction before a perceived blur occurs. On the negative relative accommodation (NRA) test, plus lenses are added binocularly in 0.25 D steps to decrease accommodation until the patient reports a blur. On the positive relative accommodation (PRA) test, minus lenses are added until a blur is noted. Poor performance on relative accommodation can indicate a problem with either accommodation or vergence. The PRA is often low when the patient has esophoria at near. A low NRA test result can be secondary to exophoria. (In esophoria, when fusion is broken the eyes converge toward a point closer than the object being viewed. In exophoria, when fusion is broken the eyes diverge toward a point farther than the object being viewed.)

ACCOMMODATION WITH SPECTACLES AND CONTACT LENSES

The amount of accommodation required for a given near-point distance varies depending on whether individuals wear spectacles or contact lenses for their refractive correction. To demonstrate this, we will consider three examples: Example 1, an eye corrected with a contact lens (the amount or sign of the refractive correction does not matter); Example 2, an eye with a –5.00 D spectacle lens correction; and Example 3, an eye with a +5.00 D spectacle lens correction. In each case, we will determine the amount of principal plane accommodation required for an object located 40 cm from the spectacle plane. We will assume that the first principal plane of each eye is 1.35 mm behind the anterior surface of the cornea, and we will assume that the spectacle plane is 14 mm in front of the cornea. Therefore, the spectacle plane will be 15.35 mm from the first principal plane. In each case the amount of principal plane accommodation will be the difference between (a) the vergence of light at the first principal plane from an object infinitely distant from the eye, and (b) the vergence of light at the first principal plane from the object located 40 cm from the spectacle plane.

Example 1. Eye corrected with a contact lens. A contact lens is so close to the first principal plane

of the eye that the principal plane for the combined contact lens-eye system does not differ significantly from the principal plane for the eye alone. This is true for ametropic eyes of any amount, as well as emmetropic eyes. Figure 9.4 shows this example diagrammatically.

For a distant object, the vergence of light in the principal plane is 0.00 D. The near object is 41.535 cm from the principal plane (40 cm from the object to the spectacle plane plus 1.535 cm from the spectacle plane to the principal plane). So the vergence of light in the principal plane for the near object is:

$$L = 1/(-0.41535 \text{ m}) = -2.41 \text{ D}$$

The amount of principal plane accommodation required is:

$$A = 0 - (-2.41 \text{ D}) = 2.41$$

Example 2. Eye with a spectacle correction of –5.00 D (Figure 9.5).

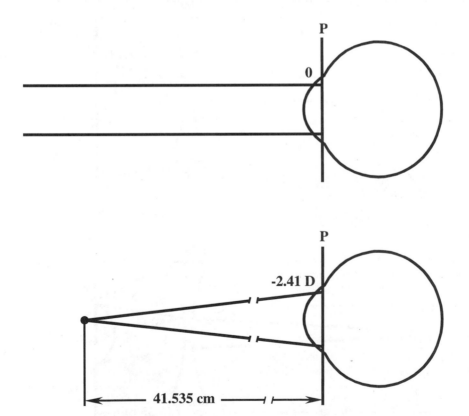

Figure 9.4. The amount of principal plane accommodation required for a contact lens–corrected eye to view an object at 40 cm from the spectacle plane is 2.41 D. See text for explanation. (Modified from Goss DA, Eskridge JB. Myopia. In: JF Amos, ed. *Diagnosis and Management in Vision Care*. Boston: Butterworth-Heinemann, 1987;157.)

When light from infinity leaves the lens its vergence is –5.00 D:

$$L_1' = 0 + (-5.00 \text{ D}) = -5.00 \text{ D}$$

$$\ell_1' = \frac{1}{(-5.00 \text{ D})} = -0.2 \text{ m}$$

For the vergence of light in the first principal plane:

$$\ell_2 = \ell_1' + (-0.01535 \text{ m}) = -0.2 \text{ m}$$
$$+ (-0.01535 \text{ m}) = -0.21535 \text{ m}$$

$$L_2 = \frac{1}{(-0.21535 \text{ m})} = -4.64 \text{ D}$$

Now for the near-point object, the vergence of light leaving the spectacle lens would be –7.50 D:

$$L_1' = -2.50 \text{ D} + (-5.00 \text{ D}) = -7.50 \text{ D}$$

$$\ell_1' = \frac{1}{(-7.50 \text{ D})} = -0.13333 \text{ m}$$

The calculation of the vergence of light in the principal plane yields:

$$\ell_2 = (-0.13333 \text{ m}) + (-0.01535 \text{ m})$$
$$= -0.14868 \text{ m}$$

$$L_2 = \frac{1}{(-0.14868 \text{ m})} = -6.73 \text{ D}$$

The amount of principal plane accommodation is therefore:

$$A = -4.64 \text{ D} - (-6.73 \text{ D}) = 2.09 \text{ D}$$

Example 3: Eye with a spectacle lens correction of +5.00 D (Figure 9.6).

$$L_1' = 0 + (+5.00 \text{ D}) = +5.00 \text{ D}$$

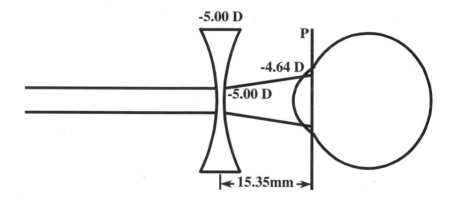

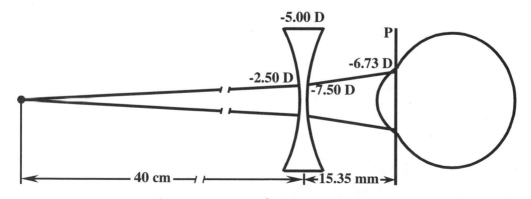

Figure 9.5. The amount of principal plane accommodation required of an eye with a spectacle correction of –5.00 D to view an object 40 cm from the spectacle plane is 2.09 D. See text for explanation. (Modified from Goss DA, Eskridge JB. Myopia. In: JF Amos, ed. *Diagnosis and Management in Vision Care.* Boston: Butterworth-Heinemann, 1987;157.)

$$\ell_1' = \frac{1}{(+5.00 \text{ D})} = +0.2 \text{ m}$$

For the vergence of light in the first principal plane:

$$\ell_2 = \ell_1' + (-0.01535 \text{ m}) = +0.2 \text{ m} + (-0.01535 \text{ m}) = +0.18465 \text{ m}$$

$$L_2 = \frac{1}{(+0.18465 \text{ m})} = +5.42 \text{ D}$$

For the near-point object, the vergence of light leaving the spectacle lens would be +2.50 D:

$$L_1' = -2.50 \text{ D} + (+5.00 \text{ D}) = +2.50 \text{ D}$$

$$\ell_1' = \frac{1}{(+2.50 \text{ D})} = +0.4 \text{ m}$$

Then when we calculate the vergence of light in the principal plane we get:

$$\ell_2 = (+0.4 \text{ m}) + (-0.01535 \text{ m}) = +0.38465 \text{ m}$$

$$L_2 = \frac{1}{(+0.38465 \text{ m})} = +2.60 \text{ D}$$

Therefore, the amount of principal plane accommodation is:

$$A = +5.42 \text{ D} - (+2.60 \text{ D}) = 2.82 \text{ D}$$

To summarize, the principal plane accommodations required for an object 40 cm from the spectacle plane in the three examples are:

Example 1: Contact lens–corrected eye (any amount of ametropia): 2.41 D.

Example 2: Myopic eye with a spectacle correction of –5.00 D: 2.09 D.

Example 3: Hyperopic eye with a spectacle correction of +5.00 D: 2.82 D.

Based on examples 1 and 2, we can see that a 5.00-D myope will have to accommodate 0.32 D more with contact lenses than with spectacle lenses.

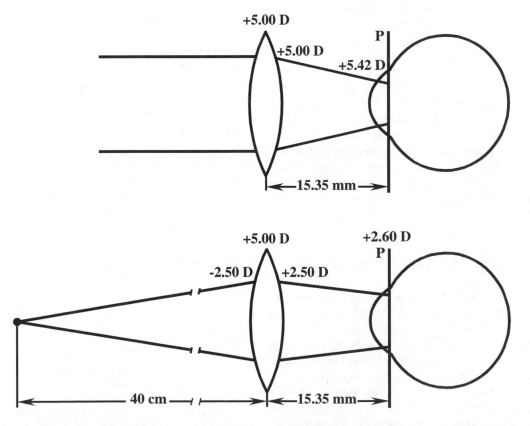

Figure 9.6. The amount of principal plane accommodation required of an eye with a spectacle correction of +5.00 D to view an object 40 cm from the spectacle plane is 2.82 D. See text for explanation.

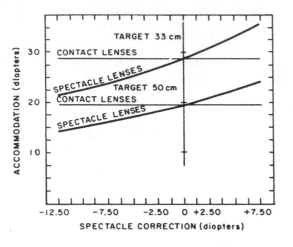

Figure 9.7. Principal plane accommodation required with contact lenses and with spectacle lenses as a function of spectacle correction for viewing objects at 33 cm and 50 cm. The spectacle plane vertex distance is 14 mm from the corneal apex. (Reprinted with permission from Westheimer G. The visual world of the new contact lens wearer. *J Am Optom Assoc.* 1962;34:137.)

The difference increases as the amount of ametropia increases (Figure 9.7). A consequence is that moderate to high myopes who are approaching presbyopia may have more difficulty reading with contact lenses than they have when reading with spectacles.

If we compare examples 2 and 3, we can observe that the spectacle-corrected hyperope has to accommodate more than the spectacle-corrected myope. So we can expect hyperopes who wear glasses to have presbyopic symptoms earlier than myopes who wear glasses. Some myopes further forestall getting bifocals or progressive addition lenses by taking their glasses off to read, although this may not provide the optimal correction.

SURGICAL TREATMENT OF PRESBYOPIA

Up until now the loss of accommodation with age has been untreatable, with the only options being the use of spectacles or contact lenses. However, several techniques are currently being considered for the surgical correction of presbyopia by which the ability to accommodate itself might be restored.

A technique that is currently undergoing FDA clinical trials is that of Presbycorp, a company formed by Ronald Schachar, who was mentioned earlier in this chapter for his novel theory about the mechanism of accommodation. Recall that his theory assumes that the increase in lens power during accommodation is caused by a pulling on the lens by the zonules rather than a relaxation as the Helmholtz theory maintains. According to Schachar the space between the ciliary muscle and the crystalline lens decreases with age so that the zonules become slack and pull on the lens less effectively during accommodation. In Schachar's surgical procedure four small plastic implants are embedded in the sclera posterior to the ciliary attachments. This is claimed to expand the diameter of the sclera anterior to the implants and increase the space between ciliary muscle and the edge of the lens so that the zonules can again exert useful tension on the lens during accommodation.

Another technique is anterior ciliary sclerotomy (ACS) that places radial incisions in the sclera. This is similar to radial keratotomy but it is applied posterior to the cornea. Although this technique seems to reduce presbyopia the effect undergoes regression and is short lived. A company called SurgiLight uses a similar technique whose effect they claim is longer lasting. In this procedure, a short-pulsed infrared laser is used to produce eight radial incisions about 3- to 5-mm long and 500-μm deep in the sclera posterior to the lens. As of this writing, clinical trials are being conducted outside the United States.

Other techniques assume that accommodation is lost due to a loss of elasticity in the crystalline lens. One procedure undergoing experimental tests replaces the crystalline lens with an elastic artificial lens that is then attached to the ciliary muscle. Alternatively, it has been contemplated that the crystalline lens could be removed from its capsule and that the capsule could then serve as a mold to be injected with an elastic polymer that would then take up the form of the removed lens. As of this writing, neither of these techniques are close to being marketed.

REFERENCES

1. Adler-Grinberg D. Questioning our classical understanding of accommodation and presbyopia. *Am J Optom Physiol Opt.* 1986;63:571–580.
2. Duke-Elder S, Abrams D. Ophthalmic Optics and Refraction. In: S Duke-Elder, ed. *System of Ophthalmology, 5.* Mosby: St. Louis, 1970;153–161.

3. Coleman DJ. Unified model for accommodative mechanism. *Am J Ophthalmol.* 1970;69:1063–1079.
4. Schachar RA, Anderson DA. The mechanism of ciliary muscle function. *Ann Ophthalmol.* 1995;27:126–132.
5. Schachar RA. Histology of the ciliary muscle-zonular connections. *Ann Ophthalmol.* 1996;28:70–79.
6. Glasser A, Kaufman PL. The mechanism of accommodation in primates. *Ophthalmol.* 1999;106:863–872.
7. Leibowitz HW, Owens DA. New evidence for the intermediate position of relaxed accommodation. *Doc Ophthalmol.* 1978;46:133–147.
8. Hofstetter HW. A longitudinal study of amplitude changes in presbyopia. *Am J Optom Arch Am Acad Optom.* 1965;42:3–8.
9. Ramsdale C, Charman WN. A longitudinal study of the changes in the static accommodation response. *Ophthal Physiol Opt.* 1989;9:255–263.
10. Hofstetter HW. A comparison of Duane's and Donders' tables of the amplitude of accommodation. *Am J Optom Arch Am Acad Optom.* 1944;21:345–363.
11. Hofstetter HW. A useful age-amplitude formula. *Pennsylvania Optom.* 1947;7:5–8.
12. Stark L. Presbyopia in light of accommodation. *Am J Optom Physiol Opt.* 1988;65:407–416.
13. Kaufman PL. Accommodation and presbyopia: neuromuscular and biophysical aspects. In: WM Hart Jr, ed. *Adler's Physiology of the Eye.* 9th ed. St. Louis: Mosby, 1992;391–411.
14. Pierscionek BK. What we know and understand about presbyopia. *Clin Exp Optom.* 1993;76:83–90.
15. Atchison DA. Accommodation and presbyopia. *Ophthal Physiol Opt.* 1995;15:255–272.
16. Gilmartin B. The aetiology of presbyopia: a summary of the role of lenticular and extralenticular structures. *Ophthal Physiol Opt.* 1995;15:431–437.
17. Ciuffreda KJ, Kenyon RV. Accommodative vergence and accommodation in normals, amblyopes, and strabismics. In: CM Schor, KJ Ciuffreda, eds. *Vergence Eye Movements: Basic and Clinical Aspects.* Boston: Butterworth-Heinemann, 1983;101–173.
18. Ward PA. A review of some factors affecting accommodation. *Clin Exp Optom.* 1987;70:23–32.
19. Wick B, Hall P. Relation between accommodative facility, lag, and amplitude in elementary school children. *Am J Optom Physiol Opt.* 1987;64:593–598.
20. Jackson TW, Goss DA. Variation and correlation of clinical tests of accommodative function in a sample of school-age children. *J Am Optom Assoc.* 1991;62:857–866.
21. Goss DA. *Ocular Accommodation, Convergence, and Fixation Disparity: A Manual of Clinical Analysis.* 2nd ed. Boston: Butterworth-Heinemann, 1995;135–141.

FURTHER READING

Ciuffreda KJ. Accommodation, the pupil, and presbyopia. In: WJ Benjamin, ed. *Borish's Clinical Refraction.* Philadelphia: Saunders, 1998;77–120.
Cooper J. Accommodative dysfunction. In: JF Amos, ed. *Diagnosis and Management in Vision Care.* Boston: Butterworth-Heinemann, 1987;431–459.

Chapter 10

Developments in Visual Optics and Some of the People Who Made Them Possible

To many of its early practitioners [the science of optics] . . . appeared . . . to be the most fundamental of the natural sciences, the key that would unlock nature's door and reveal her innermost secrets. —David C. Lindberg, 1976 (From Lindberg DC. *Theories of Vision from Al-Kindi to Kepler.* Chicago: University of Chicago Press, 1976;ix.)

Issues that have fascinated natural philosophers since time immemorial . . . can now be examined with an experimental sophistication that has not previously been matched, but it is arrogant in the extreme to consider that technological advance is a substitute for theoretical insight. —Nicholas J. Wade, 1998. (From Wade NJ. *A Natural History of Vision.* Cambridge, MA: MIT Press, 1998;xiii.)

In this chapter we discuss some of the significant developments in knowledge of the optics of the eye, with emphasis on discoveries up to the twentieth century. We also present some short biographical sketches of selected persons who made classic contributions to visual optics.

IMAGE FORMATION BY THE EYE

The earliest known theories of the optics of vision are from the ancient Greeks. In about 450 B.C., Empedocles proposed that a *visual ray* is sent out by the eye.[1] The visual ray then contacts the rays emanating from an object, and upon the return of the visual ray to the eye somehow an image in the mind is produced. An analogy from the sense of touch is that the visual ray reaches out like one's hand to touch an object. The theory of the visual ray has also been attributed to Pythagoras in about 600 B.C.[2] The visual ray theories have also been referred to as *extramission* or *emanation* theories.

The extramission theory of vision was accepted and written about in various forms by Euclid in third-century B.C. Greece, by the astronomer Ptolemy in A.D. second-century Alexandria, by the Greek anatomist Galen (c. A.D. 130–200), and by the Arab philosopher Alkindi (c. A.D. 801–866).

A second category of early theories of vision is the *intromission* theories, in which some form of radiation enters the eye.[3] At about the same time as Empedocles proposed an extramission theory, Leucippus and his student Democritus proposed an intromission theory. They suggested that when objects are acted upon by light they emit thin skins or veils of matter in all directions. These *eidola* (or as they were called later in the Middle Ages, *species*) keep the shape of the object from which they originated. The eidola then enter the eye and stimulate it.

A third category of early theories of vision has been referred to as *mediumistic* theories.[3] Aristotle proposed that an object sends its properties through the air (or other transparent medium). In doing so, changes occur in the medium. These changes are transmitted to the transparent humors (media) of the eye. The media of the eye then are transformed to resemble the object. In thirteenth-century Europe, Albertus Magnus (c.1206–1280) championed the Aristotelian theory, and as a result it was a constituent of the medieval university arts curriculum.

Each of the theories had its proponents in ancient and medieval times. Generally different writers used the different theories as part of an explanation of some mathematical, physical, or physiological aspect of vision. For example, Euclid used the extramission theory in his attempt to describe the geometry of space perception mathematically.[3]

The extramission theory was eventually shown to be false by ibn al-Haitham or Alhazen (965–c.1041). Alhazen was born south of Baghdad and moved to Cairo, where he supported himself by producing copies of Euclid's and Ptolemy's books.[4] Alhazen himself wrote more than 100 commentaries and books, one of them being *The Book of Optics*. In it Alhazen presented observations showing the extramission theory to be incorrect, and he suggested a different theory. Alhazen knew the anatomy of the eye from existing anatomy books. He proposed that light rays travel in straight lines and one ray from each point on an object passes through the cornea and pupil to stimulate the crystalline humor (which we now call the crystalline lens). He thought the crystalline humor initiated the visual sensation. In about 1200, Alhazen's book was translated into Latin under the title *On Vision*. The theories of vision it presented would predominate for the next few hundred years. The English mathematician Robert Grosseteste (1175–1253), the German/Polish natural philosopher Vitello (c.1220–1270), the English scholar Roger Bacon (c.1214–c.1294), and the monk John Peckham (c.1228–1294) wrote influential books that emphasized the work of Alhazen.

Works in the late sixteenth and early seventeenth centuries correctly identified the crystalline lens as part of the image-forming apparatus of the eye and the retina as the light sensitive element.[5,6] Francesco Maurolico (1494–1575), a mathematician from Italy, studied the optics of lenses and showed that rays from a point object are projected in all directions and are focused to a point image by convex lenses. He then reasoned that the image formation in the eye worked in the same way. The Swiss anatomist Felix Plater (1536–1614), noting that vision persisted after the zonules were cut and the crystalline lens displaced, suggested that the retina was the light-sensitive portion of the eye. Evidence for image formation on the retina came from experimentation on sheep and ox eyes by Christoph Scheiner (1573–1650). Scheiner removed sclera and choroid from the back of the eye and found that an inverted image was formed on the remaining retinal tissue (1619). Scheiner also corrected mistakes in "knowledge" about the structure of the image forming parts of the eye. He noted that the radius of curvature of the cornea was less than that of the sclera, and that the crystalline lens was located just behind the iris instead of in the middle of the eye. Also during this time, the remarkable astronomer and mathematician Johannes Kepler (1571–1630) produced many important works.

Kepler was the first to describe accurately the optics of image formation on the retina and the function of the pupil.[6–8] His books on optics were *Supplements to Vitello* (1604) and *Dioptrics* (1611). It has been suggested that what is taught in geometrical optics today is simply the refinement of the basic elements put forward by Kepler. In *Dioptrics*, Kepler describes the optics of lenses, as well as the optics of the eye and how it is corrected by spectacles. Kepler showed that the image formed on the retina is inverted, and explained how that occurs. Kepler suggested the existence of accommodation, but didn't know how the eye changed to make it possible. Kepler was the first to correctly explain the optics of spherical refractive errors and their correction with lenses, and the epigram from Kepler given at the beginning of Chapter 8 in this book may have been the first published connection between myopia and near work. (Kepler, for those readers who haven't guessed from the epigram, was nearsighted!) The contributions of Kepler in the seventeenth century made possible the next series of important works in the second half of the nineteenth century.

Bendikt Listing (1808–1882), who studied mathematics and optics with the great mathematician Karl Friedrich Gauss (1777–1855), appears to have been the first to calculate an accurate schematic eye, published in 1853. Listing's schematic eye, with a few modifications, was incorporated into the *Treatise on Physiological Optics* by the noted German physiologist and physicist Hermann von Helmholtz (1821–1894). The volumes of the first edition of Helmholtz's work were published in 1856 to 1867, and the second edition was published in 1885. In it Helmholtz covered ocular dioptrics, ocular structure, ocular motility, visual sensation, and visual perception. A measure of the importance of this work may be that additions were made to assemble a third edition after his death. The additions were composed by Allvar Gullstrand, J. von Kries, and W. Nagel, and it was published in 1909 to 1910. The third edition was translated into English in 1924 by James P. C. Southall. With its three editions, Helmholtz's

Physiological Optics was the standard reference on ocular dioptrics for decades. Allvar Gullstrand (1862–1930) published his schematic eyes in the first volume of the third edition of Helmholtz's *Physiological Optics*. His contribution to that treatise also included the analysis of the heterogeneous media of the crystalline lens.

Dutch ophthalmologist Frans Cornelis Donders (1818–1889) published *On the Anomalies of Accommodation and Refraction of the Eye* in 1864. Donders analyzed the types of refractive errors, elucidating their signs and symptoms and clarifying their clinical management with spectacles. Donders may have been the first to clearly explain the difference between hyperopia and presbyopia, and to show the clinical importance of astigmatism. Donders understood the basic relationship between accommodation and convergence and discussed their clinical significance. His book is one of the most influential books in the history of optometry and ophthalmology.

Although we often take the term *diopter* for granted, it was not yet in use when Donders wrote his book. The French ophthalmologist Felix Monoyer proposed the term *diopter* in 1872.

While the underlying principles of image formation by the eye were laid down by the nineteenth century, the twentieth century saw enormous advances in knowledge in areas such as aberrations of the eye, corneal topography, the nature of refractive errors, and methods of measuring refractive errors and the ocular dioptric components.

SPECTACLES

The exact origin and inventor of spectacles are unknown.[9–15] Artifacts that appear to be lenses have been excavated from sites that date back as early as 1550 B.C.[9,16] The Greek author Aristophanes wrote about a burning lens in his play *The Comedy of the Clouds* in about 434 B.C.

The invention of spectacles, however, appears to have been much later according to evidence pointing to the late thirteenth century, probably in Italy. Sometimes it has been attributed to the English scholar Roger Bacon (c.1214–c.1294). Bacon wrote about the ability of convex lenses to magnify, and appears to have used a segment of a glass sphere to aid in reading. However, it seems unlikely that he mounted such lenses in a spectacle frame or held them close to his eye. Attention has been drawn to a grave in Florence, Italy, that has the inscription "Here lies Salvino of the family Armati from Florence, inventor of spectacles. May God forgive his sins. In the year A.D. 1317." Collective opinion is that this inscription was a deliberate fabrication of more recent origin. Another person sometimes connected to the invention of spectacles was an Italian monk named Alessandro della Spina (?–1313). A manuscript from Pisa says that he was a good and humble man who made spectacles for himself and his friends. There are conflicting writings as to whether he was the inventor of spectacles or learned from someone else. In a sermon dated February 23, 1305, a monk from Pisa, Giordano da Rivalto, stated, "It is not yet 20 years since there was discovered the art of making eyeglasses." This would place the invention of spectacles around 1285. Most likely, the first person to make spectacles was an unknown artisan, who tried to keep his methods secret to avoid economic competition.

Once spectacles appeared, they must have caught on quickly. Spectacle-manufacturing businesses appeared by A.D. 1300 in Nuremberg in Germany, Haarlem in the Netherlands, and Venice in Italy. The rapid manufacture of durable paper also developed at about this time, and not long thereafter the invention of the printing press. Both of these developments must have stimulated literacy, and as literacy increased, the demand for spectacles must have increased as well. Early spectacles contained convex lenses and were used for reading. The first known written description of the use of concave lenses in spectacles appeared in 1450 in a book entitled *De Beryllo* by Nicolaus Cusanus (1401–1464).

ASTIGMATISM

Thomas Young was the first to describe and measure astigmatism (1801). He describes how he used an optometer of his own design to measure the far points of the horizontal and vertical meridians for his own eyes. He had myopia and against-the-rule astigmatism. In one of his eyes there was 3.94 D of myopia in the vertical meridian and 5.62 D of myopia in the horizontal meridian.[17] Young also described how some objects appeared elongated to him. It has been reported that Young did not commonly wear spectacles, but rather sometimes used a concave monocle, which he would sometimes tilt and look through obliquely to correct his astigmatism.[18]

The first person to design and wear a spherocylindrical correction for astigmatism was the English astronomer and mathematician, George Biddell Airy (1801–1892). Airy had always had poor visual acuity in his left eye and he observed that a star seen by his left eye appeared elongated, which he correctly recognized as being caused by astigmatism. He published a description of his astigmatism in 1827. Like Young, Airy had myopia and against-the-rule astigmatism, but Airy's astigmatism was greater than Young's. In 1825, the year of his first measurements, Airy had 4.69 D of astigmatism. Fuller, an optician of Ipswich, England, made a spherocylindrical lens for Airy. Airy named the condition astigmatism in 1849 at the suggestion of his colleague at Cambridge, William Whewell (1794–1866). The term *interval of Sturm,* the astigmatic interval in image space, comes from the description of astigmatic imagery by the French mathematician Jacques Charles François Sturm (1803–1855).

In the same year that Airy described his astigmatism, an American minister and scientist, Chauncey E. Goodrich, discovered his own astigmatism and used spherocylindrical lenses to correct it. It is thought that his lenses were made by John McAllister, Jr., of the McAllister family of opticians in Philadelphia.

The correction of astigmatism became common clinical practice after Frans Cornelis Donders wrote about the optics and importance of astigmatism in his book *On the Anomalies of Accommodation and Refraction of the Eye* (1864). According to a paper published in the same year that Donders published his book, there had been only about 11 cases of astigmatism reported in the literature up to that time.[18]

ACCOMMODATION

The existence of ocular accommodation, an actual change in the refractive power of the eye to achieve clear focus of objects at different distances, was first shown by Christoph Scheiner in 1619.[19] He demonstrated this by holding multiple pinholes close to his eye while he held a small, near object in front of him. When he looked at the near object he saw one, but when he focused so that distant objects were clear, the near object appeared multiple (see the epigram at the beginning of Chapter 9). Through the ensuing years, there were numerous theories given to try to explain how accommodation occurred. Thomas Young was the first to show that accommodation was due to a change in the crystalline lens (1801).[20] He ruled out a change in axial length of the eye by noting a lack of change in pressure phosphenes during accommodation. (He produced a phosphene by turning his eye inward maximally so that the retina near the posterior pole was accessible beneath the lateral sclera and then pressed a key against it.) He ruled out corneal changes by observing that the amplitude of accommodation did not change when he held a bath of water against the eye, which effectively negated the corneal refractive surface. With the optometer he invented, Young corroborated an earlier report in 1759 by William Porterfield (c.1700–1771) that persons who had no crystalline lens were not capable of accommodation. Young was also able to demonstrate that the spherical aberration of the eye changed during accommodation. Young correctly assumed that the crystalline lens changed its power by changing its shape, but incorrectly proposed that it could do this because it was muscular. The change in shape was supported by Langenbeck (1849) and Helmholtz (1853 to 1856) who noted that the Purkinje images formed by reflection from the crystalline lens surfaces changed during accommodation.

Cramer (1851) showed that electrical stimulation of the eyes of animals would cause accommodation and suggested that it was the ciliary muscle that acted on the crystalline lens. Hensen and Völckers (1873), in an often-noted experiment, convincingly proved that the ciliary muscle contracted during accommodation by observing the movement of needles inserted through the sclera into the ciliary muscle of cats and apes.[19]

Today we know that the ciliary muscle acts on the crystalline lens to produce changes in its radii of curvature, particularly on the anterior surface. The exact mechanism by which this occurs is not known for certain, but the Helmholtz theory of accommodation is the most accepted theory. (The Helmholtz theory and some competing theories are discussed in Chapter 9.) The experimental work to establish the general acceptance of the basic aspects of the Helmholtz theory was largely done by Edgar F. Fincham (1893–1963).[21]

OPTICS OF THE EYE AND PATIENT CARE

Although some refractive anomalies of the eye had been described before A.D. 1300, their basic nature was not understood, and they were left uncorrected. During about 1300 to 1900 the basic principles of optics in general and also the optics of the eye were elucidated. It is likely that spectacles were first developed around A.D. 1285. During this period the art and craft of spectacle lens making developed. Methods to measure lens power were delineated. The idea that sight testing should be done to determine appropriate lens power slowly took root, and methods of testing evolved.

Tannebaum[22,23] has suggested that this era could be subdivided into two periods: before and after the publication of the first two significant optometry books in the seventeenth century. These books were written by Benito Daza de Valdes of Seville, Spain (1623) and William Molyneux of Dublin, Ireland (1692).

Daza de Valdes (1591–c.1636), a Jacobian Friar, wrote a practical and systematic book on optics, ocular anatomy and the use and fitting of spectacles.[24,25] He described convex, concave, and plano lenses, and included a system of lens numbering or lens grades to indicate lens powers. Among other things, he presented a table of lens grades for the correction of presbyopia at various ages. He suggested slightly stronger presbyopic lenses for women than for men. Daza de Valdes also was of the opinion that lenses used for myopia should not be so powerful as to cause a perceived reduction in the size of objects being viewed.

William Molyneux has been described as a philosopher, mathematician, astronomer, and politician.[26] In his book Molyneux described image formation by convex and concave lenses, the origin and use of spectacles, the occasional near-point problems of myopes after correction of their distance vision, and selection of lenses for presbyopia.[27] He noted that the weakest lens that remedies a problem should be the one that is used. He also discussed the use of telescopes and microscopes to aid persons with diminished vision.

Opticianry

Opticians are persons who manufacture and/or dispense spectacles. The first opticians were the early spectacle makers. As testing methods for the determination of refractive errors and the prescription of spectacles developed, a distinction could be made between refracting opticians and dispensing opticians. In the late nineteenth and early twentieth centuries in the United States, refracting opticians started calling themselves optometrists.

Optometry

The profession that has identified itself more than anything else as the group of practitioners who examine for and ameliorate optical and related defects of the eye is optometry. It is often stated that optometry began about a hundred years ago when the first licensure laws were passed, as if it suddenly sprang into being by legislative fiat. In reality, optometry has been practiced for hundreds of years. As evidence of this, one need only examine the contents of the 1623 book by Daza deValdes. In speaking of a portion of this book devoted to case reports, Hofstetter[25] notes that "the procedural pattern of optometric practice is quite evident, namely: (1) preliminary findings and case history, (2) refractive and functional measurements, (3) visual task analysis and prescribing, (4) eyewear selection and dispensing, and (5) explanatory and counseling services."

The beginnings of optometry can be traced to fourteenth- and fifteenth-century spectacle makers and early vision scientists. The first use of the term *optometer* as a device to measure refractive error appears to have been by Porterfield in 1750.[28] The word *optometry* was used by Verschoor in Holland in 1865 and by Landolt in France in 1877 to describe the determination of ocular refraction.[28] As with any profession, the sophistication of optometry's diagnostic methods, treatment regimens, and educational programs have increased dramatically since its origin.

The earliest laws for the licensure of optometrists in the United States were passed in the early 1900s, the first being in Minnesota in 1901. The American Association of Opticians was formed in 1898 and has since evolved into the

American Optometric Association, the latter name of the organization being adopted officially in 1919.[29] Charles F. Prentice (1854–1946) and other optometrists started charging a fee for examinations in the late 1880s, a sign of professionalism as opposed to the mercantilism of making an income exclusively from the sale of glasses. The use of the term *optometrist,* rather than *optician,* to describe persons who examined for and fitted glasses, became more common in the early 1900s.

The profession of optometry changed radically in the twentieth century, including the introduction of formal university programs in optometry. Prior to the university programs, the development of vision-examination procedures was largely through the accumulated experience of generations of practitioners. The development of the university programs has enhanced formalized research on optometric procedures and care. Twentieth-century optometry has gradually expanded to offer therapy for binocular vision and accommodation disorders, fitting of contact lenses, low-vision care, and management or comanagement of ocular disease.

Ophthalmology

The other profession that examines patients for optical defects of the eye is ophthalmology, a field of medicine. Ophthalmology had its origins in the barber-surgeons of the Middle Ages. Throughout its history, ophthalmology has emphasized surgery and eye disease over refractive anomalies of the eye. Until the middle nineteenth century ophthalmologists typically did not practice refraction or prescribe spectacles and, if they felt spectacles were necessary, they suggested that their patients go to an optician.[30] In spite of this fact, many eminent ophthalmologists have been responsible for advances in our knowledge of the optics of the eye. Of particular note is Allvar Gullstrand who won a Nobel Prize in 1911 for his work in optics. A very important factor, which increased interest in the management of refractive errors by ophthalmology, was the publication of the ground-breaking book *On the Anomalies of Accommodation and Refraction of the Eye* by Dutch ophthalmologist Frans Cornelis Donders in 1864. Although management of refractive errors had its origins outside of the field of medicine, many noted ophthalmologists,

such as Duke-Elder, have recognized its importance, as shown by the epigram at the beginning of the preface of this book.

BIOGRAPHICAL SKETCHES

Johannes Kepler

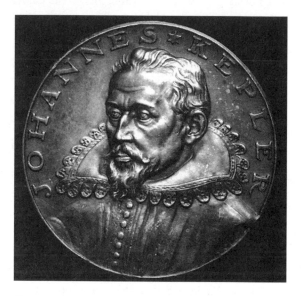

Figure 10.1. Silver medal commemorating Johannes Kepler, produced in Germany in 1930. (Courtesy Jay M. Galst.)

Johannes Kepler[6–8,31,32] (Figure 10.1) was born to German Lutheran parents in December of 1571. When he was a small child he barely survived smallpox, and it left him with impaired vision and an affected hand. His academic talents were recognized early and he attended a Latin school and a preparatory school before beginning studies at the University of Tübingen in Germany in 1589. It was there that he learned about the Copernican theory of the solar system. Kepler was in the last year of his studies to become a Lutheran minister in 1594 when he was assigned to be teacher and mathematician at a seminary in Graz, Austria. His duties included teaching mathematics, astronomy, Virgil and rhetoric, doing surveying, and producing an annual almanac. The almanac included various prognostications, several of which in Kepler's first almanac turned out to be correct. The success of his early predictions was noted, and he continued to produce calendars and almanacs for needed income through much of his life.

After a few years in Graz, Kepler moved to work with the Danish astronomer Tycho Brahe, who was living in exile in Prague. It was there that Kepler did much of his noted astronomical work. Brahe died less than a year after Kepler arrived to work with him, and Kepler replaced him as King Rudolph's imperial mathematician. Kepler moved several times in his lifetime, often as a consequence of war and the religious turmoil between Catholics and Protestants prevalent at that time.

Kepler is best known for the three laws of planetary motion that bear his name. He showed mathematically that the Copernican theory of the solar system was correct, and he is often considered the founder of modern astronomy. He is credited as the first to calculate latitude and longitude correctly, and he formulated the inverse squares law expressing the decrease in illuminance with distance from a source. Kepler was a prodigious writer in astronomy, physics, and mathematics. His works have been collected in 24 large volumes.

The books Kepler wrote on optics were *Supplements to Vitello* (1604) and *Dioptrics* (1611). Various aspects of optics were contained in those books, but perhaps the most significant parts of them were the portions on the optics of the eye. The important contributions of these books to the optics of vision are discussed in the preceding section on image formation of the eye.

Descartes was quoted as saying, "Kepler was my principal teacher in optics, and I think that he knew more about this subject than all those who preceded him." Science historian David Lindberg strongly emphasized the importance of Kepler's work in visual optics when he stated: "All early natural philosophers acknowledged that vision is man's most noble and dependable sense, and the struggle to understand its workings occupied large numbers of scholars for some two thousand years. Kepler's successful solution of the problem of vision early in the seventeenth century was a theoretical triumph comparable in significance to other, far more celebrated developments of the scientific revolution."[33]

Kepler was profoundly religious, and this was a driving force in his work. He believed that God had produced the universe with mathematical harmony and perfection, and he sought to understand the mathematical relations that existed therein. While in Graz, he wrote to his former mentor in astronomy at the University of Tübingen: "I wanted to become a theologian. For a long time I was restless. Now, however, behold how through my effort God is being celebrated in astronomy."

Kepler in many ways can be portrayed as a tragic figure. His father was absent from home for extended periods of time as a mercenary soldier, and he abandoned the family forever when Johannes was 16 years old. Kepler's first wife died. He had twelve children with his two wives; only four of the children survived to adulthood. He was distracted from 1615–1621 by having to defend his mother from charges of witchcraft, of which she was finally acquitted. Kepler had difficulty collecting his salary as court astronomer to King Ferdinand II and King Ferdinand III. Kepler died of a fever in November of 1630, 6 weeks short of his fifty-ninth birthday, after a journey to petition for the salary that had been promised to him. Despite his troubles, Kepler was remarkably productive and insightful in his work

Christoph Scheiner

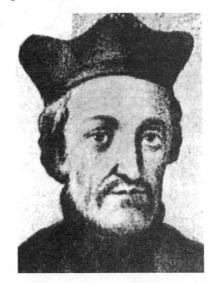

Figure 10.2. Christoph Scheiner. (Reprinted with permission from Albert DM, Edwards DD, eds. *The History of Ophthalmology.* Cambridge, MA: Blackwell Science, 1996;51.)

Christoph Scheiner[34,35] (Figure 10.2) was born in 1573 in Germany. He attended Jesuit schools, and he entered the Society of the Jesuits in 1595.

Scheiner then studied philosophy, mathematics, and theology, and underwent training as a teacher. His first professorial position was as a professor of Hebrew and mathematics at Ingolstadt in 1610. In 1611 Scheiner built a telescope and observed sunspots, one of several people to independently discover them. Scheiner authored several works on astronomy. Most of his studies on the eye were published in 1619 in a book entitled *Oculus, hoc est: fundamentum opticum*. Scheiner showed that the sclera had a flatter radius of curvature than the cornea by comparing the images reflected from these two surfaces to the size of images reflected from glass balls of varying diameters. Scheiner described the principle of image formation with a multiple aperture disc, a system that bears his name and that has been incorporated into the design of many autorefractors and other optical equipment. He then used the multiple aperture to demonstrate the existence of accommodation.

Scheiner reported studies in ocular anatomy that corrected some errors in existing knowledge. He found that the optic nerve is situated nasal to the posterior pole of the eye rather than at the posterior pole and he observed that the crystalline lens was just behind the iris instead of in the middle of the eye. He described the change in pupillary size to light and accommodation. Scheiner also wrote about cutting away the sclera and choroid from the back of animal eyes and finding an inverted image. From 1620 to his death of a stroke in 1650, Scheiner lived variously in Freiburg, Neisse, and Vienna; served as a professor and administrator of Jesuit colleges; and did astronomical studies.

Thomas Young

Thomas Young[36–38] (Figure 10.3) was born in June of 1773, at Milverton, Somersetshire, England. His exceptional intelligence manifested itself at an early age. He started reading at the age of 2, and had read the Bible from front to back twice and begun the study of Latin by the age of 6. He studied medicine in London, Edinburgh, and Göttingen, received the M.D. degree at Cambridge in 1808, and was elected to the Royal College of Physicians in 1809. In his thesis he developed a phonetic alphabet, based on the analysis of the sounds produced in speech. He studied linguistics and languages extensively. Latin,

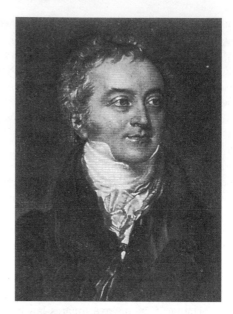

Figure 10.3. Thomas Young. (Reprinted with permission from Albert DM, Edwards DD, eds. *The History of Oph-thalmology*. Cambridge, MA: Blackwell Science, 1996;109.)

Greek, Hebrew, French, German, Italian, Arabic, Chaldean, Aramaic, and Persian were among the languages he knew.

Young received a substantial inheritance from an uncle. Young was not particularly busy in his medical practice, so the inheritance allowed him the time to be a gentleman scholar. He was undoubtedly a very competent physician, but it is said that he didn't gain the confidence of his patients because he was too formal and distant. In 1811 he became a physician at St. George's Hospital. He held various public offices related to science, some of which were paid positions. He was foreign secretary of the Royal Society, a consultant to the Admiralty, secretary to the Royal Commission on Weights and Measures, secretary of the Board of Longitude, and superintendent of the Nautical Almanac.

Young published his physiological optics studies in two extensive papers published in 1793 and 1801. His contributions to vision science are among the most important in the field. They include the demonstration that the crystalline lens was responsible for accommodation, the first description of astigmatism, and the first presentation of a trichromatic theory of color vision. Young published extensively in clinical medicine. Among his writings were a comprehensive medical bibliography, a textbook on consumption, an analysis of motions of the heart and arteries, and various contributions to therapeutic methods, such as Young's rule for pediatric doses. Young is noted for his textbook on physics, entitled *Lectures in Natural Philosophy and the Mechanical Arts,* first published in 1807. It conveyed physical explanations and engineering principles for numerous machines, structures, and natural phenomena. Some of the major contributions to physics presented in the book were Young's modulus of elasticity, his experiments on interference, and his development of a wave theory of light.

Young obtained significant income from writings on a number of topics for various periodicals. He also made extensive contributions to *Encyclopedia Britannica.* He wrote on topics in physics, mathematics, languages, optics, engineering, as well as topics outside of science, including many biographical essays. Around 1812 Young became interested in the Rosetta stone, the tablet discovered in Egypt in 1799 that contains writing in Greek, Egyptian demotics, and Egyptian hieroglyphics. By insight gained from his studies on the varying structures of languages, he was able to provide the first translation of Egyptian hieroglyphics. Young died of a heart ailment in May of 1829 at 55 years of age.

Jan Evangelista Purkinje

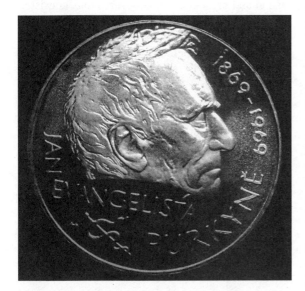

Figure 10.4. Medal commemorating Jan Evangelista Purkinje, made in Czechoslovakia in 1969, one hundred years after his death. (Courtesy Jay M. Galst.)

Jan Purkinje[39,40] (Purkyně in his native Czech) was born in 1787. A likeness of Purkinje is shown in Figure 10.4. Purkinje's father died when he was 6 years old, but a local teacher and parson recognized his scholastic abilities and helped arrange for his education. Purkinje spent his academic career as a professor of physiology at Breslau and then at Prague. Much of Purkinje's work was in sensory physiology, but he also made contributions to histology, tissue preparation techniques for microscopy, and physiological pharmacology. There are several structures and phenomena that are associated with his name: Purkinje cells in the cerebellum, Purkinje fibers in the heart, the Purkinje shift for the change in relative sensitivity of the retina to different wavelengths under photopic and scotopic conditions, the Purkinje tree for the entoptic visualization of the retinal blood vessels, and of course, the Purkinje images for the images reflected from the surfaces of the eye.

Purkinje's most important publication on vision was *Physiologic Examination of the Organ of Vision* (1823). In it Purkinje covered the effects of illumination and refractive error on visual acuity, the limits of the visual field, and his observations of the anterior segment of the eye with a microscope. He also wrote about the examination of the vitreous and retina that he had achieved with a candle. He thus showed how ophthalmoscopy could be done, and suggested that clinicians should find it useful in the diagnosis of ocular conditions. Perhaps because Purkinje didn't do anything else to promote ophthalmoscopy, he generally is not credited with the invention of the ophthalmoscope. In this publication, Purkinje also described the images reflected from the surfaces of cornea and crystalline lens, the images now known as the Purkinje images. The reflection from the anterior surface of the cornea had been known for many years, but the others had not. Purkinje suggested that the sizes of the reflected images could be used to measure the radii of curvature of the surfaces, which was done later in keratometry and phakometry.

Purkinje is recognized for his important efforts in the latter part of his life in promoting science education among the Czech people. For example, he started publication of a science periodical in the Czech language in 1853. He also worked toward the acceptance of Czech as a teaching language at the University of Prague, and he emphasized the importance of science in daily life. Purkinje died in Prague in 1869.

Hermann von Helmholtz

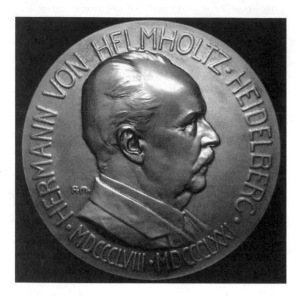

Figure 10.5. Medal depicting Hermann von Helmholtz made in Austria in 1894 for the 66th Natural Science Meeting in Vienna. (Courtesy Jay M. Galst.)

Hermann von Helmholtz[40-43] (Figure 10.5) was born at Potsdam, Germany on August 31, 1821. His father, August Ferdinand Helmholtz, was a teacher of classical languages and philosophy. His mother, Caroline Penn, was a descendant of William Penn, who founded Pennsylvania. In school Helmholtz excelled in mathematics and physics. Helmholtz wanted to pursue university studies in physics, but his family couldn't afford it. His father convinced him to study medicine because the state would pay for his education. Helmholtz studied for 5 years at the Friedrich Wilhelm Institute in Berlin and the University of Berlin in exchange for 8 years of service as a physician and surgeon in the Prussian army. In 1849 he became professor of physiology at Königsberg. His subsequent appointments were professor of anatomy and physiology at Bonn (1855), professor of physiology at Heidelberg (1858), and professor of physics and director of the Physical Institute at Berlin (1871).

Helmholtz made important fundamental contributions in both physiology and physics, including

papers on the conservation of energy and the laws of thermodynamics. He did experiments to show that chemical changes occur in contracting muscle and that muscles generate heat when they contract. Helmholtz was the first to measure nerve conduction velocity. Because of his extensive work on the physiology of hearing, he is held with the same esteem by persons who study hearing as those who study vision. Among his publications on hearing is a tome on the application of the physiology of hearing to music theory. Helmholtz brought mathematical precision to all his physiological studies. After he became professor of physics in Berlin, much of his research was on electrodynamic phenomena. Helmholtz is known for the many notable scientists he trained, and he is recognized as one of the leading scientists of his time.

The first volume of Helmholtz's *Treatise on Physiological Optics* appeared in 1856. It was this volume that dealt with ocular anatomy and the optics of the eye. In it Helmholtz noted that the line of sight of the eye is not coincident with the optical axis, he presented his theory of accommodation, and he discussed the invention of his ophthalmometer, which was the keratometer upon which subsequent keratometer designs were based. In Volume 2 Helmholtz dealt with various aspects of visual sensation. In this volume Helmholtz drew attention to Young's trichromatic theory of color vision and presented some observations consistent with it. Volume 3 was published in 1867 and covered eye movements, binocular vision, and various aspects of visual perception. A second edition of the three volumes was published in 1885, and a third edition in 1909 to 1910 after Helmholtz's death with additions by Gullstrand, von Kries, and Nagel. This three-volume set of books did more to establish physiological optics as a separate discipline of science than any other publication.

Helmholtz is generally credited with the invention of the ophthalmoscope in late 1850. Purkinje made an ophthalmoscope for his physiological studies in the 1820s, but his work with an ophthalmoscope was largely overlooked. The English mathematician Charles Babbage (1792–1871) also made an ophthalmoscope in 1847, but the physician to whom he showed it didn't realize its potential significance, and Babbage did not publish anything on it. Helmholtz apparently discovered the principle of ophthalmoscopy independently, and he certainly was the first to show its importance and how it could be used. Helmholtz published a monograph describing his ophthalmoscope in October of 1851. He had a machinist make one for him, and by the end of 1851 the machinist had received 18 orders for ophthalmoscopes.

Late in his life Helmholtz experienced occasional migraine and depression. In 1893, at 72 years of age, Helmholtz made a trip to the United States, as a representative of the German government to the world Columbian Exposition in Chicago. On July 12, 1894, he suffered what may have been a stroke, and he died 2 months later in Berlin on September 8.

Frans Cornelis Donders

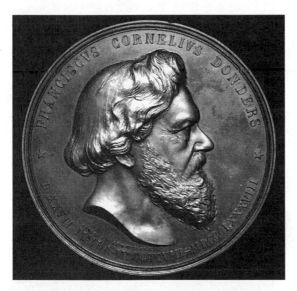

Figure 10.6. Medal honoring the 70th birthday of Frans Cornelis Donders in 1888. (Courtesy Jay M. Galst.)

Frans Cornelis Donders[44–46] (Figure 10.6) was born on May 27, 1818, in Tilburg, Holland, the youngest and only boy of nine children. His father, a merchant who studied chemistry, music, and literature, died when Frans was an infant. From 1835 to 1840 Frans Donders attended the military medical school in Utrecht, Holland, and the medical school at the University of Utrecht. In 1840 Donders passed the examinations for the degree doctor of medicine at the University of Leiden and com-

pleted a doctoral dissertation on meningitis. In 1842 he took a position at the University of Utrecht, where he served until his retirement in 1888. Donders was very industrious, being active in research, teaching, clinical work, journal editing, translation work, and administration. He completed more than 340 publications. In addition to his native Dutch, Donders knew Latin, and he was fluent in English, German, and French.

Much of Donders's work was in physiology. Some of the topics he studied were the formation of blood and lymph, intestinal function and the digestion of fat, metabolism, and heat regulation. He wrote a widely used textbook on physiology. In his first few years at the University of Utrecht, he taught six different courses. One of them was a course in physiological optics, which he taught so well that he was urged to work in ophthalmology. In 1851 Donders started the practice of ophthalmology. In 1855 he became a co-editor of *Archiv für Ophthalmologie* with von Graefe and von Arlt. In 1858 he opened a charity eye hospital for indigent patients.

Donders published many papers in ophthalmology, but his best-known work was his classical book *On the Anomalies of Accommodation and Refraction of the Eye* published in 1864. This book, more than anything else, put the practice of refraction on a firm foundation. It covered refractive and accommodative problems comprehensively. Most of the concepts in Donders's book have stood the test of time, and frequently ideas presented as new in the twentieth century were actually discussed there.

Donders's personal attributes earned him the admiration and endearment of his colleagues. He was said to be erudite and intelligent, but modest. He enjoyed teaching, and his writings were popular for their clear and simple style. His clinic was visited by ophthalmologists from all over the world. He received many awards from ophthalmological organizations, but he was also honored by his country. A statue of Donders stands in Utrecht and his portrait was featured on a Dutch postage stamp. When Donders reached the Dutch professors' retirement age of 70, he appeared to be in excellent health and capable of many more years of productive work. However, just a few months after his retirement he was found to have a brain disease, possibly a tumor. He declined rapidly, and died in Utrecht on March 24, 1889.

Allvar Gullstrand

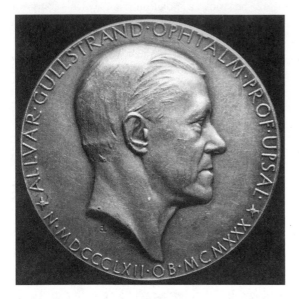

Figure 10.7. Silver medal depicting Allvar Gullstrand, produced in 1935 for the Royal Swedish Academy of Science. (Courtesy Jay M. Galst.)

Allvar Gullstrand[47–49] was born on June 5, 1862, in Landskrona, Sweden, the son of the town physician. Gullstrand is depicted in Figure 10.7. In school Gullstrand showed an aptitude in mathematics, and for a while was undecided between a career in engineering and a career in medicine. Influenced by his father, he chose medicine. After receiving his doctorate degree in 1890, Gullstrand worked as an ophthalmologist and as a lecturer at the Royal Caroline Institute in Stockholm. From 1894–1914 he was a professor of ophthalmology at the University of Uppsala in Sweden, and from 1914–1927 he was a research professor of physiological and physical optics at the University of Uppsala.

Gullstrand published on the topics of astigmatism, monochromatic aberrations, optical image formation, optics of the crystalline lens, ophthalmic lens design, theories of accommodation and presbyopia, the analysis of photokeratoscopy images, the use of the first Purkinje image in the diagnosis of ocular motility disorders, and other areas. He developed a reflexless ophthalmoscope and a slit lamp illumination system that was incorporated into a slit lamp biomicroscope. Gullstrand is probably best known for the five new chapters he

added to the first volume of Helmholtz's *Treatise on Physiological Optics* (1909). This material included the schematic eyes that bear his name.

Gullstrand received the Nobel Prize in physiology or medicine in 1911. Gullstrand was awarded honorary degrees from the University of Uppsala, University of Jena, and University of Dublin. Gullstrand has been described as tall and slender, very reserved, and as a tireless worker who regularly worked late into the night. Gullstrand retired in 1927. He died of a hemorrhagic stroke in Uppsala on July 21, 1930.

Glenn Ansel Fry

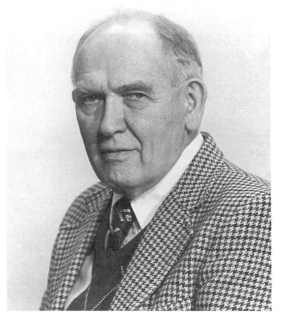

Figure 10.8. Glenn A. Fry. (Courtesy of The Ohio State University.)

Glenn A. Fry[50–53] (Figure 10.8) was born on September 10, 1908, in Wellford, South Carolina. Fry received a B.A. degree from Davidson College in 1929, and was then trained in psychology at Duke University, where he received M.A. (1931) and Ph.D. (1933) degrees. He then worked as a Research Fellow at the Washington University Department of Ophthalmology in St. Louis. He was the director of the optometry program at The Ohio State University from 1935 to 1966, when he

Developments in Visual Optics and Some of the People Who Made Them Possible **225**

was made Regents Professor at Ohio State. Fry started the physiological optics graduate program at Ohio State, the first university Ph.D. program associated with an optometry school.

Fry published more than 250 papers in many areas of optometry and vision science, including color vision, space perception, accommodation and convergence relationships, visual ergonomics, ophthalmic optics, geometrical optics, and visual optics. His book *Blur of the Retinal Image* (1955) is considered a classic. Fry's work was meticulous, often done with complicated apparatus that he constructed himself. He was equally adept at studying fundamental and practical clinical concepts. He was known for his service on numerous standards committees of the American Optometric Association, American National Standards Institute, and the Illuminating Engineering Society. The awards Fry received include the Tillyer Medal of the Optical Society of America, Distinguished Service Award from the American Optometric Association, the Gold Medal from the Illuminating Engineering Society, and the Prentice Award from the American Academy of Optometry. He received seven honorary degrees, the optometry building was named for him at Ohio State, and an award given by the American Academy of Optometry bears his name.

Henry Hofstetter wrote, "I think of him as the 'American Helmholtz,' and when I say this to others they always agree." Perhaps his most enduring legacy is the many persons who have gone on to distinguished careers after his tutelage and who have, in turn, trained others. His Ph.D. students would make a good start on a who's who list in optometric science and optometric education: Henry Hofstetter (1942), Vincent Ellerbrock (1947), Merrill Allen (1949), Mathew Alpern (1950), Henry Knoll (1950), Charles R. Stewart (1951), Gerald Westheimer (1953), Neal J. Bailey (1954), Jay Enoch (1956), Theodore Grosvenor (1956), Bradford Wild (1959), Earl F. Miller II (1961), Jess Boyd Eskridge (1964), Vincent King (1971), John P. Schoessler (1971), Ronald Jones (1972), William Brown (1977), David Loshin (1977), James E. Sheedy (1977), William W. Somers (1977), and Kent M. Daum (1979) (personal communication from JP Schoessler, February 1999). Students of Fry tell stories of his indefatigable energy in the laboratory, and his ability to refresh himself late at night by taking catnaps. He retired in 1979, but he continued to make regular

contributions to literature, publishing his last paper only months before his death on January 5, 1996, at 87 years of age.

REFERENCES

1. Park D. *The Fire within the Eye: A Historical Essay on the Nature and Meaning of Light.* Princeton, NJ: Princeton University Press, 1997;35–38.
2. Duke-Elder S, Gloster J, Weale RA. The Physiology of the Eye and of Vision. In: S Duke-Elder, ed. *System of Ophthalmology, 4.* Mosby: St. Louis, 1968;435–446.
3. Lindberg DC. The science of optics. In: DC Lindberg, ed. *Studies in the History of Medieval Optics.* London: Variorum Reprints, 1983;338–368.
4. Park D. *The Fire within the Eye: A Historical Essay on the Nature and Meaning of Light.* Princeton, NJ: Princeton University Press, 1997;76–87.
5. Hirsch MJ, Wick RE. *The Optometric Profession.* Philadelphia: Chilton, 1968;93–100.
6. Duke-Elder S, Abrams D. Ophthalmic Optics and Refraction. In: S Duke-Elder, ed. *System of Ophthalmology, 4.* St. Louis: Mosby, 1970;12–21.
7. Ronchi V. *Optics: The Science of Vision* (trans. E Rosen). New York: New York University Press, 1957;41–54.
8. Park D. *The Fire within the Eye: A Historical Essay on the Nature and Meaning of Light.* Princeton, NJ: Princeton University Press, 1997;153–171.
9. Hofstetter HW. *Optometry: Professional, Economic, and Legal Aspects.* St. Louis: Mosby, 1948;17–35.
10. Rosen E. The invention of spectacles. *J Hist Med Allied Sci.* 1956;11:13–46,183–218.
11. Hirsch MJ, Wick RE. *The Optometric Profession.* Philadelphia: Chilton, 1968;75–88.
12. Duke-Elder S, Abrams D. Ophthalmic Optics and Refraction. In: S Duke-Elder, ed. *System of Ophthalmology, 5.* St. Louis: Mosby, 1970;609–624.
13. Albert DM. Ocular refraction and the development of spectacles. In: DM Albert, DD Edwards, eds. *The History of Ophthalmology.* Cambridge, MA: Blackwell Science, 1996;107–123.
14. Rosenthal JW. *Spectacles and Other Vision Aids: A History and Guide to Collecting.* San Francisco: Norman Publishing, 1996;35–49,489–495.
15. Park D. *The Fire within the Eye: A Historical Essay on the Nature and Meaning of Light.* Princeton, NJ: Princeton University Press, 1997;121–125.
16. Enoch JM. Early lens use: lenses found in context with their original objects. *Optom Vis Sci.* 1996;73:707–715.
17. Duke-Elder S, Abrams D. Ophthalmic Optics and Refraction. In: S Duke-Elder, ed. *System of Ophthalmology, 5.* St. Louis: Mosby, 1970;18, 208.
18. Levene JR. *Clinical Refraction and Visual Science.* London: Butterworths, 1977;203–285.

19. Duke-Elder S, Abrams D. Ophthalmic Optics and Refraction. In: S Duke-Elder, ed. *System of Ophthalmology, 5.* St. Louis: Mosby, 1970;153–161.

20. Levene JR. *Clinical Refraction and Visual Science.* London: Butterworth-Heinemann, 1977;119–140.

21. Fincham EF. The mechanism of accommodation. *Brit J Ophthalmol.* Monograph Supplement 8, 1937.

22. Tannebaum S. The puzzle of our optometric past. *J Am Optom Assoc.* 1972;43:443–451.

23. Tannebaum S. A case history: the development of optometry. *J Am Optom Assoc.* 1974;45:1251–1255.

24. Guerra CT. Benito Daza de Valdes: a seventeenth-century optometrist. *J Am Optom Assoc.* 1961;32: 541–545.

25. Hofstetter HW. Optometry of Daza de Valdes (1591–c.1636). *Am J Optom Physiol Opt.* 1988;65: 354–357.

26. Hirsch MJ, Wick RE. *The Optometric Profession.* Philadelphia: Chilton, 1968;113–114.

27. Tannebaum S. William Molyneux: Dioptrica, a 17th century classic. *J Am Optom Assoc.* 1972;43:566–570.

28. Hofstetter HW. *Optometry: Professional, Economic, and Legal Aspects.* St. Louis: Mosby, 1948;90–91.

29. Koetting RA. *The American Optometric Association's First Century.* St. Louis: American Optometric Association, 1997.

30. Duke-Elder S, Abrams D. Ophthalmic Optics and Refraction. In: S Duke-Elder, ed. *System of Ophthalmology, 5.* St. Louis: Mosby, 1970;823.

31. Gingerich O. Johannes Kepler. In: CC Gillispie, ed. *Dictionary of Scientific Biography.* New York: Charles Scribner's Sons, 1973;7:289–312.

32. Lindberg DC. *Theories of Vision from Al-Kindi to Kepler.* Chicago: University of Chicago Press, 1976;185–208.

33. Lindberg DC. *Theories of Vision from Al-Kindi to Kepler.* Chicago: University of Chicago Press, 1976;x.

34. Shea WR. Christoph Scheiner. In: CC Gillispie, ed. *Dictionary of Scientific Biography.* New York: Charles Scribner's Sons, 1975;12:151–152.

35. Daxecker F. Christoph Scheiner's eye studies. *Doc Ophthalmol.* 1992;81;27–35.

36. Levene JR. Thomas Young, 1773–1829. In: RC Olby, ed. *Early Nineteenth Century European Scientists.* Oxford: Pergamon Press, 1967;67–93.

37. Morse EW. Thomas Young. In: CC Gillispie, ed. *Dictionary of Scientific Biography.* New York: Charles Scribner's Sons, 1976;14:562–572.

38. Gauger GE. The great mind of Thomas Young (1773–1829). *Doc Ophthalmol.* 1997;94:113–121.

39. Kruta V. Jan Evangelista Purkyně (Purkinje). In: CC Gillispie, ed. *Dictionary of Scientific Biography.* New York: Charles Scribner's Sons, 1975;11:213–217.

40. Albert DM. The ophthalmoscope and retinovitreous surgery. In: DM Albert, DD Edwards, eds. *The History of Ophthalmology.* Cambridge, MA: Blackwell Science, 1996;177–202.

41. Duke-Elder S, Abrams D. Ophthalmic Optics and Refraction. In: S Duke-Elder, ed. *System of Ophthalmology, 5.* St. Louis: Mosby, 1970;92–93.

42. Turner RS. Hermann von Helmholtz. In: CC Gillispie, ed. *Dictionary of Scientific Biography.* New York: Charles Scribner's Sons, 1972;6;241–253.

43. Henkes HE. Helmholtz, the first reformer of ophthalmology. *Doc Ophthalmol.* 1992;81:17–25.

44. Pfeiffer RL. Frans Cornelis Donders Dutch physiologist and ophthalmologist. *Bull New York Acad Med.* 1936;566–581.

45. ter Laage RJChV. Franciscus Cornelis Donders. In: CC Gillispie, ed. *Dictionary of Scientific Biography.* New York: Charles Scribner's Sons, 1971;4:162–164.

46. Duke-Elder S, Abrams D. Ophthalmic Optics and Refraction. In: S Duke-Elder, ed. *System of Ophthalmology, 5.* St. Louis: Mosby, 1970;254–255.

47. Duke-Elder S, Abrams D. Ophthalmic Optics and Refraction. In: S Duke-Elder, ed. *System of Ophthalmology, 5.* St. Louis: Mosby, 1970;94–95.

48. Herzberger MJ. Allvar Gullstrand. In: CC Gillispie, ed. *Dictionary of Scientific Biography.* New York: Charles Scribner's Sons, 1972;5:590–591.

49. Albert DM. Allvar Gullstrand, 1862–1930: A lonesome giant of optical theory. *Trends Neurosci.* 1980; 3:4–6.

50. MacNeille SM. Glenn A. Fry: Edgar D. Tillyer Medalist for 1961. *J Opt Soc Am.* 1961;51:1045.

51. Enoch JM. Glenn Ansel Fry: An 80th birthday celebration: Introduction. *Optom Vis Sci.* 1990;67:577.

52. Anonymous. Dr. Fry's art, science transformed optometry. *Am Optom Assoc News.* January 22, 1996;5–6.

53. Augusburger A. A celebration of the life of Glenn Ansel Fry, September 10, 1908–January 5, 1996. *Optom Vis Sci.* 1996;73:223–224.

Index